World report on violence and health

Edited by
Etienne G. Krug, Linda L. Dahlberg, James A. Mercy,
Anthony B. Zwi and Rafael Lozano

World Health Organization
Geneva
2002

WHO Library Cataloguing-in-Publication Data

World report on violence and health / edited by Etienne G. Krug ... [et al.].
    1.Violence 2.Domestic violence 3.Suicide 4.Sex offenses 5.War
    6.Public health 7.Risk factors I.Krug, Etienne G.

    ISBN 92 4 154561 5   (NLM classification: HV 6625)

Suggested citation: Krug EG et al., eds. *World report on violence and health*. Geneva, World Health Organization, 2002.

Photograph of Nelson Mandela reproduced with permission from the African National Congress.

The World Health Organization welcomes requests for permission to reproduce or translate its publications, in part or in full. Applications and enquiries should be addressed to the Office of Publications, World Health Organization, Geneva, Switzerland, which will be glad to provide the latest information on any changes made to the text, plans for new editions, and reprints and translations already available.

The designations employed and the presentation of the material in this publication do not imply the expression of any opinion whatsoever on the part of the Secretariat of the World Health Organization concerning the legal status of any country, territory, city or area or of its authorities, or concerning the delimitation of its frontiers or boundaries.

The mention of specific companies or of certain manufacturers' products does not imply that they are endorsed or recommended by the World Health Organization in preference to others of a similar nature that are not mentioned. Errors and omissions excepted, the names of proprietary products are distinguished by initial capital letters.

Where the designation "country or area" appears in the headings of tables, it covers countries, territories, cities or areas.

Designed by minimum graphics
Typeset and printed in Switzerland
2002/14323—Stratcom—20 000

Contents

Foreword

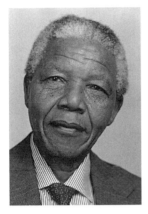

The twentieth century will be remembered as a century marked by violence. It burdens us with its legacy of mass destruction, of violence inflicted on a scale never seen and never possible before in human history. But this legacy – the result of new technology in the service of ideologies of hate – is not the only one we carry, nor that we must face up to.

Less visible, but even more widespread, is the legacy of day-to-day, individual suffering. It is the pain of children who are abused by people who should protect them, women injured or humiliated by violent partners, elderly persons maltreated by their caregivers, youths who are bullied by other youths, and people of all ages who inflict violence on themselves. This suffering – and there are many more examples that I could give – is a legacy that reproduces itself, as new generations learn from the violence of generations past, as victims learn from victimizers, and as the social conditions that nurture violence are allowed to continue. No country, no city, no community is immune. But neither are we powerless against it.

Violence thrives in the absence of democracy, respect for human rights and good governance. We often talk about how a "culture of violence" can take root. This is indeed true – as a South African who has lived through apartheid and is living through its aftermath, I have seen and experienced it. It is also true that patterns of violence are more pervasive and widespread in societies where the authorities endorse the use of violence through their own actions. In many societies, violence is so dominant that it thwarts hopes of economic and social development. We cannot let that continue.

Many who live with violence day in and day out assume that it is an intrinsic part of the human condition. But this is not so. Violence can be prevented. Violent cultures can be turned around. In my own country and around the world, we have shining examples of how violence has been countered. Governments, communities and individuals can make a difference.

I welcome this first *World report on violence and health*. This report makes a major contribution to our understanding of violence and its impact on societies. It illuminates the different faces of violence, from the "invisible" suffering of society's most vulnerable individuals to the all-too-visible tragedy of societies in conflict. It advances our analysis of the factors that lead to violence, and the possible responses of different sectors of society. And in doing so, it reminds us that safety and security don't just happen: they are the result of collective consensus and public investment.

The report describes and makes recommendations for action at the local, national and international levels. It will thus be an invaluable tool for policy-makers, researchers, practitioners, advocates and volunteers involved in violence prevention. While violence traditionally has been the domain of the criminal justice system, the report strongly makes the case for involving all sectors of society in prevention efforts.

We owe our children – the most vulnerable citizens in any society – a life free from violence and fear. In order to ensure this, we must be tireless in our efforts not only to attain peace, justice and prosperity for countries, but also for communities and members of the same family. We must address the roots of violence. Only then will we transform the past century's legacy from a crushing burden into a cautionary lesson.

Nelson Mandela

Preface

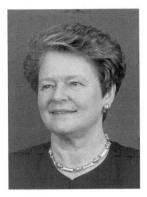

Violence pervades the lives of many people around the world, and touches all of us in some way. To many people, staying out of harm's way is a matter of locking doors and windows and avoiding dangerous places. To others, escape is not possible. The threat of violence is behind those doors – well hidden from public view. And for those living in the midst of war and conflict, violence permeates every aspect of life.

This report, the first comprehensive summary of the problem on a global scale, shows not only the human toll of violence – over 1.6 million lives lost each year and countless more damaged in ways that are not always apparent – but exposes the many faces of interpersonal, collective and self-directed violence, as well as the settings in which violence occurs. It shows that where violence persists, health is seriously compromised.

The report also challenges us in many respects. It forces us to reach beyond our notions of what is acceptable and comfortable – to challenge notions that acts of violence are simply matters of family privacy, individual choice, or inevitable facets of life. Violence is a complex problem related to patterns of thought and behaviour that are shaped by a multitude of forces within our families and communities, forces that can also transcend national borders. The report urges us to work with a range of partners and to adopt an approach that is proactive, scientific and comprehensive.

We have some of the tools and knowledge to make a difference – the same tools that have successfully been used to tackle other health problems. This is evident throughout the report. And we have a sense of where to apply our knowledge. Violence is often predictable and preventable. Like other health problems, it is not distributed evenly across population groups or settings. Many of the factors that increase the risk of violence are shared across the different types of violence and are modifiable.

One theme that is echoed throughout this report is the importance of primary prevention. Even small investments here can have large and long-lasting benefits, but not without the resolve of leaders and support for prevention efforts from a broad array of partners in both the public and private spheres, and from both industrialized and developing countries.

Public health has made some remarkable achievements in recent decades, particularly with regard to reducing rates of many childhood diseases. However, saving our children from these diseases only to let them fall victim to violence or lose them later to acts of violence between intimate partners, to the savagery of war and conflict, or to self-inflicted injuries or suicide, would be a failure of public health.

While public health does not offer all of the answers to this complex problem, we are determined to play our role in the prevention of violence worldwide. This report will contribute to shaping the global response to violence and to making the world a safer and healthier place for all. I invite you to read the report carefully, and to join me and the many violence prevention experts from around the world who have contributed to it in implementing its vital call for action.

Gro Harlem Brundtland
Director-General
World Health Organization

Contributors

Editorial guidance

Editorial Committee

Etienne G. Krug, Linda L. Dahlberg, James A. Mercy, Anthony B. Zwi, Rafael Lozano.

Executive Editor

Linda L. Dahlberg.

Advisory Committee

Nana Apt, Philippe Biberson, Jacquelyn Campbell, Radhika Coomaraswamy, William Foege, Adam Graycar, Rodrigo Guerrero, Marianne Kastrup, Reginald Moreels, Paulo Sergio Pinheiro, Mark L. Rosenberg, Terezinha da Silva, Mohd Sham Kasim.

WHO Secretariat

Ahmed Abdullatif, Susan Bassiri, Assia Brandrup-Lukanow, Alberto Concha-Eastman, Colette Dehlot, Antonio Pedro Filipe, Viviana Mangiaterra, Hisahi Ogawa, Francesca Racioppi, Sawat Ramaboot, Pang Ruyan, Gyanendra Sharma, Safia Singhateh, Yasuhiro Suzuki, Nerayo Tecklemichael, Tomris Turmen, Madan Upadhyay, Derek Yach.

Regional consultants

WHO African Region

Nana Apt, Niresh Bhagwandin, Chiane Esther, Helena Zacarias Pedro Garinne, Rachel Jewkes, Naira Khan, Romilla Maharaj, Sandra Marais, David Nyamwaya, Philista Onyango, Welile Shasha, Safia Singhateh, Isseu Diop Touré, Greer van Zyl.

WHO Region of the Americas

Nancy Cardia, Arturo Cervantes, Mariano Ciafardini, Carme Clavel-Arcas, Alberto Concha-Eastman, Carlos Fletes, Yvette Holder, Silvia Narvaez, Mark L. Rosenberg, Ana Maria Sanjuan, Elizabeth Ward.

WHO South-East Asia Region

Srikala Bharath, Vijay Chandra, Gopalakrishna Gururaj, Churnrutai Kanchanachitra, Mintarsih Latief, Panpimol Lotrakul, Imam Mochny, Dinesh Mohan, Thelma Narayan, Harsaran Pandey, Sawat Ramaboot, Sanjeeva Ranawera, Poonam Khetrapal Singh, Prawate Tantipiwatanaskul.

WHO European Region

Franklin Apfel, Assia Brandrup-Lukanow, Kevin Browne, Gani Demolli, Joseph Goicoechea, Karin Helweg-Larsen, Mária Herczog, Joseph Kasonde, Kari Killen, Viviana Mangiaterra, Annemiek Richters, Tine Rikke, Elisabeth Schauer, Berit Schei, Jan Theunissen, Mark Tsechkovski, Vladimir Verbitski, Isabel Yordi.

WHO Eastern Mediterranean Region

Saadia Abenaou, Ahmed Abdullatif, Abdul Rahman Al-Awadi, Shiva Dolatabadi, Albert Jokhadar, Hind Khattab, Lamis Nasser, Asma Fozia Qureshi, Sima Samar, Mervat Abu Shabana.

WHO Western Pacific Region

Liz Eckermann, Mohd Sham Kasim, Bernadette Madrid, Pang Ruyan, Wang Yan, Simon Yanis.

Authors and reviewers
Chapter 1. Violence — a global public health problem
Authors: Linda L. Dahlberg, Etienne G. Krug.
Boxes: Alberto Concha-Eastman, Rodrigo Guerrero (1.1); Alexander Butchart (1.2); Vittorio Di Martino (1.3).

Chapter 2. Youth violence
Authors: James A. Mercy, Alexander Butchart, David Farrington, Magdalena Cerdá.
Boxes: Magdalena Cerdá (2.1); Alexander Butchart (2.2).
Peer reviewers: Nancy Cardia, Alberto Concha-Eastman, Adam Graycar, Kenneth E. Powell, Mohamed Seedat, Garth Stevens.

Chapter 3. Child abuse and neglect by parents and other caregivers
Authors: Desmond Runyan, Corrine Wattam, Robin Ikeda, Fatma Hassan, Laurie Ramiro.
Boxes: Desmond Runyan (3.1); Akila Belembaogo, Peter Newell (3.2); Philista Onyango (3.3); Magdalena Cerdá, Mara Bustelo, Pamela Coffey (3.4).
Peer reviewers: Tilman Furniss, Fu-Yong Jiao, Philista Onyango, Zelided Alma de Ruiz.

Chapter 4. Violence by intimate partners
Authors: Lori Heise, Claudia Garcia-Moreno.
Boxes: Mary Ellsberg (4.1); Pan American Health Organization (4.2); Lori Heise (4.3).
Peer reviewers: Jill Astbury, Jacquelyn Campbell, Radhika Coomaraswamy, Terezinha da Silva.

Chapter 5. Abuse of the elderly
Authors: Rosalie Wolf, Lia Daichman, Gerry Bennett.
Boxes: HelpAge International Tanzania (5.1); Yuko Yamada (5.2); Elizabeth Podnieks (5.3).
Peer reviewers: Robert Agyarko, Nana Apt, Malgorzata Halicka, Jordan Kosberg, Alex Yui-Huen Kwan, Siobhan Laird, Ariela Lowenstein.

Chapter 6. Sexual violence
Authors: Rachel Jewkes, Purna Sen, Claudia Garcia-Moreno.
Boxes: Rachel Jewkes (6.1); Ivy Josiah (6.2); Fatma Khafagi (6.3); Nadine France, Maria de Bruyn (6.4).
Peer reviewers: Nata Duvvury, Ana Flávia d'Oliveira, Mary P. Koss, June Lopez, Margarita Quintanilla Gordillo, Pilar Ramos-Jimenez.

Chapter 7. Self-directed violence
Authors: Diego DeLeo, José Bertolote, David Lester.
Boxes: Ernest Hunter, Antoon Leenaars (7.1); Danuta Wasserman (7.2).
Peer reviewers: Annette Beautrais, Michel Grivna, Gopalakrishna Gururaj, Ramune Kalediene, Arthur Kleinman, Paul Yip.

Chapter 8. Collective violence

Authors: Anthony B. Zwi, Richard Garfield, Alessandro Loretti.

Boxes: James Welsh (8.1); Joan Serra Hoffman, Jose Teruel, Sylvia Robles, Alessandro Loretti (8.2); Rachel Brett (8.3).

Peer reviewers: Suliman Baldo, Robin Coupland, Marianne Kastrup, Arthur Kleinman, David Meddings, Paulo Sergio Pinheiro, Jean Rigal, Michael Toole.

Chapter 9. The way forward: recommendations for action

Authors: Etienne G. Krug, Linda L. Dahlberg, James A. Mercy, Anthony B. Zwi, Andrew Wilson.

Boxes: Tyrone Parks, Shereen Usdin, Sue Goldstein (9.1); Joan Serra Hoffman, Rodrigo Guerrero, Alberto Concha-Eastman (9.2); Laura Sminkey, Etienne G. Krug (9.3).

Statistical annex

Colin Mathers, Mie Inoue, Yaniss Guigoz, Rafael Lozano, Lana Tomaskovic.

Resources

Laura Sminkey, Alexander Butchart, Andrés Villaveces, Magdalena Cerdá.

Acknowledgements

The World Health Organization and the Editorial Committee would like to pay a special tribute to the principal author of the chapter on abuse of the elderly, Rosalie Wolf, who passed away in June 2001. She made an invaluable contribution to the care and protection of the elderly from abuse and neglect, and showed an enduring commitment to this particularly vulnerable and often voiceless population.

The World Health Organization acknowledges with thanks the many authors, peer reviewers, advisers and consultants whose dedication, support and expertise made this report possible.

The report also benefited from the contributions of a number of other people. In particular, acknowledgement is made to Tony Kahane, who revised the draft manuscript, and to Caroline Allsopp and Angela Haden, who edited the final text. Thanks are also due to the following: Sue Armstrong and Andrew Wilson for preparing the summary of the report; Laura Sminkey, for providing invaluable assistance to the Editorial Committee in the day-to-day management and coordination of the project; Marie Fitzsimmons, for editorial assistance; Catherine Currat, Karin Engstrom, Nynke Poortinga, Gabriella Rosen and Emily Rothman, for research assistance; Emma Fitzpatrick, Helen Green, Reshma Prakash, Angela Raviglione, Sabine van Tuyll van Serooskerken and Nina Vugman, for communications; and Simone Colairo, Pascale Lanvers, Angela Swetloff-Coff and Stella Tabengwa, for administrative support.

The World Health Organization also wishes to thank the California Wellness Foundation, the Global Forum for Health Research, the Governments of Belgium, Finland, Japan, Sweden and the United Kingdom, the Rockefeller Foundation and the United States Centers for Disease Control and Prevention, for their generous financial support for the development and publication of this report.

Introduction

In 1996, the Forty-Ninth World Health Assembly adopted Resolution WHA49.25, declaring violence a major and growing public health problem across the world (see Box overleaf for full text).

In this resolution, the Assembly drew attention to the serious consequences of violence – both in the short-term and the long-term – for individuals, families, communities and countries, and stressed the damaging effects of violence on health care services.

The Assembly asked Member States to give urgent consideration to the problem of violence within their own borders, and requested the Director-General of the World Health Organization (WHO) to set up public health activities to deal with the problem.

This, the first *World report on violence and health*, is an important part of WHO's response to Resolution WHA49.25. It is aimed mainly at researchers and practitioners. The latter include health care workers, social workers, those involved in developing and implementing prevention programmes and services, educators and law enforcement officials. A summary of the report is also available.[1]

Goals

The goals of the report are to raise awareness about the problem of violence globally, and to make the case that violence is preventable and that public health has a crucial role to play in addressing its causes and consequences.

More specific objectives are to:
— describe the magnitude and impact of violence throughout the world;
— describe the key risk factors for violence;
— give an account of the types of intervention and policy responses that have been tried and summarize what is known about their effectiveness;
— make recommendations for action at local, national and international levels.

Topics and scope

This report examines the types of violence that are present worldwide, in the everyday lives of people, and that constitute the bulk of the health burden imposed by violence. Accordingly, the information has been arranged in nine chapters, covering the following topics:
1. Violence – a global public health problem
2. Youth violence
3. Child abuse and neglect by parents and other caregivers
4. Violence by intimate partners

---

[1] *World report on violence and health: a summary.* Geneva, World Health Organization, 2002.

Preventing violence: a public health priority (Resolution WHA49.25)

The Forty-ninth World Health Assembly,

Noting with great concern the dramatic worldwide increase in the incidence of intentional injuries affecting people of all ages and both sexes, but especially women and children;

Endorsing the call made in the Declaration of the World Summit for Social Development for the introduction and implementation of specific policies and programmes of public health and social services to prevent violence in society and mitigate its effect;

Endorsing the recommendations made at the International Conference on Population and Development (Cairo, 1994) and the Fourth World Conference on Women (Beijing, 1995) urgently to tackle the problem of violence against women and girls and to understand its health consequences;

Recalling the United Nations Declaration on the elimination of violence against women;

Noting the call made by the scientific community in the Melbourne Declaration adopted at the Third International Conference on Injury Prevention and Control (1996) for increased international cooperation in ensuring the safety of the citizens of the world;

Recognizing the serious immediate and future long-term implications for health and psychological and social development that violence represents for individuals, families, communities and countries;

Recognizing the growing consequences of violence for health care services everywhere and its detrimental effect on scarce health care resources for countries and communities;

Recognizing that health workers are frequently among the first to see victims of violence, having a unique technical capacity and benefiting from a special position in the community to help those at risk;

Recognizing that WHO, the major agency for coordination of international work in public health, has the responsibility to provide leadership and guidance to Member States in developing public health programmes to prevent self-inflicted violence and violence against others;

1. DECLARES that violence is a leading worldwide public health problem;

2. URGES Member States to assess the problem of violence on their own territory and to communicate to WHO their information about this problem and their approach to it;

3. REQUESTS the Director-General, within available resources, to initiate public health activities to address the problem of violence that will:

   (1) characterize different types of violence, define their magnitude and assess the causes and the public health consequences of violence using also a "gender perspective" in the analysis;

   (2) assess the types and effectiveness of measures and programmes to prevent violence and mitigate its effects, with particular attention to community-based initiatives;

   (3) promote activities to tackle this problem at both international and country level including steps to:

   (a) improve the recognition, reporting and management of the consequences of violence;

   (b) promote greater intersectoral involvement in the prevention and management of violence;

   (c) promote research on violence as a priority for public health research;

   (d) prepare and disseminate recommendations for violence prevention programmes in nations, States and communities all over the world;

(continued)

      (4) ensure the coordinated and active participation of appropriate WHO technical programmes;

      (5) strengthen the Organization's collaboration with governments, local authorities and other organizations of the United Nations system in the planning, implementation and monitoring of programmes of violence prevention and mitigation;

    4. FURTHER REQUESTS the Director-General to present a report to the ninety-ninth session of the Executive Board describing the progress made so far and to present a plan of action for progress towards a science-based public health approach to violence prevention.

5. Abuse of the elderly
6. Sexual violence
7. Self-directed violence
8. Collective violence
9. The way forward: recommendations for action

Because it is impossible to cover all types of violence fully and adequately in a single document, each chapter has a specific focus. For example, the chapter on youth violence examines interpersonal violence among adolescents and young adults in the community. The chapter on child abuse discusses physical, sexual and psychological abuse, as well as neglect by parents and other caregivers; other forms of maltreatment of children, such as child prostitution and the use of children as soldiers, are covered in other parts of the report. The chapter on abuse of the elderly focuses on abuse by caregivers in domestic and institutional settings, while that on collective violence discusses violent conflict. The chapters on intimate partner violence and sexual violence focus primarily on violence against women, though some discussion of violence directed at men and boys is included in the chapter on sexual violence. The chapter on self-directed violence focuses primarily on suicidal behaviour. The chapter is included in the report because suicidal behaviour is one of the external causes of injury and is often the product of many of the same underlying social, psychological and environmental factors as other types of violence.

The chapters follow a similar structure. Each begins with a brief discussion of definitions for the specific type of violence covered in the chapter, followed by a summary of current knowledge about the extent of the problem in different regions of the world. Where possible, country-level data are presented, as well as findings from a range of research studies. The chapters then describe the causes and consequences of violence, provide summaries of the interventions and policy responses that have been tried, and make recommendations for future research and action. Tables, figures and boxes are included to highlight specific epidemiological patterns and findings, illustrate examples of prevention activities, and draw attention to specific issues.

The report concludes with two additional sections: a statistical annex and a list of Internet resources. The statistical annex contains global, regional and country data derived from the WHO mortality and morbidity database and from Version 1 of the WHO Global Burden of Disease project for 2000. A description of data sources and methods is provided in the annex to explain how these data were collected and analysed.

The list of Internet resources includes web site addresses for organizations involved in violence research, prevention and advocacy. The list includes metasites (each site offers access to hundreds of organizations involved in violence research, prevention and advocacy), web sites that focus on specific types of violence, web sites that address broader contextual issues related to violence, and web sites that offer surveillance tools for improving the understanding of violence.

How the report was developed

This report benefited from the participation of over 160 experts from around the world, coordinated by a small Editorial Committee. An Advisory Committee, comprising representatives of all the WHO regions, and members of WHO staff, provided guidance to the Editorial Committee at various stages during the writing of the report.

Chapters were peer-reviewed individually by scientists from different regions of the world. These reviewers were asked to comment not only on the scientific content of the chapter but also on the relevance of the chapter within their own culture.

As the report progressed, consultations were held with members of the WHO regional offices and diverse groups of experts from all over the world. Participants reviewed an early draft of the report, providing an overview of the problem of violence in their regions and making suggestions on what was needed to advance regional violence prevention activities.

Moving forward

This report, while comprehensive and the first of its kind, is only a beginning. It is hoped that the report will stimulate discussion at local, national and international levels and that it will provide a platform for increased action towards preventing violence.

CHAPTER 1

Violence — a global public health problem

Background

Violence has probably always been part of the human experience. Its impact can be seen, in various forms, in all parts of the world. Each year, more than a million people lose their lives, and many more suffer non-fatal injuries, as a result of self-inflicted, interpersonal or collective violence. Overall, violence is among the leading causes of death worldwide for people aged 15–44 years.

Although precise estimates are difficult to obtain, the cost of violence translates into billions of US dollars in annual health care expenditures worldwide, and billions more for national economies in terms of days lost from work, law enforcement and lost investment.

The visible and the invisible

The human cost in grief and pain, of course, cannot be calculated. In fact, much of it is almost invisible. While satellite technology has made certain types of violence – terrorism, wars, riots and civil unrest – visible to television audiences on a daily basis, much more violence occurs out of sight in homes, workplaces and even in the medical and social institutions set up to care for people. Many of the victims are too young, weak or ill to protect themselves. Others are forced by social conventions or pressures to keep silent about their experiences.

As with its impacts, some causes of violence are easy to see. Others are deeply rooted in the social, cultural and economic fabric of human life. Recent research suggests that while biological and other individual factors explain some of the predisposition to aggression, more often these factors interact with family, community, cultural and other external factors to create a situation where violence is likely to occur.

A preventable problem

Despite the fact that violence has always been present, the world does not have to accept it as an inevitable part of the human condition. As long as there has been violence, there have also been systems – religious, philosophical, legal and communal – which have grown up to prevent or limit it. None has been completely successful, but all have made their contribution to this defining mark of civilization.

Since the early 1980s, the field of public health has been a growing asset in this response. A wide range of public health practitioners, researchers and systems have set themselves the tasks of understanding the roots of violence and preventing its occurrence.

Violence can be prevented and its impact reduced, in the same way that public health efforts have prevented and reduced pregnancy-related complications, workplace injuries, infectious diseases, and illness resulting from contaminated food and water in many parts of the world. The factors that contribute to violent responses – whether they are factors of attitude and behaviour or related to larger social, economic, political and cultural conditions – can be changed.

Violence can be prevented. This is not an article of faith, but a statement based on evidence. Examples of success can be found around the world, from small-scale individual and community efforts to national policy and legislative initiatives.

What can a public health approach contribute?

By definition, public health is not about individual patients. Its focus is on dealing with diseases and with conditions and problems affecting health, and it aims to provide the maximum benefit for the largest number of people. This does not mean that public health ignores the care of individuals. Rather, the concern is to prevent health problems and to extend better care and safety to entire populations.

The public health approach to any problem is interdisciplinary and science-based (1). It draws upon knowledge from many disciplines, including medicine, epidemiology, sociology, psychology, criminology, education and economics. This has allowed the field of public health to be innovative and responsive to a wide range of diseases, illnesses and injuries around the world.

The public health approach also emphasizes collective action. It has proved time and again that cooperative efforts from such diverse sectors as health, education, social services, justice and policy are necessary to solve what are usually assumed to be purely "medical" problems. Each sector has an important role to play in addressing the problem of violence and, collectively, the approaches taken by each have the potential to produce important reductions in violence (see Box 1.1).

The public health approach to violence is based on the rigorous requirements of the scientific method. In moving from problem to solution, it has four key steps (*1*):

- Uncovering as much basic knowledge as possible about all the aspects of violence – through systematically collecting data on the magnitude, scope, characteristics and consequences of violence at local, national and international levels.

- Investigating why violence occurs – that is, conducting research to determine:
  — the causes and correlates of violence;
  — the factors that increase or decrease the risk for violence;
  — the factors that might be modifiable through interventions.
- Exploring ways to prevent violence, using the information from the above, by designing, implementing, monitoring and evaluating interventions.
- Implementing, in a range of settings, interventions that appear promising, widely disseminating information and determining the cost-effectiveness of programmes.

Public health is above all characterized by its emphasis on prevention. Rather than simply accepting or reacting to violence, its starting point

---

BOX 1.1

The public health approach in action: DESEPAZ in Colombia

In 1992, the mayor of Cali, Colombia – himself a public health specialist – helped the city set up a comprehensive programme aimed at reducing the high levels of crime there. Rates of homicide in Cali, a city of some 2 million inhabitants, had risen from 23 per 100 000 population in 1983 to 85 per 100 000 in 1991. The programme that ensued was called DESEPAZ, an acronym for *Desarrollo, Seguridad, Paz* (development, security, peace).

In the initial stages of the city's programme, epidemiological studies were conducted so as to identify the principal risk factors for violence and shape the priorities for action. Special budgets were approved to strengthen the police, the judicial system and the local human rights office.

DESEPAZ undertook education on civil rights matters for both the police and the public at large, including television advertising at peak viewing times highlighting the importance of tolerance for others and self-control. A range of cultural and educational projects were organized for schools and families in collaboration with local nongovernmental organizations, to promote discussions on violence and help resolve interpersonal conflicts. There were restrictions on the sale of alcohol, and the carrying of handguns was banned on weekends and special occasions.

In the course of the programme, special projects were set up to provide economic opportunities and safe recreational facilities for young people. The mayor and his administrative team discussed their proposals to tackle crime with local people, and the city administration ensured the continuing participation and commitment of the community.

With the programme in operation, the homicide rate in Cali declined from an all-time high of 124 per 100 000 to 86 per 100 000 between 1994 and 1997, a reduction of 30%. In absolute numbers, there were approximately 600 fewer homicides between 1994 and 1997 compared with the previous 3-year period, which allowed the law enforcement authorities to devote scarce resources to combating more organized forms of crime. Furthermore, public opinion in Cali shifted strongly from a passive attitude towards dealing with violence to a vociferous demand for more prevention activities.

is the strong conviction that violent behaviour and its consequences can be prevented.

Defining violence

Any comprehensive analysis of violence should begin by defining the various forms of violence in such a way as to facilitate their scientific measurement. There are many possible ways to define violence. The World Health Organization defines violence (2) as:

> The intentional use of physical force or power, threatened or actual, against oneself, another person, or against a group or community, that either results in or has a high likelihood of resulting in injury, death, psychological harm, maldevelopment or deprivation.

The definition used by the World Health Organization associates intentionality with the committing of the act itself, irrespective of the outcome it produces. Excluded from the definition are unintentional incidents – such as most road traffic injuries and burns.

The inclusion of the word "power", in addition to the phrase "use of physical force", broadens the nature of a violent act and expands the conventional understanding of violence to include those acts that result from a power relationship, including threats and intimidation. The "use of power" also serves to include neglect or acts of omission, in addition to the more obvious violent acts of commission. Thus, "the use of physical force or power" should be understood to include neglect and all types of physical, sexual and psychological abuse, as well as suicide and other self-abusive acts.

This definition covers a broad range of outcomes – including psychological harm, deprivation and maldevelopment. This reflects a growing recognition among researchers and practitioners of the need to include violence that does not necessarily result in injury or death, but that nonetheless poses a substantial burden on individuals, families, communities and health care systems worldwide. Many forms of violence against women, children and the elderly, for instance, can result in physical, psychological and social problems that do not necessarily lead to injury, disability or death. These conse-

quences can be immediate, as well as latent, and can last for years after the initial abuse. Defining outcomes solely in terms of injury or death thus limits the understanding of the full impact of violence on individuals, communities and society at large.

Intentionality

One of the more complex aspects of the definition is the matter of intentionality. Two important points about this should be noted. First, even though violence is distinguished from unintended events that result in injuries, the presence of an intent to use force does not necessarily mean that there was an intent to cause damage. Indeed, there may be a considerable disparity between intended behaviour and intended consequence. A perpetrator may intentionally commit an act that, by objective standards, is judged to be dangerous and highly likely to result in adverse health effects, but the perpetrator may not perceive it as such.

As examples, a youth may be involved in a physical fight with another youth. The use of a fist against the head or the use of a weapon in the dispute certainly increases the risk of serious injury or death, though neither outcome may be intended. A parent may vigorously shake a crying infant with the intent to quieten it. Such an action, however, may instead cause brain damage. Force was clearly used, but without the intention of causing an injury.

A second point related to intentionality lies in the distinction between the intent to injure and the intent to "use violence". Violence, according to Walters & Parke (3), is culturally determined. Some people mean to harm others but, based on their cultural backgrounds and beliefs, do not perceive their acts as violent. The definition used by the World Health Organization, however, defines violence as it relates to the health or well-being of individuals. Certain behaviours – such as hitting a spouse – may be regarded by some people as acceptable cultural practices, but are considered violent acts with important health implications for the individual.

Other aspects of violence, though not explicitly stated, are also included in the definition. For example, the definition implicitly includes all acts of violence, whether they are public or private, whether they are reactive (in response to previous events such as provocation) or proactive (instrumental for or anticipating more self-serving outcomes) (*4*), or whether they are criminal or non-criminal. Each of these aspects is important in understanding the causes of violence and in designing prevention programmes.

Typology of violence

In its 1996 resolution WHA49.25, declaring violence a leading public health problem, the World Health Assembly called on the World Health Organization to develop a typology of violence that characterized the different types of violence and the links between them. Few typologies exist already and none is very comprehensive (*5*).

Types of violence

The typology proposed here divides violence into three broad categories according to characteristics of those committing the violent act:

— self-directed violence;

— interpersonal violence;

— collective violence.

This initial categorization differentiates between violence a person inflicts upon himself or herself, violence inflicted by another individual or by a small group of individuals, and violence inflicted by larger groups such as states, organized political groups, militia groups and terrorist organizations (see Figure 1.1).

These three broad categories are each divided further to reflect more specific types of violence.

Self-directed violence

Self-directed violence is subdivided into suicidal behaviour and self-abuse. The former includes suicidal thoughts, attempted suicides – also called "parasuicide" or "deliberate self-injury" in some countries – and completed suicides. Self-abuse, in contrast, includes acts such as self-mutilation.

Interpersonal violence

Interpersonal violence is divided into two sub-categories:

- Family and intimate partner violence – that is, violence largely between family members and intimate partners, usually, though not exclusively, taking place in the home.
- Community violence – violence between individuals who are unrelated, and who may or may not know each other, generally taking place outside the home.

The former group includes forms of violence such as child abuse, intimate partner violence and abuse of the elderly. The latter includes youth violence, random acts of violence, rape or sexual assault by strangers, and violence in institutional settings such as schools, workplaces, prisons and nursing homes.

Collective violence

Collective violence is subdivided into social, political and economic violence. Unlike the other two broad categories, the subcategories of collective violence suggest possible motives for violence committed by larger groups of individuals or by states. Collective violence that is committed to advance a particular social agenda includes, for example, crimes of hate committed by organized groups, terrorist acts and mob violence. Political violence includes war and related violent conflicts, state violence and similar acts carried out by larger groups. Economic violence includes attacks by larger groups motivated by economic gain – such as attacks carried out with the purpose of disrupting economic activity, denying access to essential services, or creating economic division and fragmentation. Clearly, acts committed by larger groups can have multiple motives.

The nature of violent acts

Figure 1.1 illustrates the nature of violent acts, which can be:

— physical;

— sexual;

— psychological;

— involving deprivation or neglect.

The horizontal array in Figure 1.1 shows who is affected, and the vertical array describes how they are affected.

FIGURE 1.1

A typology of violence

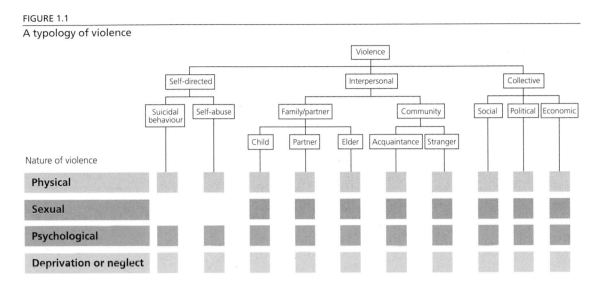

These four types of violent acts occur in each of the broad categories and their subcategories described above – with the exception of self-directed violence. For instance, violence against children committed within the home can include physical, sexual and psychological abuse, as well as neglect. Community violence can include physical assaults between young people, sexual violence in the workplace and neglect of older people in long-term care facilities. Political violence can include such acts as rape during conflicts, and physical and psychological warfare.

This typology, while imperfect and far from being universally accepted, does provide a useful framework for understanding the complex patterns of violence taking place around the world, as well as violence in the everyday lives of individuals, families and communities. It also overcomes many of the limitations of other typologies by capturing the nature of violent acts, the relevance of the setting, the relationship between the perpetrator and the victim, and – in the case of collective violence – possible motivations for the violence. However, in both research and practice, the dividing lines between the different types of violence are not always so clear.

Measuring violence and its impact
Types of data

Different types of data are needed for different purposes, including:

— describing the magnitude and impact of violence;
— understanding which factors increase the risk for violent victimization and perpetration;
— knowing how effective violence prevention programmes are.

Some of these types of data and sources are described in Table 1.1.

Mortality data

Data on fatalities, particularly through homicide, and on suicide and war-related deaths can provide an indication of the extent of lethal violence in a particular community or country. When compared to statistics on other deaths, such data are useful indicators of the burden created by violence-related injuries. These data can also be used for monitoring changes over time in fatal violence, identifying groups and communities at high risk of violence, and making comparisons within and between countries.

Other types of data

Mortality figures, however, are only one possible type of data for describing the magnitude of the problem. Since non-fatal outcomes are much more common than fatal outcomes and because certain types of violence are not fully represented by mortality data, other types of information are

TABLE 1.1
Types of data and potential sources for collecting information

Type of data	Data sources	Examples of information collected
Mortality	Death certificates, vital statistics registries, medical examiners', coroners' or mortuary reports	Characteristics of the decedent, cause of death, location, time, manner of death
Morbidity and other health data	Hospital, clinic or other medical records	Diseases, injuries, information on physical, mental or reproductive health
Self-reported	Surveys, special studies, focus groups, media	Attitudes, beliefs, behaviours, cultural practices, victimization and perpetration, exposure to violence in the home or community
Community	Population records, local government records, other institutional records	Population counts and density, levels of income and education, unemployment rates, divorce rates
Crime	Police records, judiciary records, crime laboratories	Type of offence, characteristics of offender, relationship between victim and offender, circumstances of event
Economic	Programme, institutional or agency records, special studies	Expenditures on health, housing or social services, costs of treating violence-related injuries, use of services
Policy or legislative	Government or legislative records	Laws, institutional policies and practices

necessary. Such information can help in understanding the circumstances surrounding specific incidents and in describing the full impact of violence on the health of individuals and communities. These types of data include:

— health data on diseases, injuries and other health conditions;

— self-reported data on attitudes, beliefs, behaviours, cultural practices, victimization and exposure to violence;

— community data on population characteristics and levels of income, education and unemployment;

— crime data on the characteristics and circumstances of violent events and violent offenders;

— economic data related to the costs of treatment and social services;

— data describing the economic burden on health care systems and possible savings realized from prevention programmes;

— data on policy and legislation.

Sources of data

Potential sources of the various types of information include:

— individuals;

— agency or institutional records;

— local programmes;

— community and government records;

— population-based and other surveys;

— special studies.

Though not listed in Table 1.1, almost all sources include basic demographic information – such as a person's age and sex. Some sources – including medical records, police records, death certificates and mortuary reports – include information specific to the violent event or injury. Data from emergency departments, for instance, may provide information on the nature of an injury, how it was sustained, and when and where the incident occurred. Data collected by the police may include information on the relationship between the victim and the perpetrator, whether a weapon was involved, and other circumstances related to the offence.

Surveys and special studies can provide detailed information about the victim or perpetrator, and his or her background, attitudes, behaviours and possible previous involvement in violence. Such sources can also help uncover violence that is not reported to the police or other agencies. For example, a household survey in South Africa showed that between 50% and 80% of victims of violence received medical treatment for a violence-related injury without reporting the incident to the police (6). In another study, conducted in the United States of America, 46% of victims who sought emergency treatment did not make a report to the police (7).

Problems with collecting data

The availability, quality and usefulness of the different data sources for comparing types of violence within and between countries vary considerably. Countries around the world are at very different stages with regard to their capacity for data collection.

Availability of data

Mortality data are the most widely collected and available of all sources of data. Many countries maintain birth and death registries and keep basic counts of homicides and suicides. Calculating rates from these basic counts, however, is not always possible because population data are often unavailable or unreliable. This is especially true where populations are in flux – in areas, for instance, experiencing conflict or continuous movements among population groups – or where populations are difficult to count, as is the case in densely populated or very remote areas.

Systematic data on non-fatal outcomes are not available in most countries of the world, though systems to collect such data are currently being developed. A number of documents providing guidance for measuring different types of violence in a range of settings have also been published in recent years (8–14).

Quality of data

Even when data are available, the quality of the information may be inadequate for research purposes and for identifying strategies for prevention. Given that agencies and institutions keep records for their own purposes, following their own internal procedures for record-keeping, their data may be incomplete or lack the kind of information necessary for a proper understanding of violence.

Data from health care facilities, for instance, are collected with a view to providing optimal treatment for the patient. The medical record may contain diagnostic information about the injury and course of treatment, but not the circumstances surrounding the injury. These data may also be confidential and thus not available for research purposes. Surveys, on the other hand, contain more detailed information about the person and his or her background and involvement in violence. They are limited, though, by the extent to which a person recalls events and admits to engaging in certain behaviours, and also by the manner in which questions are asked and by whom they are asked – as well as when, where and how well the interview is conducted.

Other obstacles

Linking data across sources is one of the more difficult problems in research on violence. Data on violence generally come from a variety of organizations that operate independently of one another. As such, data from medical examiners and coroners cannot usually be linked to data collected by the police. Also, there is a general lack of uniformity in the way data on violence are collected, which makes it very difficult to compare data across communities and nations.

Although they are beyond the scope of this discussion, a number of other problems in collecting violence-related data should be mentioned. They include:

— the difficulty of developing measures that are relevant and specific to subpopulation groups and different cultural contexts (8, 9, 11, 14);
— devising appropriate protocols to protect the confidentiality of victims and ensure their safety (15);
— a range of other ethical considerations associated with research into violence.

An overview of current knowledge

The prevention of violence, according to the public health approach, begins with a description of the magnitude and impact of the problem. This section describes what is currently known about global patterns of violence, using data compiled for this report from the World Health Organization's mortality database and Version 1 of the World Health Organization's Global Burden of Disease project for 2000, as well as data from surveys and special studies of violence.

Estimates of mortality

In 2000, an estimated 1.6 million people worldwide died as a result of self-inflicted, interpersonal or collective violence, for an overall age-adjusted rate of 28.8 per 100 000 population (see Table 1.2).

TABLE 1.2

Estimated global violence-related deaths, 2000

Type of violence	Number[a]	Rate per 100 000 population[b]	Proportion of total (%)
Homicide	520 000	8.8	31.3
Suicide	815 000	14.5	49.1
War-related	310 000	5.2	18.6
Total[c]	1 659 000	28.8	100.0
Low- to middle-income countries	1 510 000	32.1	91.1
High-income countries	149 000	14.4	8.9

Source: WHO Global Burden of Disease project for 2000, Version 1 (see Statistical annex).

[a] Rounded to the nearest 1000.

[b] Age-standardized.

[c] Includes 14 000 intentional injury deaths resulting from legal intervention.

The vast majority of these deaths occurred in low- to middle-income countries. Less than 10% of all violence-related deaths occurred in high-income countries.

Nearly half of these 1.6 million violence-related deaths were suicides, almost one-third were homicides and about one-fifth were war-related.

Mortality according to sex and age

Like many other health problems in the world, violence is not distributed evenly among sex or age groups. In 2000, there were an estimated 520 000 homicides, for an overall age-adjusted rate of 8.8 per 100 000 population (see Table 1.2). Males accounted for 77% of all homicides and had rates that were more than three times those of females (13.6 and 4.0, respectively, per 100 000) (see Table 1.3). The highest rates of homicide in the

TABLE 1.3

Estimated global homicide and suicide rates by age group, 2000

Age group (years)	Homicide rate (per 100 000 population)		Suicide rate (per 100 000 population)	
	Males	Females	Males	Females
0–4	5.8	4.8	0.0	0.0
5–14	2.1	2.0	1.7	2.0
15–29	19.4	4.4	15.6	12.2
30–44	18.7	4.3	21.5	12.4
45–59	14.8	4.5	28.4	12.6
⩾60	13.0	4.5	44.9	22.1
Total[a]	13.6	4.0	18.9	10.6

Source: WHO Global Burden of Disease project for 2000, Version 1 (see Statistical annex).

[a] Age-standardized.

world are found among males aged 15–29 years (19.4 per 100 000), followed closely by males aged 30–44 years (18.7 per 100 000).

Worldwide, suicide claimed the lives of an estimated 815 000 people in 2000, for an overall age-adjusted rate of 14.5 per 100 000 (see Table 1.2). Over 60% of all suicides occurred among males, over half of these occurring among those aged 15–44 years. For both males and females, suicide rates increase with age and are highest among those aged 60 years and older (see Table 1.3). Suicide rates, though, are generally higher among males than females (18.9 per 100 000 as against 10.6 per 100 000). This is especially true among the oldest age groups, where worldwide, male suicide rates among those aged 60 years and older are twice as high as female suicide rates in the same age category (44.9 per 100 000 as against 22.1 per 100 000).

Mortality according to country income level and region

Rates of violent death vary according to country income levels. In 2000, the rate of violent death in low- to middle-income countries was 32.1 per 100 000 population, more than twice the rate in high-income countries (14.4 per 100 000) (see Table 1.2).

There are also considerable regional differences in rates of violent death. These differences are evident, for example, among the WHO regions (see Figure 1.2). In the African Region and the Region of the Americas, homicide rates are nearly three times greater than suicide rates. However, in the European and South-East Asia Regions, suicide rates are more than double homicide rates (19.1 per 100 000 as against 8.4 per 100 000 for the European Region, and 12.0 per 100 000 as against 5.8 per 100 000 for the South-East Asia Region), and in the Western Pacific Region, suicide rates are nearly six times greater than homicide rates (20.8 per 100 000 as against 3.4 per 100 000).

Within regions there are also large differences between countries. For example, in 1994 the homicide rate among males in Colombia was reported to be 146.5 per 100 000, while the corresponding rates in Cuba and Mexico were 12.6

FIGURE 1.2

Homicide and suicide rates by WHO region, 2000

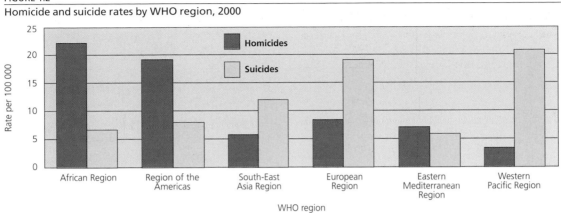

and 32.3 per 100 000, respectively (*16*). Large differences within countries also exist between urban and rural populations, between rich and poor groups, and between different racial and ethnic groups. In the United States in 1999, for instance, African-American youths aged 15–24 years had a rate of homicide (38.6 per 100 000) more than twice that of their Hispanic counterparts (17.3 per 100 000), and over 12 times the rate of their Caucasian, non-Hispanic counterparts (3.1 per 100 000) (*17*).

Estimates of non-fatal violence

The above-mentioned mortality figures are almost certainly underestimates of the true burden of violence. In all parts of the world, deaths represent the "tip of the iceberg" as far as violence is concerned. Physical and sexual assaults occur daily, though precise national and international estimates of each are lacking. Not all assaults result in injuries severe enough to require medical attention and – even among those that do result in serious injuries – surveillance systems for reporting and compiling these injuries are in many countries either lacking or are still being developed.

Much of what is known about non-fatal violence comes from surveys and special studies of different population groups. For example, in national surveys, the percentage of women who reported ever being physically assaulted by an intimate partner ranged from 10% in Paraguay and the Philippines, to 22.1% in the United States, 29.0% in Canada and 34.4% in Egypt (*18–21*). The proportion of women from various cities or provinces around the world reporting ever having been sexually assaulted (including victims of attempted assault) varied from 15.3% in Toronto, Canada, to 21.7% in León, Nicaragua, 23.0% in London, England, and 25.0% in one province in Zimbabwe (*21–25*). Among adolescent males in secondary schools, the percentage reporting involvement in physical fighting in the past year ranged from 22.0% in Sweden and 44.0% in the United States to 76.0% in Jerusalem, Israel (*26–28*).

An important point here is that these data are based largely on self-reports. It is difficult to know whether they overestimate or underestimate the true extent of physical and sexual assaults among these population groups. Certainly, in those countries with strong cultural pressures to keep violence "behind closed doors" or simply to accept it as "natural", non-fatal violence is likely to be underreported. Victims may be reluctant to discuss violent experiences not only out of shame and because of taboos, but through fear. Admitting to having experienced certain violent events, such as rape, may in some countries result in death. In certain cultures, the preservation of family honour is a traditional motive for killing women who have been raped (so-called "honour killings").

The costs of violence

Violence exacts both a human and an economic toll on nations, and costs economies many billions of US dollars each year in health care, legal costs, absenteeism from work and lost productivity. In the United

States, a 1992 study estimated the direct and indirect annual costs of gunshot wounds at US$ 126 billion. Cutting or stab wounds cost an additional US$ 51 billion (*29*). In a 1996 study in the Canadian province of New Brunswick, the mean total cost per suicide death was over US$ 849 000. The total direct and indirect costs, including costs for health care services, autopsies, police investigations and lost productivity resulting from premature death, amounted to nearly US$ 80 million (*30*).

The high cost of violence is not unique to Canada and the United States. Between 1996 and 1997, the Inter-American Development Bank sponsored studies on the magnitude and economic impact of violence in six Latin American countries (*31*). Each study examined expenditures, as a result of violence, for health care services, law enforcement and judicial services, as well as intangible losses and losses from the transfer of assets. Expressed as a percentage of the gross domestic product (GDP) in 1997, the cost of health care expenditures arising from violence was 1.9% of the GDP in Brazil, 5.0% in Colombia, 4.3% in El Salvador, 1.3% in Mexico, 1.5% in Peru and 0.3% in Venezuela.

It is difficult to calculate the precise burden of all types of violence on health care systems, or their effects on economic productivity around the world. The available evidence shows that victims of domestic and sexual violence have more health problems, significantly higher health care costs and more frequent visits to emergency departments throughout their lives than those without a history of abuse (see Chapters 4 and 6). The same is true for victims of childhood abuse and neglect (see Chapter 3). These costs contribute substantially to annual health care expenditures.

Since national cost estimates are also generally lacking for other health problems, such as depression, smoking, alcohol and drug abuse, unwanted pregnancy, human immunodeficiency virus/acquired immunodeficiency syndrome (HIV/AIDS), other sexually transmitted diseases and other infections (all of which have been linked to violence in small-scale studies) (*32–37*), it is not yet possible to calculate the global economic burden of these problems as they relate to violence.

Examining the roots of violence: an ecological model

No single factor explains why some individuals behave violently toward others or why violence is more prevalent in some communities than in others. Violence is the result of the complex interplay of individual, relationship, social, cultural and environmental factors. Understanding how these factors are related to violence is one of the important steps in the public health approach to preventing violence.

Multiple levels

The chapters in this report apply an ecological model to help understand the multifaceted nature of violence. First introduced in the late 1970s (*38, 39*), this ecological model was initially applied to child abuse (*38*) and subsequently to youth violence (*40, 41*). More recently, researchers have used it to understand intimate partner violence (*42, 43*) and abuse of the elderly (*44, 45*). The model explores the relationship between individual and contextual factors and considers violence as the product of multiple levels of influence on behaviour (see Figure 1.3).

Individual

The first level of the ecological model seeks to identify the biological and personal history factors that an individual brings to his or her behaviour. In addition

FIGURE 1.3

Ecological model for understanding violence

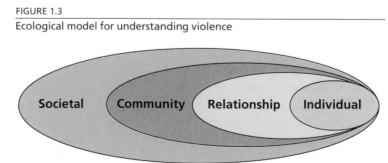

to biological and demographic factors, factors such as impulsivity, low educational attainment, substance abuse, and prior history of aggression and abuse are considered. In other words, this level of the ecological model focuses on the characteristics of the individual that increase the likelihood of being a victim or a perpetrator of violence.

Relationship

The second level of the ecological model explores how proximal social relationships – for example, relations with peers, intimate partners and family members – increase the risk for violent victimization and perpetration of violence. In the cases of partner violence and child maltreatment, for instance, interacting on an almost daily basis or sharing a common domicile with an abuser may increase the opportunity for violent encounters. Because individuals are bound together in a continuing relationship, it is likely in these cases that the victim will be repeatedly abused by the offender (46). In the case of interpersonal violence among youths, research shows that young people are much more likely to engage in negative activities when those behaviours are encouraged and approved by their friends (47, 48). Peers, intimate partners and family members all have the potential to shape an individual's behaviour and range of experience.

Community

The third level of the ecological model examines the community contexts in which social relationships are embedded – such as schools, workplaces and neighbourhoods – and seeks to identify the characteristics of these settings that are associated with being victims or perpetrators of violence. A high level of residential mobility (where people do not stay for a long time in a particular dwelling, but move many times), heterogeneity (highly diverse population, with little of the social "glue" that binds communities together) and high population density are all examples of such characteristics and each has been associated with violence. Similarly, communities characterized by problems such as drug trafficking, high levels of unemployment or

widespread social isolation (for example, people not knowing their neighbours or having no involvement in the local community) are also more likely to experience violence. Research on violence shows that opportunities for violence are greater in some community contexts than others – for instance, in areas of poverty or physical deterioration, or where there are few institutional supports.

Societal

The fourth and final level of the ecological model examines the larger societal factors that influence rates of violence. Included here are those factors that create an acceptable climate for violence, those that reduce inhibitions against violence, and those that create and sustain gaps between different segments of society – or tensions between different groups or countries. Larger societal factors include:

— cultural norms that support violence as an acceptable way to resolve conflicts;
— attitudes that regard suicide as a matter of individual choice instead of a preventable act of violence;
— norms that give priority to parental rights over child welfare;
— norms that entrench male dominance over women and children;
— norms that support the use of excessive force by police against citizens;
— norms that support political conflict.

Larger societal factors also include the health, educational, economic and social policies that maintain high levels of economic or social inequality between groups in society (see Box 1.2).

The ecological framework highlights the multiple causes of violence and the interaction of risk factors operating within the family and broader community, social, cultural and economic contexts. Placed within a developmental context, the ecological model also shows how violence may be caused by different factors at different stages of life.

Complex linkages

While some risk factors may be unique to a particular type of violence, the various types of violence more commonly share a number of risk

---

BOX 1.2

Globalization: the implications for violence prevention

Through an ever more rapid and widespread movement and exchange of information, ideas, services and products, globalization has eroded the functional and political borders that separated people into sovereign states. On the one hand, this has driven a massive expansion in world trade accompanied by a demand for increased economic output, creating millions of jobs and raising living standards in some countries in a way previously unimaginable. On the other, the effects of globalization have been remarkably uneven. In some parts of the world, globalization has led to increased inequalities in income and helped destroy factors such as social cohesion that had protected against interpersonal violence.

The benefits and the obstacles for violence prevention arising from globalization can be summarized as follows.

The positive effects

The huge increase in information-sharing provoked by globalization has produced new international networks and alliances that have the potential to improve the scope and quality of data collected on violence. Where globalization has raised living standards and helped reduce inequalities, there is a greater possibility of economic interventions being used to lessen tensions and conflicts both within and between states. Furthermore, globalization creates new ways of using global mechanisms:

- To conduct research on violence – especially on social, economic and policy factors that transcend national boundaries.
- To stimulate violence prevention activities on a regional or global scale.
- To implement international laws and treaties designed to reduce violence.
- To support violence prevention efforts within countries, particularly those with a limited capacity to conduct such activities.

The negative effects

Societies with already high levels of inequality, which experience a further widening of the gap between rich and poor as a result of globalization, are likely to witness an increase in interpersonal violence. Rapid social change in a country in response to strong global pressures – as occurred, for instance, in some of the states of the former Soviet Union – can overwhelm existing social controls over behaviour and create conditions for a high level of violence. In addition, the removal of market constraints, and increased incentives for profit as a result of globalization can lead, for example, to much freer access to alcohol, drugs and firearms, despite efforts to reduce their use in violent incidents.

The need for global responses

Violence can no longer remain the preserve of national politics, but must be vigorously addressed also on the global level – through groupings of states, international agencies and international networks of governmental and nongovernmental organizations. Such international efforts must aim to harness the positive aspects of globalization for the greater good, while striving to limit the negative aspects.

---

factors. Prevailing cultural norms, poverty, social isolation and such factors as alcohol abuse, substance abuse and access to firearms are risk factors for more than one type of violence. As a result, it is not unusual for some individuals at risk of violence to experience more than one type of violence. Women at risk of physical violence by intimate partners, for example, are also at risk of sexual violence (*18*).

It is also not unusual to detect links between different types of violence. Research has shown that exposure to violence in the home is associated with being a victim or perpetrator of violence in adolescence and adulthood (*49*). The experience of being rejected, neglected or suffering indifference at the hands of parents leaves children at greater risk for aggressive and antisocial behaviour, including abusive behaviour as adults (*50–52*). Associations have been found between suicidal behaviour and several types of violence, including child maltreatment (*53, 54*), intimate partner violence (*33, 55*), sexual assault (*53*) and abuse of the elderly (*56, 57*). In Sri Lanka, suicide rates were shown to decrease during wartime, only to increase again after the violent conflict ended (*58*). In many countries that have suffered violent conflict, the rates of interpersonal violence remain high even after the cessation of hostilities – among other reasons because of the way violence has become more socially accepted and the availability of weapons.

The links between violence and the interaction between individual factors and the broader social, cultural and economic contexts suggest that addressing risk factors across the various levels of the ecological model may contribute to decreases in more than one type of violence.

How can violence be prevented?

The first two steps of the public health model provide important information about populations requiring preventive interventions, as well as on the risk and protective factors that need addressing. Putting this knowledge into practice is a central goal of public health.

Types of prevention

Public health interventions are traditionally characterized in terms of three levels of prevention:

- Primary prevention – approaches that aim to prevent violence before it occurs.
- Secondary prevention – approaches that focus on the more immediate responses to violence, such as pre-hospital care, emergency services

or treatment for sexually transmitted diseases following a rape.
- Tertiary prevention – approaches that focus on long-term care in the wake of violence, such as rehabilitation and reintegration, and attempts to lessen trauma or reduce the long-term disability associated with violence.

These three levels of prevention are defined by their temporal aspect – whether prevention takes place before violence occurs, immediately afterwards or over the longer term. Although traditionally they are applied to victims of violence and within health care settings, secondary and tertiary prevention efforts have also been regarded as having relevance to the perpetrators of violence, and applied in judicial settings in response to violence.

Researchers in the field of violence prevention have increasingly turned to a definition of prevention that focuses on the target group of interest. This definition groups interventions as follows (*59*):

- Universal interventions – approaches aimed at groups or the general population without regard to individual risk; examples include violence prevention curricula delivered to all students in a school or children of a particular age and community wide media campaigns.
- Selected interventions – approaches aimed at those considered at heightened risk for violence (having one or more risk factors for violence); an example of such an intervention is training in parenting provided to low-income, single parents.
- Indicated interventions – approaches aimed at those who have already demonstrated violent behaviour, such as treatment for perpetrators of domestic violence.

Many efforts to date, in both industrialized and developing countries, have focused on secondary and tertiary responses to violence. Understandably, priority is often given to dealing with the immediate consequences of violence, providing support to victims and punishing the offenders. Such responses, while important and in need of strengthening, should be accompanied by a greater investment in primary prevention. A comprehensive response to violence is one that not only protects and supports victims of violence, but also promotes non-violence, reduces the perpetration of violence, and changes the circumstances and conditions that give rise to violence in the first place.

Multifaceted responses

Because violence is a multifaceted problem with biological, psychological, social and environmental roots, it needs to be confronted on several different levels at once. The ecological model serves a dual purpose in this regard: each level in the model represents a level of risk and each level can also be thought of as a key point for intervention.

Dealing with violence on a range of levels involves addressing all of the following:

- Addressing individual risk factors and taking steps to modify individual risk behaviours.
- Influencing close personal relationships and working to create healthy family environments, as well as providing professional help and support for dysfunctional families.
- Monitoring public places such as schools, workplaces and neighbourhoods and taking steps to address problems that might lead to violence.
- Addressing gender inequality, and adverse cultural attitudes and practices.
- Addressing the larger cultural, social and economic factors that contribute to violence and taking steps to change them, including measures to close the gap between the rich and poor and to ensure equitable access to goods, services and opportunities.

Documenting effective responses

A general ground rule for the public health approach to violence is that all efforts, whether large or small, should be rigorously evaluated. Documenting existing responses and encouraging a strictly scientific assessment of interventions in different settings is valuable for everyone. It is particularly needed by others trying to determine the most effective responses to violence and the strategies likely to make a difference.

Bringing together all available evidence and experience is also an extremely useful part of advocacy, as it assures decision-makers that something can be done. Even more importantly, it provides them with valuable guidance as to which efforts are likely to reduce violence.

Balancing public health action

Rigorous research takes time to produce results. The impulse to invest only in proven approaches should not be an obstacle to supporting promising ones. Promising approaches are those that have been evaluated but require more testing in a range of settings and with different population groups.

There is also wisdom in trying out and testing a variety of programmes, and in using the initiatives and ideas of local communities. Violence is far too pressing a problem to delay public health action while waiting to gain perfect knowledge.

Addressing cultural norms

In various parts of the world, cultural specificity and tradition are sometimes given as justifications for particular social practices that perpetuate violence. The oppression of women is one of the most widely quoted examples, but many others can also be given.

Cultural norms must be dealt with sensitively and respectfully in all prevention efforts – sensitively because of people's often passionate attachment to their traditions, and respectfully because culture is often a source of protection against violence. Experience has shown that it is important to conduct early and ongoing consultations with religious and traditional leaders, lay groups and prominent figures in the community, such as traditional healers, when designing and implementing programmes.

Actions against violence at all levels

Long-term successes in the prevention of violence will increasingly depend on comprehensive approaches at all levels.

Local level

At the local level, partners may include health care providers, police, educators, social workers, employers and government officials. Much can be done here to promote violence prevention. Small-scale pilot programmes and research projects can provide a means for ideas to be tried out and – perhaps as important – for a range of partners to become used to working together. Structures such as working groups or commissions that draw together the different sectors and maintain both formal and informal contacts are essential for the success of this type of collaboration.

National level

Multisectoral partnerships are highly desirable at the national level as much as at the local level. A variety of government ministries – and not only those concerned with law enforcement, social services and health – have important contributions to make in preventing violence. Education ministries are obvious partners, given the importance of intervening in schools. Ministries of labour can do much to reduce violence in the workplace, especially in collaboration with trade unions and employers (see Box 1.3). Defence ministries can positively shape the attitudes towards violence of large numbers of young men under their control, by encouraging discipline, promoting codes of honour, and impressing a strong awareness of the lethalness of weapons. Religious leaders and organizations have a role to play in their pastoral work and, in appropriate cases, by offering their good offices to mediate in specific problems.

Global level

As has been shown, for instance, in the international response to AIDS and in the field of disaster relief, cooperation and exchange of information between organizations globally can produce significant benefits – in the same way as partnerships at the national and local levels. The World Health Organization clearly has an important global role to play in this respect as the United Nations agency responsible for health. Other international agencies, though, also have a considerable amount to offer in their specialized fields. These include the Office of the United Nations High Commissioner for Human Rights (in relation to human rights), the Office of the United Nations High Commissioner for Refu-

gees (refugees), the United Nations Children's Fund (children's well-being), the United Nations Development Fund for Women and the United Nations Population Fund (women's health), the United Nations Development Programme (human development), the United Nations Interregional Crime and Justice Research Institute (crime) and the World Bank (financing and governance), to name just a few. A variety of international donors, bilateral programmes, nongovernmental organizations and religious organizations are already involved in violence prevention activities around the world.

Problems for national decision-makers

If violence is largely preventable, the question arises: why are there not more efforts to prevent it, particularly at national or provincial and state level?

A major obstacle is simply an absence of knowledge. For many decision-makers, the idea that violence is a public health problem is new – and indeed rather contrary to their belief that violence is a crime problem. This is particularly the case for the less visible forms of violence, such as abuse of children, women and the elderly. The notion that violence is preventable is also new or questionable for decision-makers. To many people in authority, a violence-free society seems unobtainable; an "acceptable" level of violence, especially on the streets where they live, appears far more realistic. To others, paradoxically, the inverse is true: since much of violence is hidden, distant or sporadic, peace and security seem to them the prevalent state. In the same way that clean air is taken for granted until the sky becomes full of smog, violence only has to be dealt with when it arrives on the doorstep. It is not surprising then that some of the most innovative solutions have come from the community and municipal levels of government – precisely those that are closest to the problem on a daily basis.

A second problem relates to the feasibility of policy options to tackle the problem. Not enough decision-makers have seen the evidence that many forms of violence are preventable. Too many of

BOX 1.3

A comprehensive approach to preventing violence at work

Violence in the workplace is a major contributor to death and injury in many parts of the world. In the United States of America, official statistics have placed homicide as the second single leading cause of death in the workplace – after road traffic injuries – for men, and the first for women. In the European Union, an estimated 3 million workers (2% of the labour force) have been subjected to physical violence at work. Studies on female migrant workers from the Philippines have shown that many, especially those working in domestic service or the entertainment industry, are disproportionately affected by violence within their work.

Violence at work involves not only physical but also psychological behaviour. Many workers are subjected to bullying, sexual harassment, threats, intimidation and other forms of psychological violence. Research in the United Kingdom has found that 53% of employees have suffered bullying at work and 78% have witnessed such behaviour. In South Africa, workplace hostilities have been reported as "abnormally high" and a recent study showed that 78% of those surveyed had at some time experienced bullying within the workplace.

Repeated acts of violence – from bullying, sexual harassment, and threats to humiliate and undermine workers – may also develop cumulatively into very serious cases. In Sweden, it is estimated that such behaviour has been a factor in 10–15% of suicides.

The costs

Violence in the workplace causes immediate and often long-term disruption to interpersonal relationships and to the whole working environment. The costs of such violence include:

- Direct costs – stemming from such things as:
  - accidents;
  - illness;
  - disability and death;
  - absenteeism;
  - turnover of staff.
- Indirect costs, including:
  - reduced work performance;
  - a lower quality of products or service and slower production;
  - decreased competitiveness.
- More intangible costs, including:
  - damage to the image of an organization;
  - decreased motivation and morale;
  - diminished loyalty to the organization;
  - lower levels of creativity;
  - an environment that is less conducive to work.

The responses

As in dealing with violence in other settings, a comprehensive approach is required. Violence at work is not simply an individual problem that happens from time to time, but a structural problem with much wider socioeconomic, cultural and organizational causes.

The traditional response to violence at work, based exclusively on the enforcement of regulations, fails to reach many situations in the workplace. A more comprehensive approach focuses on the causes of violence in the workplace. Its aim is to make the health, safety and well-being of workers integral parts of the development of the organization.

> **BOX 1.3 (continued)**
>
> The type of systematic and targeted package to prevent violence at work that is being increasingly adopted includes:
>
> — the active collaboration of workers' and employers' organizations in formulating clear anti-violence workplace policies and programmes;
> — supporting legislation and guidelines from national and local government;
> — the dissemination of case studies of good practice in preventing violence at work;
> — improvements to the working environment, styles of management and the organization of work;
> — greater opportunities for training;
> — counselling and support for those affected.
>
> By directly linking health and safety with the management and development of an organization, this comprehensive approach offers the means of prompt and sustainable action to eliminate violence in the workplace.

them feel that the traditional approaches of the criminal justice system are the only ones that "work". Such a view fails to acknowledge the range of violence in society. It perpetuates the concentration on certain highly visible forms of violence – notably youth violence – while paying much less attention to other types, such as intimate partner violence and abuse of children and the elderly, where the criminal justice system is less responsive and less effective.

A third problem is one of determination. Violence is an extremely emotional issue and many countries tend to be reluctant to take initiatives challenging long-established attitudes or practices. It can take considerable political courage to try new approaches in areas such as policing and public security.

With all three of these problems, there is a strong role to be played by public health practitioners, academic institutions, nongovernmental organizations and international organizations, to help governments increase their knowledge of and confidence in workable interventions. Part of this role is advocacy, using education and science-based information. The other part is as a partner or consultant, helping to develop policies and design or implement interventions.

Conclusion

Public health is concerned with the health and well-being of populations as a whole. Violence imposes a major burden on that well-being. The objective of public health is to create safe and healthy communities around the world. A major priority today is to persuade all the various sectors – at the global, national and community levels – to commit themselves to this objective. Public health officials can do much to establish national plans and policies to prevent violence, building important partnerships between sectors and ensuring a proper allocation of resources to prevention efforts.

While public health leadership need not and indeed cannot direct all the actions to prevent and respond to violence, it has a significant role to play. The data at the disposal of public health and other agencies, the insights and understanding developed through scientific method, and the dedication to finding effective responses are important assets that the field of public health brings to the global response to violence.

References

1. Mercy JA et al. Public health policy for preventing violence. *Health Affairs*, 1993, 12:7–29.
2. WHO Global Consultation on Violence and Health. *Violence: a public health priority*. Geneva, World Health Organization, 1996 (document WHO/EHA/SPI.POA.2).
3. Walters RH, Parke RD. Social motivation, dependency, and susceptibility to social influence. In: Berkowitz L, ed. *Advances in experimental social psychology. Vol. 1.* New York, NY, Academic Press, 1964:231–276.

4. Dodge KA, Coie JD. Social information processing factors in reactive and proactive aggression in children's peer groups. *Journal of Personality and Social Psychology*, 1987, 53:1146–1158.

5. Foege WH, Rosenberg ML, Mercy JA. Public health and violence prevention. *Current Issues in Public Health*, 1995, 1:2–9.

6. Kruger J et al. A public health approach to violence prevention in South Africa. In: van Eeden R, Wentzel M, eds. *The dynamics of aggression and violence in South Africa*. Pretoria, Human Sciences Research Council, 1998:399–424.

7. Houry D et al. Emergency department documentation in cases of intentional assault. *Annals of Emergency Medicine*, 1999, 34:715–719.

8. *WHO multi-country study on women's health and domestic violence*. Geneva, World Health Organization, 1999 (document WHO/FCH/GWH/02.01).

9. Holder Y et al., eds. *Injury surveillance guidelines*. Geneva, World Health Organization (published in collaboration with the United States Centers for Disease Control and Prevention), 2001 (document WHO/NMH/VIP/01.02).

10. Sethi D, Krug E, eds. *Guidance for surveillance of injuries due to landmines and unexploded ordnance*. Geneva, World Health Organization, 2000 (document WHO/NMH/PVI/00.2).

11. Saltzman LE et al. *Intimate partner surveillance: uniform definitions and recommended data elements*, Version 1.0. Atlanta, GA, National Center for Injury Prevention and Control, Centers for Disease Control and Prevention, 1999.

12. *Uniform data elements for the national fatal firearm injury reporting system*. Boston, MA, Harvard Injury Control Research Center, Harvard School of Public Health, 2000.

13. *Data elements for emergency departments*. Atlanta, GA, National Center for Injury Prevention and Control, Centers for Disease Control and Prevention, 1997.

14. Dahlberg LL, Toal SB, Behrens CB. *Measuring violence-related attitudes, beliefs, and behaviors among youths: a compendium of assessment tools*. Atlanta, GA, Centers for Disease Control and Prevention, 1998.

15. *Putting women first: ethical and safety recommendations for research on domestic violence against women*. Geneva, World Health Organization, 2001 (document WHO/FCH/GWH/01.01).

16. *World health statistics annual 1996*. Geneva, World Health Organization, 1998.

17. Anderson RN. Deaths: leading causes for 1999. *National Vital Statistics Reports*, 2001, 49:1–87.

18. Heise LL, Ellsberg M, Gottemoeller M. *Ending violence against women*. Baltimore, MD, Johns Hopkins University School of Public Health, Center for Communications Programs, 1999 (Population Reports, Series L, No. 11).

19. Tjaden P, Thoennes N. *Full report of the prevalence, incidence, and consequences of violence against women: findings from the National Violence Against Women Survey*. Washington, DC, National Institute of Justice, Office of Justice Programs, United States Department of Justice and Centers for Disease Control and Prevention, 2000.

20. Rodgers K. Wife assault: the findings of a national survey. *Juristat Service Bulletin*, 1994, 14:1–22.

21. El-Zanaty F et al. *Egypt demographic and health survey, 1995*. Calverton, MD, Macro International, 1996.

22. Randall M et al. Sexual violence in women's lives: findings from the women's safety project, a community-based survey. *Violence Against Women*, 1995, 1:6–31.

23. Ellsberg MC et al. Candies in hell: women's experience of violence in Nicaragua. *Social Science and Medicine*, 2000, 51:1595–1610.

24. Mooney J. *The hidden figure: domestic violence in north London*. London, Middlesex University, 1993.

25. Watts C et al. Withholding sex and forced sex: dimensions of violence against Zimbabwean women. *Reproductive Health Matters*, 1998, 6:57–65.

26. Grufman M, Berg-Kelly K. Physical fighting and associated health behaviours among Swedish adolescents. *Acta Paediatrica*, 1997, 86:77–81.

27. Kann L et al. Youth risk behavior surveillance: United States, 1999. *Morbidity and Mortality Weekly Report*, 2000, 49:1–104 (CDC Surveillance Summaries, SS-5).

28. Gofin R, Palti H, Mandel M. Fighting among Jerusalem adolescents: personal and school-related factors. *Journal of Adolescent Health*, 2000, 27:218–223.

29. Miller TR, Cohen MA. Costs of gunshot and cut/stab wounds in the United States, with some Canadian comparisons. *Accident Analysis and Prevention*, 1997, 29:329–341.

30. Clayton D, Barcel A. The cost of suicide mortality in New Brunswick, 1996. *Chronic Diseases in Canada*, 1999, 20:89–95.

31. Buvinic M, Morrison A. *Violence as an obstacle to development*. Washington, DC, Inter-American Development Bank, 1999:1–8 (Technical Note 4: Economic and social consequences of violence).

32. Kaplan SJ et al. Adolescent physical abuse: risk for adolescent psychiatric disorders. *American Journal of Psychiatry*, 1998, 155:954–959.

33. Kaslow NJ et al. Factors that mediate and moderate the link between partner abuse and suicidal behavior in African-American women. *Journal of Consulting and Clinical Psychology*, 1998, 66:533–540.

34. Pederson W, Skrondal A. Alcohol and sexual victimization: a longitudinal study of Norwegian girls. *Addiction*, 1996, 91:565–581.

35. Holmes MM et al. Rape-related pregnancy: estimates and descriptive characteristics from a national sample of women. *American Journal of Obstetrics and Gynecology*, 1996, 175:320–325.

36. Kakar F et al. The consequences of landmines on public health. *Prehospital Disaster Medicine*, 1996, 11:41–45.

37. Toole MJ. Complex emergencies: refugee and other populations. In: Noji E, ed. *The public health consequences of disasters*. New York, NY, Oxford University Press, 1997:419–442.

38. Garbarino J, Crouter A. Defining the community context for parent–child relations: the correlates of child maltreatment. *Child Development*, 1978, 49:604–616.

39. Bronfenbrenner V. *The ecology of human development: experiments by nature and design*. Cambridge, MA, Harvard University Press, 1979.

40. Garbarino J. *Adolescent development: an ecological perspective*. Columbus, OH, Charles E. Merrill, 1985.

41. Tolan PH, Guerra NG. *What works in reducing adolescent violence: an empirical review of the field*. Boulder, CO, University of Colorado, Center for the Study and Prevention of Violence, 1994.

42. Chaulk R, King PA. *Violence in families: assessing prevention and treatment programs*. Washington, DC, National Academy Press, 1998.

43. Heise LL. Violence against women: an integrated ecological framework. *Violence Against Women*, 1998, 4:262–290.

44. Schiamberg LB, Gans D. An ecological framework for contextual risk factors in elder abuse by adult children. *Journal of Elder Abuse and Neglect*, 1999, 11:79–103.

45. Carp RM. *Elder abuse in the family: an interdisciplinary model for research*. New York, NY, Springer, 2000.

46. Reiss AJ, Roth JA, eds. *Violence in families: understanding and preventing violence. Panel on the understanding and control of violent behavior. Vol. 1*. Washington, DC, National Academy Press, 1993:221–245.

47. Thornberry TP, Huizinga D, Loeber R. The prevention of serious delinquency and violence: implications from the program of research on the causes and correlates of delinquency. In: Howell JC et al., eds. *Sourcebook on serious, violent and chronic juvenile offenders*. Thousand Oaks, CA, Sage, 1995:213–237.

48. Lipsey MW, Derzon JH. Predictors of serious delinquency in adolescence and early adulthood: a synthesis of longitudinal research. In: Loeber R, Farrington DP, eds. *Serious and violent juvenile offenders: risk factors and successful interventions*. Thousand Oaks, CA, Sage, 1998:86–105.

49. Maxfield MG, Widom CS. The cycle of violence: revisited 6 years later. *Archives of Pediatrics and Adolescent Medicine*, 1996, 150:390–395.

50. Farrington DP. The family backgrounds of aggressive youths. In: Hersov LA, Berger M, Shaffer D, eds. *Aggression and antisocial behavior in childhood and adolescence*. Oxford, Pergamon Press, 1978:73–93.

51. McCord J. A forty-year perspective on the effects of child abuse and neglect. *Child Abuse & Neglect*, 1983, 7:265–270.

52. Widom CS. Child abuse, neglect, and violent criminal behavior. *Criminology*, 1989, 27:251–272.

53. Paolucci EO, Genuis ML, Violato C. A meta-analysis of the published research on the effects of child sexual abuse. *Journal of Psychology*, 2001, 135:17–36.

54. Brown J et al. Childhood abuse and neglect: specificity of effects on adolescent and young adult depression and suicidality. *Journal of the American Academy of Child and Adolescent Psychiatry*, 1999, 38:1490–1496.

55. Stark E, Flitcraft A. Killing the beast within: woman battering and female suicidality. *International Journal of Health Services*, 1995, 25:43–64.

56. Bristowe E, Collins JB. Family-mediated abuse of non-institutionalised elder men and women living in British Columbia. *Journal of Elder Abuse and Neglect*, 1989, 1:45–54.

57. Pillemer KA, Prescott D. Psychological effects of elder abuse: a research note. *Journal of Elder Abuse and Neglect*, 1989, 1:65–74.

58. Somasundaram DJ, Rajadurai S. War and suicide in Northern Sri Lanka. *Acta Psychiatrica Scandinavica*, 1995, 91:1–4.

59. Tolan PH, Guerra NG. Prevention of juvenile delinquency: current status and issues. *Journal of Applied and Preventive Psychology*, 1994, 3:251–273.

CHAPTER 2

Youth violence

FIGURE 2.1

Estimated homicide rates among youths aged 10–29 years, 2000[a]

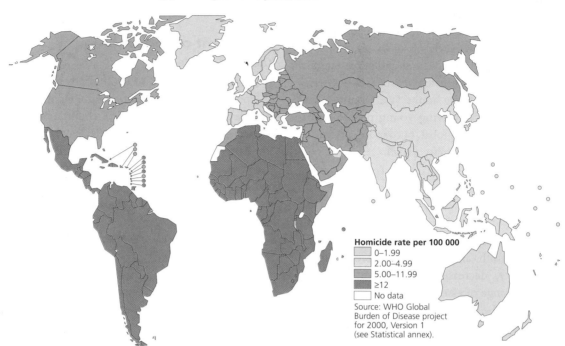

Homicide rate per 100 000
- 0–1.99
- 2.00–4.99
- 5.00–11.99
- ≥12
- No data

Source: WHO Global
Burden of Disease project
for 2000, Version 1
(see Statistical annex).

[a] Rates were calculated by WHO region and country income level and then grouped according to magnitude.

— such as in Hungary (0.9:1), and the Netherlands and the Republic of Korea (1.6:1). The variation between countries in the female homicide rate is considerably less than the variation in the male rate.

Epidemiological findings on youth homicide are scant in those countries and regions where WHO mortality data are lacking or incomplete. Where proper data on youth homicide do exist, such as in several studies in countries in Africa (including Nigeria, South Africa and the United Republic of Tanzania) and in Asia and the Pacific (such as China (including the Province of Taiwan) and Fiji) (9–16), similar epidemiological patterns have been reported, namely:

— a marked preponderance of male over female homicide victims;

— a substantial variation in rates between countries and between regions.

Trends in youth homicides

Between 1985 and 1994, youth homicide rates increased in many parts of the world, especially among youths in the 10–24-year-old age bracket.

There were also important differences between the sexes, and between countries and regions. In general, rates of homicides among youths aged 15–19 and 20–24 years increased more than the rate among 10–14-year-olds. Male rates rose more than female rates (see Figure 2.2), and increases in youth homicide rates were more pronounced in developing countries and economies in transition. Furthermore, the increases in youth homicide rates were generally associated with increases in the use of guns as the method of attack (see Figure 2.3).

While youth homicide rates in Eastern Europe and the former Soviet Union increased dramatically after the collapse of communism there in the late 1980s and early 1990s, rates in Western Europe remained generally low and stable. In the Russian Federation, in the period 1985–1994, rates in the 10–24-year-old age bracket increased by over 150%, from 7.0 per 100 000 to 18.0 per 100 000, while in Latvia there was an increase of 125%, from 4.4 per 100 000 to 9.9 per 100 000. In the same period in many of these countries there was a steep increase in the proportion of deaths from gunshot wounds — the proportion

FIGURE 2.2

Global trends in youth homicide rates among males and females aged 10–24 years, 1985–1994[a]

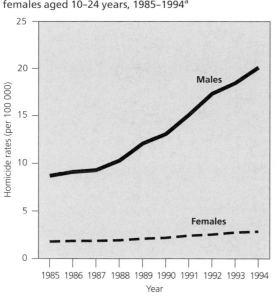

^a Based on WHO mortality data from 66 countries.

more than doubling in Azerbaijan, Latvia and the Russian Federation.

In the United Kingdom, in contrast, homicide rates for 10–24-year olds over the same 10-year period increased by 37.5% (from 0.8 per 100 000

FIGURE 2.3

Trends in method of attack in homicides among youths aged 10–24 years, 1985–1994[a]

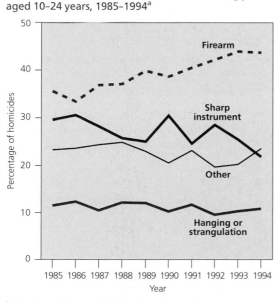

^a Based on WHO mortality data from 46 countries.

to 1.1 per 100 000). In France, youth homicide rates increased by 28.6% over the same period (from 0.7 per 100 000 to 0.9 per 100 000). In Germany, youth homicide rates increased by 12.5% between 1990 and 1994 (from 0.8 per 100 000 to 0.9 per 100 000). While rates of youth homicide increased in these countries over the period, the proportion of youth homicides involving guns remained at around 30%.

Remarkable differences in youth homicide trends for the period 1985–1994 were observed across the American continent. In Canada, where around one-third of youth homicides involve guns, rates fell by 9.5%, from 2.1 per 100 000 to 1.9 per 100 000. In the United States, the trend was exactly the reverse, with over 70% of youth homicides involving guns and an increase in homicides of 77%, from 8.8 per 100 000 to 15.6 per 100 000. In Chile, rates in the period remained low and stable, at around 2.4 per 100 000. In Mexico, where guns account for some 50% of all youth homicides, rates stayed high and stable, rising from 14.7 per 100 000 to 15.6 per 100 000. On the other hand, in Colombia, youth homicides increased by 159%, from 36.7 per 100 000 to 95.0 per 100 000 (with 80% of cases, at the end of this period, involving guns), and in Venezuela by 132%, from 10.4 per 100 000 to 24.1 per 100 000.

In Australia, the youth homicide rate declined from 2.0 per 100 000 in 1985 to 1.5 per 100 000 in 1994, while in neighbouring New Zealand it more than doubled in the same period, from 0.8 per 100 000 to 2.2 per 100 000. In Japan, rates in the period stayed low, at around 0.4 per 100 000.

Non-fatal violence

In some countries, data on youth homicide can be read alongside studies of non-fatal violence. Such comparisons give a more complete picture of the problem of youth violence. Studies of non-fatal violence reveal that for every youth homicide there are around 20–40 victims of non-fatal youth violence receiving hospital treatment. In some countries, including Israel, New Zealand and Nicaragua, the ratio is even greater (*17–19*). In Israel, among those under the age of 18 years, the annual incidence of violent injuries receiving emergency room treatment is 196 per 100 000, compared with youth homicide rates of 1.3 per 100 000 in males and 0.4 per 100 000 in females (*19*).

As with fatal youth violence, the majority of victims of non-fatal violence treated in hospitals are males (*20–26*), although the ratio of male to female cases is somewhat lower than for fatalities. A study in Eldoret, Kenya, for instance, found the ratio of male to female victims of non-fatal violence to be 2.6:1 (*22*). Other research has found a ratio of around 3:1 in Jamaica, and of 4–5:1 in Norway (*23, 24*).

The rates of non-fatal violent injuries tend to increase dramatically during mid-adolescence and young adulthood. A survey of homes in Johannesburg, South Africa, found that 3.5% of victims of violence were 13 years old or younger, compared with 21.9% aged 14–21 years and 52.3% aged 22–35 years (*27*). Studies conducted in Jamaica, Kenya, Mozambique and a number of cities in Brazil, Chile, Colombia, Costa Rica, El Salvador and Venezuela also show high rates of non-fatal injuries from violence among adolescents and young adults (*22, 28, 29*).

Compared with fatal youth violence, non-fatal injuries resulting from violence involve substantially fewer firearm attacks and a correspondingly greater use of the fists and feet, and other weapons, such as knives or clubs. In Honduras, 52% of non-fatal attacks on youths involved weapons other

TABLE 2.1

Homicide rates among youths aged 10–29 years by country or area: most recent year available[a]

Country or area	Year	Total number of deaths	Homicide rate per 100 000 population aged 10–29 years			
			Total	Males	Females	Male:female ratio
Albania	1998	325	28.2	53.5	5.5	9.8
Argentina	1996	628	5.2	8.7	1.6	5.5
Armenia	1999	26	1.9	3.1	—[b]	—[c]
Australia	1998	88	1.6	2.2	1.0	2.3
Austria	1999	7	—[b]	—[b]	—[b]	—[c]
Azerbaijan	1999	194	6.7	12.1	—[b]	—[c]
Belarus	1999	267	8.8	13.2	4.3	3.1
Belgium	1995	37	1.4	1.8	—[b]	—[c]
Bosnia and Herzegovina	1991	2	—[b]	—[b]	—[b]	—[c]
Brazil	1995	20 386	32.5	59.6	5.2	11.5
Bulgaria	1999	51	2.2	3.2	—[b]	—[c]
Canada	1997	143	1.7	2.5	0.9	2.7
Chile	1994	146	3.0	5.1	—[b]	—[c]
China						
Hong Kong SAR	1996	16	—[b]	—[b]	—[b]	—[c]
Selected rural and urban areas	1999	778	1.8	2.4	1.2	2.1
Colombia	1995	12 834	84.4	156.3	11.9	13.1
Costa Rica	1995	75	5.5	8.4	—[b]	—[c]
Croatia	1999	21	1.6	—[b]	—[b]	—[c]
Cuba	1997	348	9.6	14.4	4.6	3.2
Czech Republic	1999	36	1.2	1.4	—[b]	—[c]
Denmark	1996	20	1.5	—[b]	—[b]	—[c]
Ecuador	1996	757	15.9	29.2	2.3	12.4
El Salvador	1993	1 147	50.2	94.8	6.5	14.6
Estonia	1999	33	7.7	13.3	—[b]	—[c]
Finland	1998	19	—[b]	—[b]	—[b]	—[c]
France	1998	91	0.6	0.7	0.4	1.9
Georgia	1992	4	—[b]	—[b]	—[b]	—[c]
Germany	1999	156	0.8	1.0	0.6	1.6
Greece	1998	25	0.9	1.4	—[b]	—[c]
Hungary	1999	41	1.4	1.4	1.5	0.9
Ireland	1997	10	—[b]	—[b]	—[b]	—[c]
Israel	1997	13	—[b]	—[b]	—[b]	—[c]
Italy	1997	210	1.4	2.3	0.5	4.5
Jamaica	1991	2	—[b]	—[b]	—[b]	—[c]
Japan	1997	127	0.4	0.5	0.3	1.7
Kazakhstan	1999	631	11.5	18.0	5.0	3.6
Kuwait	1999	14	—[b]	—[b]	—[b]	—[c]
Kyrgyzstan	1999	88	4.6	6.7	2.4	2.8
Latvia	1999	55	7.8	13.1	—[b]	—[c]
Lithuania	1999	59	5.4	8.4	—[b]	—[c]
Mauritius	1999	4	—[b]	—[b]	—[b]	—[c]
Mexico	1997	5 991	15.3	27.8	2.8	9.8
Netherlands	1999	60	1.5	1.8	1.2	1.6
New Zealand	1998	20	1.8	—[b]	—[b]	—[c]
Nicaragua	1996	139	7.3	12.5	—[b]	—[c]
Norway	1997	11	—[b]	—[b]	—[b]	—[c]
Panama (excluding Canal Zone)	1997	151	14.4	25.8	—[b]	—[c]
Paraguay	1994	191	10.4	18.7	—[b]	—[c]

TABLE 2.1 *(continued)*

Country or area	Year	Total number of deaths	Homicide rate per 100 000 population aged 10-29 years			
			Total	Males	Females	Male:female ratio
Philippines	1993	3 252	12.2	22.7	1.4	16.0
Poland	1995	186	1.6	2.3	0.8	2.7
Portugal	1999	37	1.3	2.1	—[b]	—[c]
Puerto Rico	1998	538	41.8	77.4	5.3	14.5
Republic of Korea	1997	282	1.7	2.1	1.3	1.6
Republic of Moldova	1999	96	7.7	12.8	—[b]	—[c]
Romania	1999	169	2.3	3.5	1.1	3.1
Russian Federation	1998	7 885	18.0	27.5	8.0	3.4
Singapore	1998	15	—[b]	—[b]	—[b]	—[c]
Slovakia	1999	26	1.5	2.4	—[b]	—[c]
Slovenia	1999	4	—[b]	—[b]	—[b]	—[c]
Spain	1998	96	0.8	1.2	0.4	2.9
Sweden	1996	16	—[b]	—[b]	—[b]	—[c]
Switzerland	1996	17	—[b]	—[b]	—[b]	—[c]
Tajikistan	1995	124	5.5	9.7	—[b]	—[c]
Thailand	1994	1 456	6.2	10.0	2.2	4.4
The former Yugoslav Republic of Macedonia	1997	6	—[b]	—[b]	—[b]	—[c]
Trinidad and Tobago	1994	55	11.4	15.4	—[b]	—[c]
Turkmenistan	1998	131	6.9	12.4	—[b]	—[c]
Ukraine	1999	1 273	8.7	13.0	4.3	3.1
United Kingdom	1999	139	0.9	1.4	0.4	3.9
England and Wales	1999	91	0.7	1.0	0.3	3.4
Northern Ireland	1999	7	—[b]	—[b]	—[b]	—[c]
Scotland	1999	41	3.1	5.3	—[b]	—[c]
United States of America	1998	8 226	11.0	17.9	3.7	4.8
Uruguay	1990	36	3.6	4.5	—[b]	—[c]
Uzbekistan	1998	249	2.6	3.8	1.3	3.0
Venezuela	1994	2 090	25.0	46.4	2.8	16.5

SAR: Special Administrative Region.

[a] Most recent year available between 1990 and 2000 for countries with ⩾ 1 million population.

[b] Fewer than 20 deaths reported; rate not calculated.

[c] Rate ratio not calculated if fewer than 20 deaths reported for either males or females.

than guns, and in a Colombian study only 5% of non-fatal assaults were gun-related (compared with over 80% of youth homicides involving firearms) (*25, 30*). In South Africa, gunshot wounds account for some 16% of all violent injuries presenting at hospitals, as compared with 46% of all homicides (*31*). However, direct comparison between countries and subgroups within countries using data on non-fatal violence registered at health services can be misleading. Differences in the rates of emergency room presentation for gunshot wounds, for instance, may simply reflect the fact that pre-hospital and emergency medical care varies between different settings.

Risk behaviours for youth violence

Participating in physical fights, bullying and carrying of weapons are important risk behaviours for youth violence. Most studies examining these behaviours have involved primary and secondary school pupils, who differ considerably from children and adolescents who have left or dropped out of school. Consequently, the applicability of the results of these studies to youths who are no longer attending school is likely to be limited.

Involvement in physical fighting is very common among school-age children in many parts of the world (*32–38*). Around one-third of students report having been involved in fighting, with males 2–3 times more likely than females to have fought. Bullying is also prevalent among school-age children (*39, 40*). In a study of health behaviour among school-aged children in 27 countries, the majority of 13-year-olds in most countries were found to have engaged in bullying at least some of the time (see Table 2.2) (*40*). Apart from being forms of aggression, bullying and physical fighting can also lead to more serious forms of violence (*41*).

The carrying of weapons is both an important risk behaviour and a predominantly male activity among young people of school age. There are, however, major variations in the prevalence of weapon carrying as reported by adolescents in different countries. In Cape Town, South Africa, 9.8% of males and 1.3% of females in secondary schools reported carrying knives to school during the previous 4 weeks (*42*). In Scotland, 34.1% of males and 8.6% of females aged 11–16 years said that they had carried weapons at least once during

TABLE 2.2

Bullying behaviour among 13-year-olds, 1997–1998

Country	Engaged in bullying this school term?		
	Have not %	Sometimes %	Once a week %
Austria	26.4	64.2	9.4
Belgium (Flemish region)	52.2	43.6	4.1
Canada	55.4	37.3	7.3
Czech Republic	69.1	27.9	3.0
Denmark	31.9	58.7	9.5
England	85.2	13.6	1.2
Estonia	44.3	50.6	5.1
Finland	62.8	33.3	3.8
France	44.3	49.1	6.6
Germany	31.2	60.8	7.9
Greece	76.8	18.9	4.3
Greenland	33.0	57.4	9.6
Hungary	55.8	38.2	6.0
Israel	57.1	36.4	6.6
Latvia	41.2	49.1	9.7
Lithuania	33.3	57.3	9.3
Northern Ireland	78.1	20.6	1.3
Norway	71.0	26.7	2.3
Poland	65.1	31.3	3.5
Portugal	57.9	39.7	2.4
Republic of Ireland	74.2	24.1	1.7
Scotland	73.9	24.2	1.9
Slovakia	68.9	27.3	3.9
Sweden	86.8	11.9	1.2
Switzerland	42.5	52.6	5.0
United States of America	57.5	34.9	7.6
Wales	78.6	20.0	1.4

their lifetime, with drug users significantly more likely than non-drug users to have done so (*43*). In the Netherlands, 21% of secondary-school pupils admitted to possessing a weapon, and 8% had actually brought weapons to school (*44*). In the United States, a national survey of students in grades 9–12 found that 17.3% had carried a weapon in the previous 30 days and 6.9% had carried a weapon on the school premises (*32*).

The dynamics of youth violence

Patterns of behaviour, including violence, change over the course of a person's life. The period of adolescence and young adulthood is a time when violence, as well as other types of behaviours, are often given heightened expression (*45*). Under-standing when and under what conditions violent behaviour typically occurs as a person develops can

help in formulating interventions and policies for prevention that target the most critical age groups (*3*).

How does youth violence begin?

Youth violence can develop in different ways. Some children exhibit problem behaviour in early child-hood that gradually escalates to more severe forms of aggression before and during adolescence. Between 20% and 45% of boys and 47% and 69% of girls who are serious violent offenders at the age of 16–17 years are on what is termed a "life-course persistent developmental pathway" (*3, 46–50*). Young people who fit into this category commit the most serious violent acts and often continue their violent behaviour into adulthood (*51–54*).

Longitudinal studies have examined in what ways aggression can continue from childhood to adolescence and from adolescence to adulthood to create a pattern of persistent offending throughout a person's life. Several studies have shown that childhood aggression is a good predictor of violence in adolescence and early adulthood. In a study in Örebro, Sweden (*55*), two-thirds of a sample of around 1000 young males who displayed violent behaviour up to the age of 26 years had already scored highly for aggressiveness at the ages of 10 and 13 years, compared with about one-third of all boys. Similarly, in a follow-up study in Jyväskylä, Finland, of nearly 400 youths (*56*), ratings by peers of aggression at the ages of 8 and 14 years significantly predicted violence up to the age of 20.

There is also evidence of a continuity in aggressive behaviour from adolescence to adult-hood. In a study in Columbus, OH, United States, 59% of youths arrested for violent offences before the age of 18 years were rearrested as adults, and 42% of these adult offenders were charged with at least one serious violent offence, such as homicide, aggravated assault or rape (*57*). A greater propor-tion of those arrested as young people for offences involving serious violence were rearrested as adults than was the case for young people arrested for offences involving minor violence. A study on the development of delinquency in Cambridge, Eng-land, found that one-third of young males who had been convicted of offences involving violence before the age of 20 years were convicted again between the ages of 21 and 40 years, compared with only 8% of those not convicted for violent offences during their teenage years (*58*).

The existence of a life-course persistent developmental pathway helps to explain the continuity over time in aggressive and violent behaviour. That is, there are certain individuals who persist in having a greater underlying tendency than others towards aggressive or violent behaviour. In other words, those who are relatively more aggressive at a given age also tend to be relatively more aggressive later on, even though their absolute levels of violence may vary.

There may also be progressions over time from one type of aggression to another. For instance, in a longitudinal study in Pittsburgh, PA, United States, of over 1500 boys originally studied at 7, 10 and 13 years of age, Loeber et al. reported that childhood aggression tended to develop into gang fighting and later into youth violence (*59*).

Lifetime offenders, though, represent only a small proportion of those committing violence. Most violent young people engage in violent behaviour over much shorter periods. Such people are termed "adolescence-limited offenders". Results from the National Youth Survey conducted in the United States – based on a national sample of young people aged 11–17 years in 1976, who were followed until the age of 27–33 years – show that although a small proportion of youths continued to commit violence into and through adulthood, some three-quarters of young people who had committed serious violence ceased their violent behaviour after around 1–3 years (*3*). The majority of young people who become violent are adolescence-limited offenders who, in fact, show little or no evidence of high levels of aggression or other problem behaviours during their childhood (*3*).

Situational factors

Among adolescence-limited offenders, certain situational factors may play an important role in causing violent behaviour. A situational analysis – explaining the interactions between the would-be perpetrator and victim in a given situation – describes how the potential for violence might develop into actual violence. Situational factors include:

— the motives for violent behaviour;
— where the behaviour occurs;
— whether alcohol or weapons are present;
— whether people other than the victim and offender are present;
— whether other actions (such as burglary) are involved that could be conducive to violence.

Motives for youth violence vary according to the age of the participants and whether others are present. A study of delinquency in Montreal, Canada, showed that, when the perpetrators were in their teenage years or early twenties, about half of violent personal attacks were motivated by the search for excitement, often with co-offenders, and half by rational or utilitarian objectives (*60*). For all crimes, however, the main motivation switched from being thrill-seeking in the perpetrators' teenage years to utilitarian – involving prior planning, psychological intimidation and the use of weapons – in their twenties (*61*).

The National Survey of Youth in the United States found that assaults were generally committed in retaliation for a previous attack, out of revenge, or because of provocation or anger (*61*). In the study in Cambridge mentioned above, the motives for physical fights depended on whether a boy fought alone or with a group (*62*). In individual fights, a boy was usually provoked, became angry and hit to hurt his opponent or to release internal tensions. In group fights, boys often became involved to help friends or because they were attacked – rarely because they were angry. The group fights, though, were on the whole more serious. They often escalated from minor incidents, typically occurred in bars or on the street, and were more likely to involve weapons, lead to injuries, and involve the police.

Drunkenness is an important immediate situational factor that can precipitate violence. In a Swedish study, about three-quarters of violent offenders and around half the victims of violence were intoxicated at the time of the incident, and in the Cambridge study, many of the boys fought after drinking (*62, 63*).

An interesting characteristic of young violent offenders that may make them more likely to become entangled in situations leading to violence is their tendency to be involved in a broad range of crimes, as well as their usually having a range of problem behaviours. Generally, young violent offenders are versatile rather than specialized in the types of crimes they commit. In fact, violent young people typically commit more non-violent offences than violent offences (64–66). In the Cambridge study, convicted violent delinquents up to the age of 21 years had nearly three times as many convictions for non-violent offences as for violent offences (58).

What are the risk factors for youth violence?

Individual factors

At the individual level, factors that affect the potential for violent behaviour include biological, psychological and behavioural characteristics. These factors may already appear in childhood or adolescence, and to varying degrees they may be influenced by the person's family and peers and by other social and cultural factors.

Biological characteristics

Among possible biological factors, there have been studies on injuries and complications associated with pregnancy and delivery, because of the suggestion that these might produce neurological damage, which in turn could lead to violence. In a study in Copenhagen, Denmark, Kandel & Mednick (67) followed up over 200 children born during 1959–1961. Their research showed that complications during delivery were a predictor for arrests for violence up to the age of 22 years. Eighty per cent of youths arrested for committing violent offences scored in the high range for delivery complications at birth, compared with 30% of those arrested for committing property-related offences and 47% of youths with no criminal record. Pregnancy complications, on the other hand, did not significantly predict violence.

Interestingly, delivery complications were strongly associated with future violence when a parent had a history of psychiatric illness (68). In these cases, 32% of males with significant delivery complications were arrested for violence, compared with 5% of those with only minor or no delivery complications. Unfortunately, these results were not replicated by Denno in the Philadelphia Biosocial Project (69) – a study of nearly 1000 African-American children in Philadelphia, PA, United States, who were followed from birth to 22 years of age. It may therefore be that pregnancy and delivery complications predict violence only or mainly when they occur in combination with other problems within the family.

Low heart rates – studied mainly in boys – are associated with sensation-seeking and risk-taking, both characteristics that may predispose boys to aggression and violence in an attempt to increase stimulation and arousal levels (70–73). High heart rates, however, especially in infants and young children, are linked to anxiety, fear and inhibitions (71).

Psychological and behavioural characteristics

Among the major personality and behavioural factors that may predict youth violence are hyperactivity, impulsiveness, poor behavioural control and attention problems. Nervousness and anxiety, though, are negatively related to violence. In a follow-up study of over 1000 children in Dunedin, New Zealand, boys with violent convictions up to the age of 18 years were significantly more likely to have had poor scores in behavioural control (for example, impulsiveness and lack of persistence) at the age of 3–5 years, compared with boys with no convictions or with convictions for non-violent offences (74). In the same study, personality factors of constraint (such as cautiousness and the avoidance of excitement) and of negative emotionality (such as nervousness and alienation) at the age of 18 years were significantly inversely correlated with convictions for violence (75).

Longitudinal studies conducted in Copenhagen, Denmark (68), Örebro, Sweden (76), Cambridge, England (77), and Pittsburgh, PA, United States (77), also showed links between these personality traits and both convictions for violence and self-reported violence. Hyperactivity, high levels of daring or risk-taking behaviour, and poor concentration and attention difficulties before the age of 13 years all significantly predicted violence into early adulthood. High levels of anxiety and nervousness were negatively related to violence in the studies in Cambridge and in the United States.

Low intelligence and low levels of achievement in school have consistently been found to be associated with youth violence (*78*). In the Philadelphia project (*69*), poor intelligence quotient (IQ) scores in verbal and performance IQ tests at the ages of 4 and 7 years, and low scores in standard school achievement tests at 13–14 years, all increased the likelihood of being arrested for violence up to the age of 22 years. In a study in Copenhagen, Denmark, of over 12 000 boys born in 1953, low IQ at 12 years of age significantly predicted police-recorded violence between the ages of 15 and 22 years. The link between low IQ and violence was strongest among boys from lower socioeconomic groups.

Impulsiveness, attention problems, low intelligence and low educational attainment may all be linked to deficiencies in the executive functions of the brain, located in the frontal lobes. These executive functions include: sustaining attention and concentration, abstract reasoning and concept formation, goal formulation, anticipation and planning, effective self-monitoring and self-awareness of behaviour, and inhibitions regarding inappropriate or impulsive behaviours (*79*). Interestingly, in another study in Montreal – of over 1100 children initially studied at 6 years of age and followed onwards from the age of 10 years – executive functions at 14 years of age, measured with cognitive-neuropsychological tests, provided a significant means of differentiating between violent and non-violent boys (*80*). Such a link was independent of family factors, such as socioeconomic status, the parents' age at first birth, their educational level, or separation or divorce within the family.

Relationship factors

Individual risk factors for youth violence, such as the ones described above, do not exist in isolation from other risk factors. Factors associated with the interpersonal relations of young people – with their family, friends and peers – can also strongly affect aggressive and violent behaviour and shape personality traits that, in turn, can contribute to violent behaviour. The influence of families is usually the greatest in this respect during childhood, while during adolescence friends and peers have an increasingly important effect (*81*).

Family influences

Parental behaviour and the family environment are central factors in the development of violent behaviour in young people. Poor monitoring and supervision of children by parents and the use of harsh, physical punishment to discipline children are strong predictors of violence during adolescence and adulthood. In her study of 250 boys in Boston, MA, United States, McCord (*82*) found that poor parental supervision, parental aggression and harsh discipline at the age of 10 years strongly increased the risk of later convictions for violence up to 45 years of age.

Eron, Huesmann & Zelli (*83*) followed up almost 900 children in New York, NY, United States. They found that harsh, physical punishment by parents at the age of 8 years predicted not only arrests for violence up to the age of 30 years, but also – for boys – the severity of punishment of their own children and their own histories of spouse abuse. In a study of over 900 abused children and nearly 700 controls, Widom showed that recorded physical abuse and neglect as a child predicted later arrests for violence – independently of other predictors such as sex, ethnicity and age (*84*). Other studies have recorded similar findings (*77, 85, 86*).

Violence in adolescence and adulthood has also been strongly linked to parental conflict in early childhood (*77, 82*) and to poor attachment between parents and children (*87, 88*). Other factors include: a large number of children in the family (*65, 77*); a mother who had her first child at an early age, possibly as a teenager (*77, 89, 90*); and a low level of family cohesion (*91*). Many of these factors, in the absence of other social support, can affect children's social and emotional functioning and behaviour.

McCord (*87*), for example, showed that violent offenders were less likely than non-violent offenders to have experienced parental affection and good discipline and supervision.

Family structure is also an important factor for later aggression and violence. Findings from studies conducted in New Zealand, the United Kingdom and the United States show that children growing up in single-parent households are at greater risk for violence (*74, 77, 92*). In a study of 5300 children from England, Scotland and Wales, for example, experiencing parental separation between birth and the age of 10 years increased the likelihood of convictions for violence up to the age of 21 years (*92*). In the study in Dunedin, New Zealand, living with a single parent at the age of 13 years predicted convictions for violence up to the age of 18 years (*74*). The more restricted scope for support and probable fewer economic resources in these situations may be reasons why parenting often suffers and the risk of becoming involved in violence increases for youths.

In general, low socioeconomic status of the family is associated with future violence. For example, in a national survey of young people in the United States, the prevalence of self-reported assault and robbery among youths from low socioeconomic classes was about twice that among middle-class youths (*93*). In Lima, Peru, low educational levels of the mother and high housing density were both found to be associated with youth violence (*94*). A study of young adults in São Paulo, Brazil, found that, after adjusting for sex and age, the risk of being a victim of violence was significantly higher for youths from low socioeconomic classes compared with those from high socioeconomic classes (*95*). Similar results have been obtained from studies in Denmark (*96*), New Zealand (*74*) and Sweden (*97*).

Given the importance of parental supervision, family structure and economic status in determining the prevalence of youth violence, an increase in violence by young people would be expected where families have disintegrated through wars or epidemics, or because of rapid social change. Taking the case of epidemics, some 13 million children worldwide have lost one or both parents to AIDS, more than 90% of them in sub-Saharan Africa, where millions more children are likely to be orphaned in the next few years (*98*). The onslaught of AIDS on people of reproductive age is producing orphans at such a rate that many communities can no longer rely on traditional structures to care for these children. The AIDS epidemic is thus likely to have serious adverse implications for violence among young people, particularly in Africa, where rates of youth violence are already extremely high.

Peer influences

Peer influences during adolescence are generally considered positive and important in shaping interpersonal relationships, but they can also have negative effects. Having delinquent friends, for instance, is associated with violence in young people (*88*). The results of studies in developed countries (*78, 88*) are consistent with a study in Lima, Peru (*94*), which found a correlation between violent behaviour and having friends who used drugs. The causal direction in this correlation – whether having delinquent friends comes before or after being a violent offender – is, however, not clear (*99*). In their study, Elliott & Menard concluded that delinquency caused peer bonding and, at the same time, that bonding with delinquent peers caused delinquency (*100*).

Community factors

The communities in which young people live are an important influence on their families, the nature of their peer groups, and the way they may be exposed to situations that lead to violence. Generally speaking, boys in urban areas are more likely to be involved in violent behaviour than those living in rural areas (*77, 88, 93*). Within urban areas, those living in neighbourhoods with high levels of crime are more likely to be involved in violent behaviour than those living in other neighbourhoods (*77, 88*).

Gangs, guns and drugs

The presence of gangs (see Box 2.1), guns and drugs in a locality is a potent mixture, increasing

BOX 2.1

A profile of gangs

Youth gangs are found in all regions of the world. Although their size and nature may vary greatly – from mainly social grouping to organized criminal network – they all seem to answer a basic need to belong to a group and create a self-identity.

In the Western Cape region of South Africa, there are about 90 000 members of gangs, while in Guam, some 110 permanent gangs were recorded in 1993, around 30 of them hard-core gangs. In Port Moresby, Papua New Guinea, four large criminal associations with numerous subgroups have been reported. There are an estimated 30 000–35 000 gang members in El Salvador and a similar number in Honduras, while in the United States, some 31 000 gangs were operating in 1996 in about 4800 cities and towns. In Europe, gangs exist to varying extents across the continent, and are particularly strong in those countries in economic transition such as the Russian Federation.

Gangs are primarily a male phenomenon, though in countries such as the United States, girls are forming their own gangs. Gang members can range in age from 7 to 35 years, but typically are in their teens or early twenties. They tend to come from economically deprived areas, and from low-income and working-class urban and suburban environments. Often, gang members may have dropped out of school and hold low-skilled or low-paying jobs. Many gangs in high-income and middle-income countries consist of people from ethnic or racial minorities who may be socially very marginalized.

Gangs are associated with violent behaviour. Studies have shown that as youths enter gangs they become more violent and engage in riskier, often illegal activities. In Guam, over 60% of all violent crime reported to the police is committed by young people, much of it related to activities of the island's hard-core gangs. In Bremen, Germany, violence by gang members accounts for almost half of reported violent offences. In a longitudinal study of nearly 1000 youths in Rochester, NY, United States, some 30% of the sample were gang members, but they accounted for around 70% of self-reported violent crimes and 70% of drug dealing.

A complex interaction of factors leads young people to opt for gang life. Gangs seem to proliferate in places where the established social order has broken down and where alternative forms of shared cultural behaviour are lacking. Other socioeconomic, community and interpersonal factors that encourage young people to join gangs include:

— a lack of opportunity for social or economic mobility, within a society that aggressively promotes consumption;
— a decline locally in the enforcement of law and order;
— interrupted schooling, combined with low rates of pay for unskilled labour;
— a lack of guidance, supervision and support from parents and other family members;
— harsh physical punishment or victimization in the home;
— having peers who are already involved in a gang.

Actively addressing these underlying factors that encourage youth gangs to flourish, and providing safer, alternative cultural outlets for their prospective members, can help eliminate a significant proportion of violent crime committed by gangs or otherwise involving young people.

the likelihood of violence. In the United States, for example, the presence together in neighbourhoods of these three items would appear to be an important factor in explaining why the juvenile arrest rate for homicide more than doubled between 1984 and 1993 (from 5.4 per 100 000 to 14.5 per 100 000) (*97, 101, 102*). Blumstein suggested that this rise was linked to increases occurring over the same period in the carrying of guns, in the number of gangs and in battles fought over the selling of crack cocaine (*103*). In the Pittsburgh study already mentioned, initiation into dealing in drugs coincided with a significant increase in carrying weapons, with 80% of 19-year-olds who sold hard drugs (such as cocaine), also carrying a gun (*104*). In Rio de Janeiro, Brazil, where the majority of victims and perpetrators of homicide are 25 years of age or younger, drug dealing is responsible for a large proportion of homicides, conflicts and injuries (*105*). In other parts of Latin America and the Caribbean, youth gangs involved in drug trafficking display higher levels of violence than those that are not (*106*).

Social integration

The degree of social integration within a community also affects rates of youth violence. Social capital is a concept that attempts to measure such community integration. It refers, roughly speaking, to the rules, norms, obligations, reciprocity and trust that exist in social relations and institutions (*107*). Young people living in places that lack social capital tend to perform poorly in school and have a greater probability of dropping out altogether (*108*).

Moser & Holland (*109*) studied five poor urban communities in Jamaica. They found a cyclical relationship between violence and the destruction of social capital. When community violence occurred, physical mobility in the particular locality was restricted, employment and educational opportunities were reduced, businesses were reluctant to invest in the area and local people were less likely to build new houses or repair or improve existing property. This reduction in social capital – the increased mistrust resulting from the destruction of infrastructure, amenities and opportunities – increased the likelihood of violent behaviour, especially among young people. A study on the relation between social capital and crime rates in a wide range of countries during the period 1980–1994, found that the level of trust among community members had a strong effect on the incidence of violent crimes (*107*). Wilkinson, Kawachi & Kennedy (*110*) showed that indices of social capital reflecting low social cohesion and high levels of interpersonal mistrust were linked with both higher homicide rates and greater economic inequality.

Societal factors

Several societal factors may create conditions conducive to violence among young people. Much of the evidence related to these factors, though, is based on cross-sectional or ecological studies and is mainly useful for identifying important associations, rather than direct causes.

Demographic and social changes

Rapid demographic changes in the youth population, modernization, emigration, urbanization and changing social policies have all been linked with an increase in youth violence (*111*). In places that have suffered economic crises and ensuing structural adjustment policies – such as in Africa and parts of Latin America – real wages have often declined sharply, laws intended to protect labour have been weakened or discarded, and a substantial decline in basic infrastructure and social services has occurred (*112, 113*). Poverty has become heavily concentrated in cities experiencing high population growth rates among young people (*114*).

In their demographic analysis of young people in Africa, Lauras-Locoh & Lopez-Escartin (*113*) suggest that the tension between a rapidly swelling population of young people and a deteriorating infrastructure has resulted in school-based and student revolts. Diallo Co-Trung (*115*) found a similar situation of student strikes and rebellions in Senegal, where the population under 20 years of age doubled between 1970 and 1988, during a period of economic recession and the implementation of structural adjustment policies. In a survey of youths in Algeria, Rarrbo (*116*) found that rapid demographic growth and accelerating urbanization together created conditions, including unemployment and grossly inadequate housing, that in turn led to extreme frustration, anger and pent-up tensions among youths. Young people, as a result, were more likely to turn to petty crime and violence, particularly under the influence of peers.

In Papua New Guinea, Dinnen (*117*) describes the evolution of "raskolism" (criminal gangs) in the broader context of decolonization and the ensuing social and political change, including rapid population growth unmatched by economic growth. Such a phenomenon has also been cited as a concern in some of the former communist economies (*118*), where – as unemployment has soared, and the social welfare system been severely cut – young people have lacked legitimate incomes and occupations, as well as the necessary social support between leaving school and finding work. In the absence of such support, some have turned to crime and violence.

Income inequality

Research has shown links between economic growth and violence, and between income inequality and violence (*119*). Gartner, in a study of 18 industrialized countries during the period 1950–1980 (*6*), found that income inequality, as measured by the Gini coefficient, had a significant and positive effect on the homicide rate. Fajnzylber, Lederman & Loayza (*120*) obtained the same results in an investigation of 45 industrialized and developing countries between 1965 and 1995. The rate of growth of the GDP was also significantly negatively associated with the homicide rate, but this effect was in many cases offset by rising levels of income inequality. Unnithan & Whitt came to similar conclusions in their cross-national study (*121*), namely, that income inequality was strongly linked with homicide rates, and that such rates also decreased as the per capita GDP increased.

Political structures

The quality of governance in a country, both in terms of the legal framework and the policies offering social protection, is an important determinant of violence. In particular, the extent to which a society enforces its existing laws on violence, by arresting and prosecuting offenders, can act as a deterrent against violence. Fajnzylber, Lederman & Loayza (*120*) found that the arrest rate for homicides had a significant negative effect on the homicide rate. In their study, objective measures of governance (such as arrest rates) were negatively correlated with crime rates, while subjective measures (such as confidence in the judiciary and the perceived quality of governance) were only weakly correlated with crime rates.

Governance can therefore have an impact on violence, particularly as it affects young people. Noronha et al. (*122*), in their study on violence affecting various ethnic groups in Salvador, Bahia, Brazil, concluded that dissatisfaction with the police, the justice system and prisons increased the use of unofficial modes of justice. In Rio de Janeiro, Brazil, de Souza Minayo (*105*) found that the police were among the principal perpetrators of violence against young people. Police actions – particularly against young men from lower socioeconomic classes – involved physical violence, sexual abuse, rape and bribery. Sanjuán (*123*) suggested that a sense that justice depended on socioeconomic class was an important factor in the emergence of a culture of violence among marginalized youths in Caracas, Venezuela. Similarly, Aitchinson (*124*) concluded that in post-apartheid South Africa, impunity for former perpetrators of human rights abuses and the inability of the police to change their methods significantly, have contributed to a generalized feeling of insecurity and increased the number of extrajudicial actions involving violence.

Social protection by the state, another aspect of governance, is also important. In their study, Pampel & Gartner (*125*) used an indicator measuring the level of development of national institutions responsible for collective social protection. They were interested in the question of why different countries, whose 15–29-year-old age groups had grown at the same rate over a given period, nevertheless showed differing increases in their homicide rates. Pampel & Gartner concluded that strong national institutions for social protection had a negative effect on the homicide rate. Furthermore, having such institutions in place could counter the effects on homicide rates associated with increases in the 15–29-year-old age group, the group with traditionally high rates of being a victim or perpetrator of homicide.

Messner & Rosenfeld (*126*) examined the impact of efforts to protect vulnerable populations from market forces, including economic recession. Higher welfare expenditures were found to be associated with decreases in the homicide rate, suggesting that societies with economic safety nets have fewer homicides. Briggs & Cutright (*7*), in a study of 21 countries over the period 1965–1988, found that spending on social insurance, as a proportion of the GDP, was negatively correlated with homicides of children up to 14 years of age.

Cultural influences

Culture, which is reflected in the inherited norms and values of society, helps determine how people respond to a changing environment. Cultural factors can affect the amount of violence in a society – for instance, by endorsing violence as a normal method to resolve conflicts and by teaching young people to adopt norms and values that support violent behaviour.

One important means through which violent images, norms and values are propagated is the media. Exposure of children and young people to the various forms of the media has increased dramatically in recent years. New forms of media – such as video games, video tapes and the Internet – have multiplied opportunities for young people to be exposed to violence. Several studies have shown that the introduction of television into countries was associated with increases in the level of violence (*127–131*), although these studies did not usually take into account other factors that may at the same time have influenced rates of violence (*3*). The preponderance of evidence to date indicates that exposure to violence on television increases the likelihood of immediate aggressive behaviour and has an unknown effect in the longer term on serious violence (*3*) (see Box 2.2). There is insufficient evidence on the impact of some of the newer forms of media.

Cultures which fail to provide non-violent alternatives to resolve conflicts appear to have higher rates of youth violence. In their study of gangs in Medellín, Colombia, Bedoya Marín & Jaramillo Martínez (*136*) describe how low-income youths are influenced by the culture of violence, in society in general and in their particular community. They suggest that a culture of violence is fostered at the community level through the growing acceptance of "easy money" (much of it related to drug trafficking) and of whatever means are necessary to obtain

it, as well as through corruption in the police, judiciary, military and local administration.

Cultural influences across national boundaries have also been linked to rises in juvenile violence. In a survey of youth gangs in Latin America and the Caribbean, Rodgers (*106*) has shown that violent gangs, modelling themselves on those in Los Angeles, CA, United States, have emerged in northern and south-western Mexican towns, where immigration from the United States is highest. A similar process has been found in El Salvador, which has experienced a high rate of deportations of Salvadoran nationals from the United States since 1992, many of the deportees having been members of gangs in the United States.

What can be done to prevent youth violence?

In designing national programmes to prevent youth violence, it is important to address not only individual cognitive, social and behavioural factors, but also the social systems that shape these factors.

Tables 2.3 and 2.4 illustrate examples of youth violence prevention strategies as matrices, relating ecological systems through which violence can be prevented to developmental stages, from infancy to early adulthood, where violent behaviour or the risks for violent behaviour are likely to emerge. The prevention strategies in these tables are not exhaustive, nor do they necessarily represent strategies that have proved effective. Some, in fact, have been shown to be ineffective. Rather, the matrices are meant to illustrate the wide spectrum of possible solutions to the problem of youth violence, and to emphasize the need for a range of different strategies for various stages of development.

Individual approaches

The most common interventions against youth violence seek to increase the level of protective factors associated with individual skills, attitudes and beliefs.

One violence prevention strategy appropriate for early childhood – though it is not usually thought of as such – is the adoption of preschool enrichment programmes. These programmes introduce young

BOX 2.2

The impact of media on youth violence

Children and young people are important consumers of the mass media, including entertainment and advertising. Studies in the United States have found that television viewing often begins as early as 2 years of age, and that the average young person between 8 and 18 years of age watches some 10 000 violent acts a year on television. These patterns of exposure to the media are not necessarily evident in other parts of the world, especially where there is less access to television and film. All the same, there is little doubt that the exposure everywhere of children and young people to mass media is substantial and growing. It is therefore important to explore media exposure as a possible risk factor for interpersonal violence involving young people.

Researchers have been examining the impact of the media on aggressive and violent behaviour for over 40 years. Several meta-analyses of studies on the impact of the media on aggression and violence have tended to conclude that media violence is positively related to aggression toward others. However, evidence to confirm its effect on serious forms of violence (such as assault and homicide), is lacking.

A 1991 meta-analysis, involving 28 studies of children and adolescents exposed to media violence and observed in free social interaction, concluded that exposure to media violence increased aggressive behaviour towards friends, classmates and strangers (*132*). Another meta-analysis, conducted in 1994, examined 217 studies published between 1957 and 1990 concerned with the impact of media violence on aggressive behaviour, with 85% of the sample in the age range 6–21 years. The authors concluded that there was a significant positive correlation between exposure to media violence and aggressive behaviour, regardless of age (*133*).

Many of the studies included in these analytical reviews were either randomized experiments (laboratory and field) or cross-sectional surveys. Findings from the experimental studies show that brief exposure to violence on television or film, particularly dramatic presentations of violence, produces short-term increases in aggressive behaviour. Moreover, the effects seem to be greater for children and youths with aggressive tendencies and among those who have been aroused or provoked. The findings, however, may not extend to real-life situations. Indeed, real-life settings often include influences that cannot be "controlled" as in experiments – influences that might mitigate against aggressive and violent behaviour.

Findings from the cross-sectional studies also show a positive correlation between media violence and various measures of aggression – for instance, attitudes and beliefs, behaviour and emotions such as anger. The effects of media violence on the more serious forms of violent behaviour (such as assault and homicide), though, are rather small at best ($r = 0.06$) (*133*). Also, unlike experimental and longitudinal studies where causality can more easily be established, it is not possible to conclude from cross-sectional studies that exposure to media violence causes aggressive and violent behaviour.

There have also been longitudinal studies examining the link between television viewing and interpersonal aggression some years later. A 3-year longitudinal study of children aged 7–9 years in Australia, Finland, Israel, Poland and the United States produced inconsistent results (*134*), and a 1992 study of children in the Netherlands in the same age bracket failed to show any effect on aggressive behaviour (*135*). Other studies following up children in the United States over longer periods (10–15 years), however, have shown a positive correlation between television viewing in childhood and later aggression in young adulthood (*3*).

Studies examining the relationship between homicide rates and the introduction of television (primarily by looking at homicide rates in countries before and after television was introduced) have also found a positive correlation between the two (*127–131*). These studies, however, failed

BOX 2.2 (continued)

to control for confounding variables such as economic differences, social and political change, and a variety of other potential influences on homicide rates.

The scientific findings on the relationship between media violence and youth violence are thus conclusive with respect to short-term increases in aggression. The findings, however, are inconclusive with respect to longer-term effects and on the more serious forms of violent behaviour, and suggest that more research is needed. Apart from examining the extent to which media violence is a direct cause of serious physical violence, research is also required on the influence of the media on interpersonal relations and on individual traits such as hostility, callousness, indifference, lack of respect and the inability to identify with other people's feelings.

children early on to the skills necessary for success in school and they therefore increase the likelihood of future academic success. Such programmes can strengthen a child's bonds to the school and raise achievement and self-esteem (*137*). Long-term follow-up studies of prototypes of such programmes have found positive benefits for children, including less involvement in violent and other delinquent behaviours (*138–140*).

Social development programmes to reduce antisocial and aggressive behaviour in children and violence among adolescents adopt a variety of strategies. These commonly include improving competency and social skills with peers and generally promoting behaviour that is positive, friendly and cooperative (*141*). Such programmes can be provided universally or just to high-risk groups and are most frequently carried out in school settings (*142, 143*). Typically, they focus on one or more of the following (*143*):

— managing anger;
— modifying behaviour;
— adopting a social perspective;
— moral development;
— building social skills;
— solving social problems;
— resolving conflicts.

There is evidence that these social development programmes can be effective in reducing youth violence and improving social skills (*144–146*). Programmes that emphasize social and competency skills appear to be among the most effective among youth violence prevention strategies (*3*). They also appear to be more effective when delivered to children in preschool and primary school environments rather than to secondary school students.

An example of a social development programme that uses behavioural techniques in the classroom is a programme to prevent bullying introduced in elementary and junior secondary schools in Bergen, Norway. Incidents of bullying were reduced by a half within 2 years using this intervention (*147*). The programme has been reproduced in England, Germany and the United States with similar effects (*3*).

Other interventions targeting individuals that may be effective include the following, though further evidence is needed to confirm their effect on violent and aggressive behaviour (*137, 148*):

— programmes to prevent unintended pregnancies, so as to reduce child maltreatment and the risk it poses for later involvement in violent behaviour;
— for similar reasons, programmes to increase access to prenatal and postnatal care;
— academic enrichment programmes;
— incentives for youths at high risk for violence to complete secondary schooling and to pursue courses of higher education;
— vocational training for underprivileged youths and young adults.

Programmes that do not appear effective in reducing youth violence include (*3*):

— individual counselling;
— training in the safe use of guns;

TABLE 2.3

Violence prevention strategies by developmental stage (infancy to middle childhood) and ecological context

Ecological context	Developmental stage		
	Infancy (ages 0–3 years)	Early childhood (ages 3–5 years)	Middle childhood (ages 6–11 years)
Individual	• Preventing unintended pregnancies • Increasing access to prenatal and postnatal care	• Social development programmes[a] • Preschool enrichment programmes[a]	• Social development programmes[a] • Programmes providing information about drug abuse[b]
Relationship (e.g. family, peers)	• Home visitation[a] • Training in parenting[a]	• Training in parenting[a]	• Mentoring programmes • Home–school partnership programmes to promote parental involvement
Community	• Monitoring lead levels and removing toxins from homes • Increasing the availability and quality of child-care facilities	• Monitoring lead levels and removing toxins from homes • Increasing the availability and quality of preschool enrichment programmes	• Creating safe routes for children on their way to and from school or other community activities • Improving school settings, including teacher practices, school policies and security • Providing after-school programmes to extend adult supervision • Extracurricular activities
Societal	• Deconcentrating poverty • Reducing income inequality	• Deconcentrating poverty • Reducing income inequality • Reducing media violence • Public information campaigns	• Deconcentrating poverty • Reducing income inequality • Reducing media violence • Public information campaigns • Reforming educational systems

[a] Demonstrated to be effective in reducing youth violence or risk factors for youth violence.

[b] Shown to be ineffective in reducing youth violence or risk factors for youth violence.

— probation and parole programmes that include meetings with prison inmates who describe the brutality of prison life,

— trying young offenders in adult courts;

— residential programmes taking place in psychiatric institutions or correctional institutions;

— programmes providing information about drug abuse.

Programmes for delinquent young people modelled on basic military training ("boot camps") have, in some studies, been found to lead to an increase in repeat offending (3).

Relationship approaches

Another common set of prevention strategies address youth violence by attempting to influence the type of relations that young people have with others with whom they regularly interact. These programmes address such problems as the lack of emotional relations between parents and children,

powerful pressures brought to bear by peers to engage in violence and the absence of a strong relationship with a caring adult.

Home visitation

One type of family-based approach to preventing youth violence is home visitation. This is an intervention conducted in infancy (ages 0–3 years) involving regular visits by a nurse or other health care professional to the child's home. This type of programme is found in many parts of the world, including Australia, Canada, China (Hong Kong Special Administrative Region (SAR)), Denmark, Estonia, Israel, South Africa, Thailand and the United States. The objective is to provide training, support, counselling, monitoring and referrals to outside agencies for low-income mothers, for families who are expecting or have recently had their first child, and for families at increased risk of abusing their children or with other health problems (137, 146). Home visitation pro-

about the effectiveness of community-based strategies with regard to youth violence than of those focusing on individual factors or on the relationships that young people have with others.

Community policing

Community or problem-oriented policing has become an important law enforcement strategy for addressing youth violence and other criminal problems in many parts of the world (167). It can take many forms, but its core ingredients are building community partnerships and solving community problems (168). In some programmes, for instance, police collaborate with mental health professionals to identify and refer youths who have witnessed, experienced or committed violence (169). This type of programme builds on the fact that police come into daily contact with young victims or perpetrators of violence. It then provides them with special training and links them – at an early stage in the youth's development – with the appropriate mental health professionals (168). The effectiveness of this type of programme has not yet been determined, though it appears to be a useful approach.

Community policing programmes have been implemented with some success in Rio de Janeiro, Brazil, and San José, Costa Rica (170, 171). In Costa Rica, an evaluation of the programme found an association with a decline in both crime and perceived personal insecurity (171). Such programmes need to be more rigorously evaluated, but they do offer local residents better protection and make up for a lack of regular police services (170).

Availability of alcohol

Another community strategy to address crime and violence is to reduce the availability of alcohol. As already mentioned, alcohol is an important situational factor that can precipitate violence. The effect of reducing alcohol availability on rates of offending was examined in a 4-year longitudinal study conducted in a small provincial region of New Zealand (172). The rates of serious criminal offences (homicide and rape) and other offences (related to property and traffic) were compared in two experimental towns and four control towns over the study period. While both types of offence decreased in the experimental towns and increased relative to national trends in the control towns, crime rates fell significantly for 2 years in areas of reduced alcohol availability. It is not clear, though, to what extent the intervention affected violent behaviour among young people or how well such an approach might work in other settings.

Extracurricular activities

Extracurricular activities – such as sports and recreation, art, music, drama and producing newsletters – can provide adolescents with opportunities to participate in and gain recognition for constructive group activities (3). In many communities, though, either such activities are lacking or there are no places where children can safely go outside school hours to practise them (173). After-school programmes provide these facilities for children and young people. Ideally, such programmes should be (174):

— comprehensive – addressing the whole range of risk factors for youth violence and delinquency;

— developmentally appropriate;

— of long duration.

Essor, in Maputo, Mozambique (175), is an example of a community programme designed to address adolescent delinquency in two low-income neighbourhoods. The programme, which targets adolescents between the ages of 13 and 18 years, offers sports and leisure activities to promote self-expression and team-building. Programme staff also maintain contact with youths through regular home visits. An evaluation of the programme showed significant improvements in constructive behaviour and communications with parents over an 18-month period, along with a significant drop in antisocial behaviour.

Suppressing gang violence

Community programmes to prevent gang violence have taken on several forms. Preventive strategies have included attempts to suppress gangs or to organize communities affected by gang violence in such a way that youth gangs operate differently and with less criminal activities (*106*). Rehabilitative or corrective strategies include outreach and counselling programmes for gang members as well as programmes that seek to channel gang activities into socially productive directions (*106*). There is little evidence that programmes to suppress gangs, organize communities, or provide outreach or counselling services are effective. In Nicaragua, wide-ranging police efforts in 1997 to suppress gang activity met with only temporary success and may have in the end exacerbated the problem (*176*). Attempts at community organization in the United States, in Boston, MA, and Chicago, IL, have not been successful in reducing gang violence either, possibly because the affected communities were insufficiently integrated or cohesive to sustain organized efforts (*177*). Outreach and counselling efforts have had the unwanted, and unexpected, consequence of increasing gang cohesion (*178*). In Medellín, Colombia, programmes have been successfully used to encourage gang members to involve themselves in local politics and social development projects (*179*), while in Nicaragua and the United States such "opportunity" programmes have met with only limited success (*106*).

Other strategies

Other interventions targeting communities that may prove effective include (*148, 180*):

- Monitoring lead levels and removing toxins from the home environment so as to reduce the risk of brain damage in children, something that may lead indirectly to youth violence.

- Increasing the availability and quality of child-care facilities and preschool enrichment programmes to promote healthy development and facilitate success in school.

- Attempts to improve school settings – including changing teaching practices and school policies and rules, and increasing security (for instance, by installing metal detectors or surveillance cameras).

- Creating safe routes for children on their way to and from school or other community activities.

Health care systems can contribute considerably both to responding to and preventing youth violence, by:

— improving the response and performance of emergency services;

— improving access to health services;

— training health care workers to identify and refer young people at high risk.

One type of programme that appears to be ineffective in reducing adolescent violence is where money is offered as a reward for handing in firearms to the police or other community agencies – in what is known as a "gun buy-back programme". There is some evidence that the types of guns handed in are not the types usually used in youth homicides (*3*).

Societal approaches

Changing the social and cultural environment to reduce violence is the strategy that is least frequently employed to prevent youth violence. Such an approach seeks to reduce economic or social barriers to development – for instance, by creating job programmes or strengthening the criminal justice system – or to modify the embedded cultural norms and values that stimulate violence.

Addressing poverty

Policies to reduce the concentration of poverty in urban areas may be effective in combating youth violence. This was shown in a housing and mobility experiment, "Moving to Opportunity", conducted in Maryland, United States (*181*). In a study of the impact of this programme, families from high-poverty neighbourhoods in the city of Baltimore were divided into three groups:

— families that had received subsidies, counselling and other assistance specifically to move to communities with lower levels of poverty;

— families that had received subsidies only, but with no restrictions on where they could move;

20. Lerer LB, Matzopoulos RG, Phillips R. Violence and injury mortality in the Cape Town metropole. *South African Medical Journal*, 1997, 87:298–301.

21. Zwi KJ et al. Patterns of injury in children and adolescents presenting to a South African township health centre. *Injury Prevention*, 1995, 1:26–30.

22. Odero WO, Kibosia JC. Incidence and characteristics of injuries in Eldoret, Kenya. *East African Medical Journal*, 1995, 72:706–760.

23. Mansingh A, Ramphal P. The nature of interpersonal violence in Jamaica and its strain on the national health system. *West Indian Medical Journal*, 1993, 42:53–56.

24. Engeland A, Kopjar B. Injuries connected to violence: an analysis of data from the injury registry. *Tidsskrift for den Norske Laegeforening*, 2000, 120:714–717.

25. Tercero DM. *Caracteristicas de los pacientes con lesiones de origen violento, atendidos en Hospital Mario Catarino Rivas. [Characteristics of patients with intentional injuries, attended to in the Mario Catarino Rivas Hospital.]* San Pedro Sula, Honduras, Secretary of Health, 1999.

26. Kuhn F et al. Epidemiology of severe eye injuries. United States Eye Injury Registry (USEIR) and Hungarian Eye Injury Registry (HEIR). *Ophthalmologe*, 1998, 95:332–343.

27. Butchart A, Kruger J, Nell V. Neighbourhood safety: a township violence and injury profile. *Crime and Conflict*, 1997, 9:11–15.

28. Neveis O, Bagus R, Bartolomeos K. *Injury surveillance at Maputo Central Hospital.* Abstract for XIth Day of Health, June 2001. Maputo, 2001.

29. Cruz JM. La victimización por violencia urbana: niveles y factores asociados en ciudades de América Latina y España. [Victimization through violence: levels and associated factors in Latin American and Spanish towns.] *Revista Panamericana de Salud Publica*, 1999, 5:4–5.

30. National Referral Centre for Violence. *Forensis 1999: datos para la vida. Herramienta para la interpretación, intervención y prevención del hecho violento en Colombia. [Forensis 1999: data for life. A tool for interpreting, acting against and preventing violence in Colombia.]* Santa Fe de Bogotá, National Institute of Legal Medicine and Forensic Science, 2000.

31. Peden M. Non-fatal violence: some results from the pilot national injury surveillance system. *Trauma Review*, 2000, 8:10–12.

32. Kann L et al. Youth risk behavior surveillance: United States, 1999. *Morbidity and Mortality Weekly Report*, 2000, 49:3–9 (CDC Surveillance Summaries, SS-5).

33. Rossow I et al. Young, wet and wild? Associations between alcohol intoxication and violent behaviour in adolescence. *Addiction*, 1999, 94:1017–1031.

34. Clémense A. Violence and incivility at school: the situation in Switzerland. In: Debarbieux E, Blaya C, eds. *Violence in schools: ten approaches in Europe.* Issy-les-Moulineaux, Elsevier, 2001:163–179.

35. Grufman M, Berg-Kelly K. Physical fighting and associated health behaviours among Swedish adolescents. *Acta Paediatrica*, 1997, 86:77–81.

36. Gofin R et al. Fighting among Jerusalem adolescents: personal and school-related factors. *Journal of Adolescent Health*, 2000, 27:218–223.

37. Youssef RM, Attia MS, Kamel MI. Violence among schoolchildren in Alexandria. *Eastern Mediterranean Health Journal*, 1999, 5:282–298.

38. Parrilla IC et al. Internal and external environment of the Puerto Rican adolescent in the use of alcohol, drugs and violence. *Boletin Asociación Medica de Puerto Rico*, 1997, 89:146–149.

39. O'Moore AM et al. Bullying behaviour in Irish schools: a nationwide study. *Irish Journal of Psychology*, 1997, 18:141–169.

40. Currie C, ed. *Health behaviour in school-aged children: a WHO cross-national study.* Bergen, University of Bergen, 1998.

41. Loeber R et al. Developmental pathways in disruptive child behavior. *Development and Psychopathology*, 1993, 5:103–133.

42. Flisher AJ et al. Risk-taking behaviour of Cape Peninsula high-school students. Part VII: violent behaviour. *South African Medical Journal*, 1993, 83:490–494.

43. McKeganey N, Norrie J. Association between illegal drugs and weapon carrying in young people in Scotland: schools' survey. *British Medical Journal*, 2000, 320:982–984.

44. Mooij T. *Veilige scholen en (pro)sociaal gedrag: evaluatie van de campaghne 'De veilige school' in het voortgezet onderwijs. [Safe schools and positive social behaviour: an evaluation of the "Safe schools" campaign in continuing education.]* Nijmegen, Institute for Applied Social Sciences, University of Nijmegen, 2001.

45. Dahlberg LL, Potter LB. Youth violence: developmental pathways and prevention challenges. *American Journal of Preventive Medicine*, 2001, 20(1S):3–14.

46. D'Unger AV et al. How many latent classes of delinquent/criminal careers? Results from a mixed Poisson regression analysis. *American Sociological Review*, 1998, 103:1593–1620.

47. Huizinga D, Loeber R, Thornberry TP. *Recent findings from a program of research on the causes*

and *correlates of delinquency*. Washington, DC, United States Department of Justice, 1995.

48. Nagin D, Tremblay RE. Trajectories of boys' physical aggression, opposition, and hyperactivity on the path to physically violent and nonviolent juvenile delinquency. *Child Development*, 1999, 70:1181–1196.

49. Patterson GR, Yoerger K. A developmental model for late-onset delinquency. *Nebraska Symposium on Motivation*, 1997, 44:119–177.

50. Stattin H, Magnusson M. Antisocial development: a holistic approach. *Development and Psychopathology*, 1996, 8:617–645.

51. Loeber R, Farrington DP, Waschbusch DA. Serious and violent juvenile offenders. In: Loeber R, Farrington DP, eds. *Serious and violent juvenile offenders: risk factors and successful interventions*. Thousand Oaks, CA, Sage, 1998:13–29.

52. Moffitt TE. Adolescence-limited and life-course persistent antisocial behavior: a developmental taxonomy. *Psychological Review*, 1993, 100:674–701.

53. Tolan PH. Implications of onset for delinquency risk identification. *Journal of Abnormal Child Psychology*, 1987, 15:47–65.

54. Tolan PH, Gorman-Smith D. Development of serious and violent offending careers. In: Loeber R, Farrington DP, eds. *Serious and violent juvenile offenders: risk factors and successful interventions*. Thousand Oaks, CA, Sage, 1998:68–85.

55. Stattin H, Magnusson D. The role of early aggressive behavior in the frequency, seriousness, and types of later crime. *Journal of Consulting and Clinical Psychology*, 1989, 57:710–718.

56. Pulkkinen L. Offensive and defensive aggression in humans: a longitudinal perspective. *Aggressive Behaviour*, 1987, 13:197–212.

57. Hamparian DM et al. *The young criminal years of the violent few*. Washington, DC, Office of Juvenile Justice and Delinquency Prevention, 1985.

58. Farrington DP. Predicting adult official and self-reported violence. In: Pinard GF, Pagani L, eds. *Clinical assessment of dangerousness: empirical contributions*. Cambridge, Cambridge University Press, 2001:66–88.

59. Loeber R et al. Developmental pathways in disruptive child behavior. *Development and Psychopathology*, 1993, 5:103–133.

60. LeBlanc M, Frechette M. *Male criminal activity from childhood through youth*. New York, NY, Springer-Verlag, 1989.

61. Agnew R. The origins of delinquent events: an examination of offender accounts. *Journal of Research in Crime and Delinquency*, 1990, 27:267–294.

62. Farrington DP. Motivations for conduct disorder and delinquency. *Development and Psychopathology*, 1993, 5:225–241.

63. Wikström POH. *Everyday violence in contemporary Sweden*. Stockholm, National Council for Crime Prevention, 1985.

64. Miczek KA et al. Alcohol, drugs of abuse, aggression and violence. In: Reiss AJ, Roth JA, eds. *Understanding and preventing violence: panel on the understanding and control of violent behavior. Vol. 3. Social influences*. Washington, DC, National Academy Press, 1994:377–570.

65. Brennan P, Mednick S, John R. Specialization in violence: evidence of a criminal subgroup. *Criminology*, 1989, 27:437–453.

66. Hamparian DM et al. *The violent few: a study of dangerous juvenile offenders*. Lexington, MA, DC Heath, 1978.

67. Kandel E, Mednick SA. Perinatal complications predict violent offending. *Criminology*, 1991, 29:519–529.

68. Brennan PA, Mednick BR, Mednick SA. Parental psychopathology, congenital factors, and violence. In: Hodgins S, ed. *Mental disorder and crime*. Thousand Oaks, CA, Sage, 1993:244–261.

69. Denno DW. *Biology and violence: from birth to adulthood*. Cambridge, Cambridge University Press, 1990.

70. Raine A. *The psychopathology of crime: criminal behavior as a clinical disorder*. San Diego, CA, Academic Press, 1993.

71. Kagan J. Temperamental contributions to social behavior. *American Psychologist*, 1989, 44:668–674.

72. Wadsworth MEJ. Delinquency, pulse rates, and early emotional deprivation. *British Journal of Criminology*, 1976, 16:245–256.

73. Farrington DP. The relationship between low resting heart rate and violence. In: Raine A et al., eds. *Biosocial bases of violence*. New York, NY, Plenum, 1997:89–105.

74. Henry B et al. Temperamental and familial predictors of violent and nonviolent criminal convictions: age 3 to age 18. *Developmental Psychology*, 1996, 32:614–623.

75. Caspi A et al. Are some people crime-prone? Replications of the personality–crime relationship across countries, genders, races, and methods. *Criminology*, 1994, 32:163–195.

76. Klinteberg BA et al. Hyperactive behavior in childhood as related to subsequent alcohol problems and violent offending: a longitudinal study of male

126. Messner SF, Rosenfeld R. Political restraint of the market and levels of criminal homicide: a cross-national application of institutional-anomie theory. *Social Forces*, 1997, 75:1393–1416.

127. Centerwall BS. Television and violence: the scale of the problem and where to go from here. *Journal of the American Medical Association*, 1992, 267:3059–3063.

128. Centerwall BS. Exposure to television as a cause of violence. *Public Communication and Behaviour*, 1989, 2:1–58.

129. Centerwall BS. Exposure to television as a risk factor for violence. *American Journal of Epidemiology*, 1989, 129:643–652.

130. Joy LA, Kimball MM, Zabrack ML. Television and children's aggressive behavior. In: Williams TM, ed. *The impact of television: a natural experiment in three communities*. New York, NY, Academic Press, 1986:303–360.

131. Williams TM. *The impact of television: a natural experiment in three communities*. New York, NY, Academic Press, 1986.

132. Wood W, Wong FY, Chachere G. Effects of media violence on viewers' aggression in unconstrained social interaction. *Psychological Bulletin*, 1991, 109:307–326.

133. Paik H, Comstock G. The effects of television violence on antisocial behavior: a meta-analysis. *Communication Research*, 1994, 21:516–546.

134. Huesmann LR, Eron LD, eds. *Television and the aggressive child: a cross-national comparison*. Hillsdale, NJ, Lawrence Erlbaum, 1986.

135. Wiegman O, Kuttschreuter M, Baarda B. A longitudinal study of the effects of television viewing on aggressive and antisocial behaviours. *British Journal of Social Psychology*, 1992, 31:147–164.

136. Bedoya Marín DA, Jaramillo Martínez J. *De la barra a la banda. [From football supporter to gang member.]* Medellín, El Propio Bolsillo, 1991.

137. Kellermann AL et al. Preventing youth violence: what works? *Annual Review of Public Health*, 1998, 19:271–292.

138. Johnson DL, Walker T. Primary prevention of behavior problems in Mexican-American children. *American Journal of Community Psychology*, 1987, 15:375–385.

139. Berrueta-Clement JR et al. *Changed lives: the effects of the Perry preschool program on youth through age 19*. Ypsilanti, MI, High/Scope, 1984.

140. Schweinhart LJ, Barnes HV, Weikart DP. *Significant benefits: the High/Scope Perry preschool project study through age 27*. Ypsilanti, MI, High/Scope, 1993.

141. Tolan PH, Guerra NG. *What works in reducing adolescent violence: an empirical review of the field*. Boulder, CO, University of Colorado, Center for the Study and Prevention of Violence, 1994.

142. Richards BA, Dodge KA. Social maladjustment and problem-solving in school-aged children. *Journal of Consulting and Clinical Psychology*, 1982, 50:226–233.

143. Guerra NG, Williams KR. *A program planning guide for youth violence prevention: a risk-focused approach*. Boulder, CO, University of Colorado, Center for the Study and Prevention of Violence, 1996.

144. Hawkins JD et al. Preventing adolescent health-risk behaviors by strengthening protection during childhood. *Archives of Pediatrics & Adolescent Medicine*, 1999, 153:226–234.

145. Howell JC, Bilchick S, eds. *Guide for implementing the comprehensive strategy for serious violent and chronic juvenile offenders*. Washington, DC, United States Department of Justice, Office of Juvenile Justice and Delinquency Prevention, 1995.

146. Thornton TN et al. *Best practices of youth violence prevention: a sourcebook for community action*. Atlanta, GA, Centers for Disease Control and Prevention, 2000.

147. Olweus D, Limber S, Mihalic S. *Bullying prevention program*. Boulder, CO, University of Colorado, Center for the Study and Prevention of Violence, 1998 (Blueprints for Violence Prevention Series, Book 9).

148. Williams KR, Guerra NG, Elliott DS. *Human development and violence prevention: a focus on youth*. Boulder, CO, University of Colorado, Center for the Study and Prevention of Violence, 1997.

149. Lally JR, Mangione PL, Honig AS. The Syracuse University Family Development Research Project: long-range impact of an early intervention with low-income children and their families. In: Powell DR, ed. *Annual advances in applied developmental psychology: parent education as an early childhood intervention*. Norwood, NJ, Ablex, 1988:79–104.

150. Seitz V, Rosenbaum LK, Apfel NH. Effects of a family support intervention: a 10-year follow-up. *Child Development*, 1985, 56:376–391.

151. Olds DL et al. Long-term effects of nurse home visitation on children's criminal and antisocial behavior: 15-year follow-up of a randomized controlled trial. *Journal of the American Medical Association*, 1998, 280:1238–1244.

152. Farrington DP, Welsh BC. Delinquency prevention using family-based interventions. *Children and Society*, 1999, 13:287–303.

153. Sanders MR. Triple-P-Positive Parenting Program: towards an empirically validated multilevel parent-

ing and family support strategy for the prevention of behavior and emotional problems in children. *Clinical Child and Family Psychology Review,* 1999, 2:71–90.

154. Triple-P-Positive Parenting Program. *Triple P News*, 2001, 4:1.

155. Patterson GR, Capaldi D, Bank L. An early starter model for predicting delinquency. In: Pepler DJ, Rubin KH, eds. *The development and treatment of childhood aggression.* Hillsdale, NJ, Lawrence Erlbaum, 1991:139–168.

156. Patterson GR, Reid JB, Dishion TJ. *Antisocial boys.* Eugene, OR, Castalia, 1992.

157. Hawkins JD, Von Cleve E, Catalano RF. Reducing early childhood aggression: results of a primary prevention program. *Journal of the American Academy of Child and Adolescent Psychiatry,* 1991, 30:208–217.

158. Tremblay RE et al. Parent and child training to prevent early onset of delinquency: the Montreal longitudinal experimental study. In: McCord J, Tremblay RE, eds. *Preventing antisocial behavior: interventions from birth through adolescence.* New York, NY, Guilford, 1992:117–138.

159. Greenwood PW et al. *Diverting children from a life of crime: measuring costs and benefits.* Santa Monica, CA, Rand, 1996.

160. Mihalic SF, Grotpeter JK. *Big Brothers/Big Sisters of America.* Boulder, CO, University of Colorado, Center for the Study and Prevention of Violence, 1997 (Blueprints for Violence Prevention Series, Book 2).

161. Grossman JB, Garry EM. *Mentoring: a proven delinquency prevention strategy.* Washington, DC, United States Department of Justice, Office of Justice Programs, 1997 (Juvenile Justice Bulletin, No. NCJ 164386).

162. Shadish WR. Do family and marital psychotherapies change what people do? A meta-analysis of behavior outcomes. In: Cook TD et al., eds. *Meta-analysis for explanation: a casebook.* New York, NY, Russell Sage Foundation, 1992:129–208.

163. Hazelrigg MD, Cooper HM, Borduin CM. Evaluating the effectiveness of family therapies: an integrative review and analysis. *Psychological Bulletin,* 1987, 101:428–442.

164. Klein NC, Alexander JF, Parsons BV. Impact of family systems intervention on recidivism and sibling delinquency: a model of primary prevention and program evaluation. *Journal of Consulting and Clinical Psychology,* 1977, 45:469–474.

165. Aos S et al. *The comparative costs and benefits of programs to reduce crime: a review of national research findings with implications for Washington state.* Olympia, WA, Washington State Institute for Public Policy, 1999 (Report No. 99-05-1202).

166. Henggler SW et al. *Multisystemic treatment of antisocial behavior in children and adolescents.* New York, NY, Guilford, 1998.

167. Goldstein H. *Policing of a free society.* Cambridge, MA, Ballinger, 1977.

168. Office of Juvenile Justice and Delinquency Prevention. *Bridging the child welfare and juvenile justice systems.* Washington, DC, National Institute of Justice, 1995.

169. Marens S, Schaefer M. Community policing, schools, and mental health. In: Elliott DS, Hamburg BA, Williams KR, eds. *Violence in American schools.* Cambridge, Cambridge University Press, 1998:312–347.

170. Buvinic M, Morrison A, Shifter M. *Violence in Latin America and the Caribbean: a framework for action.* Washington, DC, Inter-American Development Bank, 1999.

171. Jarquin E, Carrillo F. *La económica política de la reforma judicial. [The political economy of judicial reform.]* Washington, DC, Inter-American Development Bank, 1997.

172. Kraushaar K, Alsop B. *A naturalistic alcohol availability experiment: effects on crime.* Washington, DC, Educational Resources Information Center, 1995 (document CG 026 940).

173. Chaiken MR. Tailoring established after-school programs to meet urban realities. In: Elliott DS, Hamburg BA, Williams KR, eds. *Violence in American schools.* Cambridge, Cambridge University Press, 1998:348–375.

174. Chaiken MR, Huizinga D. Early prevention of and intervention for delinquency and related problem behavior. *The Criminologist,* 1995, 20:4–5.

175. Babotim F et al. *Avaliação 1998 do trabalho realizado pela Essor com os adolescentes de dois bairros de Maputo/Moçambique. [1998 Evaluation of work undertaken by Essor with adolescents from two districts in Maputo, Mozambique.]* Maputo, Essor, 1999.

176. Rodgers D. *Living in the shadow of death: violence, pandillas and social disorganization in contemporary urban Nicaragua* [Dissertation]. Cambridge, University of Cambridge, 1999.

177. Finestone H. *Victims of change: juvenile delinquency in American society.* Westport, CT, Greenwood, 1976.

178. Klein MW. *A structural approach to gang intervention: the Lincoln Heights project.* San Diego, CA, Youth Studies Center, 1967.

179. Salazar A. Young assassins in the drug trade. *North American Conference on Latin America*, 1994, 27:24–28.

180. Painter KA, Farrington DP. Evaluating situational crime prevention using a young people's survey. *British Journal of Criminology*, 2001, 41:266–284.

181. Ludwig J, Duncan GJ, Hirschfield P. Urban poverty and juvenile crime: evidence from a randomized housing-mobility experiment. *Quarterly Journal of Economics*, 2001, 16:655–680.

182. Sheley JF, Wright JD. *Gun acquisition and possession in selected juvenile samples*. Washington, DC, United States Department of Justice, 1993.

183. Cook PJ, Moore MH. Guns, gun control, and homicide. In: Smith MD, Zahn MA eds. *Studying and preventing homicide: issues and challenges*. Thousand Oaks, CA, Sage, 1999:246–273.

184. Teret SP et al. Making guns safer. *Issues in Science and Technology*, 1998, Summer:37–40.

185. Loftin C et al. Effects of restrictive licensing of handguns on homicide and suicide in the District of Columbia. *New England Journal of Medicine*, 1991, 325:1615–1620.

186. Villaveces A et al. Effect of a ban on carrying firearms on homicide rates in two Colombian cities. *Journal of the American Medical Association*, 2000, 283:1205–1209.

CHAPTER 3

Child abuse and neglect by parents and other caregivers

— physical abuse;
— sexual abuse;
— emotional abuse;
— neglect.

Physical abuse of a child is defined as those acts of commission by a caregiver that cause actual physical harm or have the potential for harm. Sexual abuse is defined as those acts where a caregiver uses a child for sexual gratification.

Emotional abuse includes the failure of a caregiver to provide an appropriate and supportive environment, and includes acts that have an adverse effect on the emotional health and development of a child. Such acts include restricting a child's movements, denigration, ridicule, threats and intimidation, discrimination, rejection and other non-physical forms of hostile treatment.

Neglect refers to the failure of a parent to provide for the development of the child – where the parent is in a position to do so – in one or more of the following areas: health, education, emotional development, nutrition, shelter and safe living conditions. Neglect is thus distinguished from circumstances of poverty in that neglect can occur only in cases where reasonable resources are available to the family or caregiver.

The manifestations of these types of abuse are further described in Box 3.1.

The extent of the problem

Fatal abuse

Information on the numbers of children who die each year as a result of abuse comes primarily from death registries or mortality data. According to the World Health Organization, there were an estimated 57 000 deaths attributed to homicide among children under 15 years of age in 2000. Global estimates of child homicide suggest that infants and very young children are at greatest risk, with rates for the 0–4-year-old age group more than double those of 5–14-year-olds (see Statistical annex).

The risk of fatal abuse for children varies according to the income level of a country and region of the world. For children under 5 years of age living in high-income countries, the rate of homicide is 2.2 per 100 000 for boys and 1.8 per 100 000 for girls. In

low- to middle-income countries the rates are 2–3 times higher – 6.1 per 100 000 for boys and 5.1 per 100 000 for girls. The highest homicide rates for children under 5 years of age are found in the WHO African Region – 17.9 per 100 000 for boys and 12.7 per 100 000 for girls. The lowest rates are seen in high-income countries in the WHO European, Eastern Mediterranean and Western Pacific Regions (see Statistical annex).

Many child deaths, however, are not routinely investigated and postmortem examinations are not carried out, which makes it difficult to establish the precise number of fatalities from child abuse in any given country. Even in wealthy countries there are problems in properly recognizing cases of infanticide and measuring their incidence. Significant levels of misclassification in the cause of death as reported on death certificates have been found, for example, in several states of the United States of America. Deaths attributed to other causes – for instance, sudden infant death syndrome or accidents – have often been shown on reinvestigation to be homicides (18, 19).

Despite the apparent widespread misclassification, there is general agreement that fatalities from child abuse are far more frequent than official records suggest in every country where studies of infant deaths have been undertaken (20–22). Among the fatalities attributed to child abuse, the most common cause of death is injury to the head, followed by injury to the abdomen (18, 23, 24). Intentional suffocation has also been extensively reported as a cause of death (19, 22).

Non-fatal abuse

Data on non-fatal child abuse and neglect come from a variety of sources, including official statistics, case reports and population-based surveys. These sources, however, differ as regards their usefulness in describing the full extent of the problem.

Official statistics often reveal little about the patterns of child abuse. This is partly because, in many countries, there are no legal or social systems with specific responsibility for recording, let alone responding to, reports of child abuse and neglect (7). In addition, there are differing legal and

BOX 3.1

Manifestations of child abuse and neglect

Injuries inflicted by a caregiver on a child can take many forms. Serious damage or death in abused children is most often the consequence of a head injury or injury to the internal organs. Head trauma as a result of abuse is the most common cause of death in young children, with children in the first 2 years of life being the most vulnerable. Because force applied to the body passes through the skin, patterns of injury to the skin can provide clear signs of abuse. The skeletal manifestations of abuse include multiple fractures at different stages of healing, fractures of bones that are very rarely broken under normal circumstances, and characteristic fractures of the ribs and long bones.

The shaken infant

Shaking is a prevalent form of abuse seen in very young children. The majority of shaken children are less than 9 months old. Most perpetrators of such abuse are male, though this may be more a reflection of the fact that men, being on average stronger than women, tend to apply greater force, rather than that they are more prone than women to shake children. Intracranial haemorrhages, retinal haemorrhages and small "chip" fractures at the major joints of the child's extremities can result from very rapid shaking of an infant. They can also follow from a combination of shaking and the head hitting a surface. There is evidence that about one-third of severely shaken infants die and that the majority of the survivors suffer long-term consequences such as mental retardation, cerebral palsy or blindness.

The battered child

One of the syndromes of child abuse is the "battered child". This term is generally applied to children showing repeated and devastating injury to the skin, skeletal system or nervous system. It includes children with multiple fractures of different ages, head trauma and severe visceral trauma, with evidence of repeated infliction. Fortunately, though the cases are tragic, this pattern is rare.

Sexual abuse

Children may be brought to professional attention because of physical or behavioural concerns that, on further investigation, turn out to result from sexual abuse. It is not uncommon for children who have been sexually abused to exhibit symptoms of infection, genital injury, abdominal pain, constipation, chronic or recurrent urinary tract infections or behavioural problems. To be able to detect child sexual abuse requires a high index of suspicion and familiarity with the verbal, behavioural and physical indicators of abuse. Many children will disclose abuse to caregivers or others spontaneously, though there may also be indirect physical or behavioural signs.

Neglect

There exist many manifestations of child neglect, including non-compliance with health care recommendations, failure to seek appropriate health care, deprivation of food resulting in hunger, and the failure of a child physically to thrive. Other causes for concern include the exposure of children to drugs and inadequate protection from environmental dangers. In addition, abandonment, inadequate supervision, poor hygiene and being deprived of an education have all been considered as evidence of neglect.

BOX 3.2

Corporal punishment

Corporal punishment of children — in the form of hitting, punching, kicking or beating — is socially and legally accepted in most countries. In many, it is a significant phenomenon in schools and other institutions and in penal systems for young offenders.

The United Nations Convention on the Rights of the Child requires states to protect children from "all forms of physical or mental violence" while they are in the care of parents and others, and the United Nations Committee on the Rights of the Child has underlined that corporal punishment is incompatible with the Convention.

In 1979, Sweden became the first country to prohibit all forms of corporal punishment of children. Since then, at least 10 further states have banned it. Judgements from constitutional or supreme courts condemning corporal punishment in schools and penal systems have also been handed down — including in Namibia, South Africa and Zimbabwe — and, in 2000, Israel's supreme court declared all corporal punishment unlawful. Ethiopia's 1994 constitution asserts the right of children to be free of corporal punishment in schools and institutions of care. Corporal punishment in schools has also been banned in New Zealand, the Republic of Korea, Thailand and Uganda.

Nevertheless, surveys indicate that corporal punishment remains legal in at least 60 countries for juvenile offenders, and in at least 65 countries in schools and other institutions. Corporal punishment of children is legally acceptable in the home in all but 11 countries. Where the practice has not been persistently confronted by legal reform and public education, the few existing prevalence studies suggest that it remains extremely common.

Corporal punishment is dangerous for children. In the short term, it kills thousands of children each year and injures and handicaps many more. In the longer term, a large body of research has shown it to be a significant factor in the development of violent behaviour, and it is associated with other problems in childhood and later life.

families already mentioned found that 0.1% of parents admitted to having sexually abused their children, while 9.1% of children reported having suffered sexual abuse (*34*). This discrepancy might be explained in part by the fact that the children were asked to include sexual abuse by people other than their parents.

Among published studies of adults reporting retrospectively on their own childhood, prevalence rates of childhood sexual abuse among men range from 1% (*44*) – using a narrow definition of sexual contact involving pressure or force – to 19% (*38*), where a broader definition was employed. Lifetime prevalence rates for childhood sexual victimization among adult women range from 0.9% (*45*), using rape as the definition of abuse, to 45% (*38*) with a much wider definition. Findings reported in international studies conducted since 1980 reveal a mean lifetime prevalence rate of childhood sexual victimization of 20% among women and of 5–10% among men (*46, 47*).

These wide variations in published prevalence estimates could result either from real differences in risk prevailing in different cultures or from differences in the way the studies were conducted (*46*). Including abuse by peers in the definition of child sexual abuse can increase the resulting prevalence by 9% (*48*) and including cases where physical contact does not occur can raise the rates by around 16% (*49*).

Emotional and psychological abuse

Psychological abuse against children has been allotted even less attention globally than physical and sexual abuse. Cultural factors appear strongly to influence the non-physical techniques that parents choose to discipline their children – some of which may be regarded by people from other cultural backgrounds as psychologically harmful. Defining psychological abuse is therefore very difficult. Furthermore, the consequences of psychological abuse, however defined, are likely to differ greatly depending on the context and the age of the child.

There is evidence to suggest that shouting at children is a common response by parents across many countries. Cursing children and calling them names appears to vary more greatly. In the five countries of the WorldSAFE study, the lowest incidence rate of calling children names in the previous 6 months was 15% (see Table 3.2). The practices of threatening children with abandonment or with being locked out of the house, however, varied widely among the countries. In the Philippines, for example, threats of abandonment were frequently reported by mothers as a disciplinary measure. In Chile, the rate of using such threats was much lower, at about 8%.

Data on the extent that non-violent and non-abusive disciplinary methods are employed by caregivers in different cultures and parts of the world are extremely scarce. Limited data from the WorldSAFE project suggest that the majority of parents use non-violent disciplinary practices. These include explaining to children why their behaviour was wrong and telling them to stop, withdrawing privileges and using other non-violent methods to change problem behaviour (see Table 3.3). Elsewhere, in Costa Rica, for instance, parents acknowledged using physical punishment to discipline children, but reported it as their least preferred method (50).

Neglect

Many researchers include neglect or harm caused by a lack of care on the part of parents or other caregivers as part of the definition of abuse (29, 51–53). Conditions such as hunger and poverty are some-

TABLE 3.2

Rates of verbal or psychological punishment in the previous 6 months as reported by mothers, WorldSAFE study

Verbal or psychological punishment	Incidence (%)				
	Chile	Egypt	India[a]	Philippines	USA
Yelled or screamed at the child	84	72	70	82	85
Called the child names	15	44	29	24	17
Cursed at the child	3	51	—[b]	0	24
Refused to speak to the child	17	48	31	15	—[b]
Threatened to kick the child out of the household	5	0	—[b]	26	6
Threatened abandonment	8	10	20	48	—[b]
Threatened evil spirits	12	6	20	24	—[b]
Locked the child out of the household	2	1	—[b]	12	—[b]

[a] Rural areas.
[b] Question not asked in the survey.

times included within the definition of neglect. Because definitions vary and laws on reporting abuse do not always require the mandatory reporting of neglect, it is difficult to estimate the global dimensions of the problem or meaningfully to compare rates between countries. Little research, for instance, has been done on how children and parents or other caregivers may differ in defining neglect.

In Kenya, abandonment and neglect were the most commonly cited aspects of child abuse when adults in the community were questioned on the subject (51). In this study, 21.9% of children reported that they had been neglected by their parents. In Canada, a national study of cases reported to child welfare services found that, among the substantiated cases of neglect, 19% involved physical neglect, 12% abandonment, 11% educational neglect, and 48% physical harm resulting from a parent's failure to provide adequate supervision (54).

What are the risk factors for child abuse and neglect?

A variety of theories and models have been developed to explain the occurrence of abuse within families. The most widely adopted explanatory model is the ecological model, described in Chapter 1. As applied to child abuse and neglect, the ecological model considers a number of factors, including the characteristics of the individual child and his or her family, those of the caregiver or perpetrator, the

TABLE 3.3

Rates of non-violent disciplinary practices in the previous 6 months as reported by mothers, WorldSAFE study

Non-violent discipline	Incidence (%)				
	Chile	Egypt	India[a]	Philippines	USA
Explained why the behaviour was wrong	91	80	94	90	94
Took privileges away	60	27	43	3	77
Told child to stop	88	69	—[b]	91	—[b]
Gave child something to do	71	43	27	66	75
Made child stay in one place	37	50	5	58	75

[a] Rural areas.
[b] Question not asked in the survey.

nature of the local community, and the social, economic and cultural environment (*55, 56*).

The limited research in this area suggests that some factors are fairly consistent, over a range of countries, in conferring risk. It is important to note, though, that these factors, which are listed below, may be only statistically associated and not causally linked (*6*).

Factors increasing a child's vulnerability

A number of studies, mostly from the developed world, have suggested that certain characteristics of children increase the risk for abuse.

Age

Vulnerability to child abuse – whether physical, sexual or through neglect – depends in part on a child's age (*14, 17, 57, 58*). Fatal cases of physical abuse are found largely among young infants (*18, 20, 21, 28*). In reviews of infant deaths in Fiji, Finland, Germany and Senegal, for instance, the majority of victims were less than 2 years of age (*20, 24, 28, 59*).

Young children are also at risk for non-fatal physical abuse, though the peak ages for such abuse vary from country to country. For example, rates of non-fatal physical abuse peak for children at 3–6 years of age in China, at 6–11 years of age in India and between 6 and 12 years of age in the United States (*11, 40, 43*). Sexual abuse rates, on the other hand, tend to rise after the onset of puberty, with the highest rates occurring during adolescence (*15, 47, 60*). Sexual abuse, however, can also be directed at young children.

Sex

In most countries, girls are at higher risk than boys for infanticide, sexual abuse, educational and nutritional neglect, and forced prostitution (see also Chapter 6). Findings from several international studies show rates of sexual abuse to be 1.5–3 times higher among girls than boys (*46*). Globally, more than 130 million children between the ages of 6 and 11 years are not in school, 60% of whom are girls (*61*). In some countries, girls are either not allowed to receive schooling or else are kept at home to help look after their siblings or to assist the family economically by working.

Male children appear to be at greater risk of harsh physical punishment in many countries (*6, 12, 16, 40, 62*). Although girls are at increased risk for infanticide in many places, it is not clear why boys are subjected to harsher physical punishment. It may be that such punishment is seen as a preparation for adult roles and responsibilities, or else that boys are considered to need more physical discipline. Clearly, the wide cultural gaps that exist between different societies with respect to the role of women and the values attached to male and female children could account for many of these differences.

Special characteristics

Premature infants, twins and handicapped children have been shown to be at increased risk for physical abuse and neglect (*6, 53, 57, 63*). There are conflicting findings from studies on the importance of mental retardation as a risk factor. It is believed that low birth weight, prematurity, illness, or physical or mental handicaps in the infant or child interfere with attachment and bonding and may make the child more vulnerable to abuse (*6*). However, these characteristics do not appear to be major risk factors for abuse when other factors are considered, such as parental and societal variables (*6*).

Caregiver and family characteristics

Research has linked certain characteristics of the caregiver, as well as features of the family environment, to child abuse and neglect. While some factors – including demographic ones – are related to variation in risk, others are related to the psychological and behavioural characteristics of the caregiver or to aspects of the family environment that may compromise parenting and lead to child maltreatment.

Sex

Whether abusers are more likely to be male or female, depends, in part, on the type of abuse. Research conducted in China, Chile, Finland, India and the United States suggests that women report using more physical discipline than men (*12, 40, 43, 64, 65*). In Kenya, reports from children also show more violence by mothers than fathers (*51*). However, men are the most common perpetrators of life-threatening head injuries, abusive fractures and other fatal injuries (*66–68*).

Sexual abusers of children, in the cases of both female and male victims, are predominantly men in many countries (*46, 69, 70*). Studies have consistently shown that in the case of female victims of sexual abuse, over 90% of the perpetrators are men, and in the case of male victims, between 63% and 86% of the perpetrators are men (*46, 71, 72*).

Family structure and resources

Physically abusive parents are more likely to be young, single, poor and unemployed and to have less education than their non-abusing counterparts. In both developing and industrialized countries, poor, young, single mothers are among those at greatest risk for using violence towards their children (*6, 12, 65, 73*). In the United States, for instance, single mothers are three times more likely to report using harsh physical discipline than mothers in two-parent families (*12*). Similar findings have been reported in Argentina (*73*).

Studies from Bangladesh, Colombia, Italy, Kenya, Sweden, Thailand and the United Kingdom have also found that low education and a lack of income to meet the family's needs increase the potential of physical violence towards children (*39, 52, 62, 67, 74–76*), though exceptions to this pattern have been noted elsewhere (*14*). In a study of Palestinian families, lack of money for the child's needs was one of the primary reasons given by parents for psychologically abusing their children (*77*).

Family size and household composition

The size of the family can also increase the risk for abuse. A study of parents in Chile, for example, found that families with four or more children were three times more likely to be violent towards their children than parents with fewer children (*78*). However, it is not always simply the size of the family that matters. Data from a range of countries indicate that household overcrowding increases the risk of child abuse (*17, 41, 52, 57, 74, 79*). Unstable family environments, in which the composition of the household frequently changes as family members and others move in and out, are a feature particularly noted in cases of chronic neglect (*6, 57*).

Personality and behavioural characteristics

A number of personality and behavioural characteristics have been linked, in many studies, to child abuse and neglect. Parents more likely to abuse their children physically tend to have low self-esteem, poor control of their impulses, mental health problems, and to display antisocial behaviour (*6, 67, 75, 76, 79*). Neglectful parents have many of these same problems and may also have difficulty planning important life events such as marriage, having children or seeking employment. Many of these characteristics compromise parenting and are associated with disrupted social relationships, an inability to cope with stress and difficulty in reaching social support systems (*6*).

Abusive parents may also be uninformed and have unrealistic expectations about child development (*6, 57, 67, 80*). Research has found that abusive parents show greater irritation and annoyance in response to their children's moods and behaviour, that they are less supportive, affectionate, playful and responsive to their children, and that they are more controlling and hostile (*6, 39*).

Prior history of abuse

Studies have shown that parents maltreated as children are at higher risk of abusing their own children (*6, 58, 67, 81, 82*). The relationship here is complex, though (*81–83*), and some investigations have suggested that the majority of abusing parents were not, in fact, themselves abused (*58*). While empirical data suggest that there is indeed a relationship, the importance of this risk factor may have been overstated. Other factors that have been linked to child abuse – such as young parental age, stress, isolation, overcrowding in the home, substance abuse and poverty – may be more predictive.

Violence in the home

Increasing attention is being given to intimate partner violence and its relationship to child abuse. Data from studies in countries as geographically and culturally distinct as China, Colombia, Egypt, India, Mexico, the Philippines, South Africa and the United States have all found a strong relationship between these two forms of violence (*6, 15, 17, 37, 40, 43, 67*). In a recent study in India, the occurrence of domestic violence in the home doubled the risk of child abuse (*40*). Among known victims of child abuse, 40% or more have also reported domestic violence in the home (*84*). In fact, the relationship may be even stronger, since many agencies charged with protecting children do not routinely collect data on other forms of violence in families.

Other characteristics

Stress and social isolation of the parent have also been linked to child abuse and neglect (*6, 39, 57, 73, 85*). It is believed that stress resulting from job changes, loss of income, health problems or other aspects of the family environment can heighten the level of conflict in the home and the ability of members to cope or find support. Those better able to find social support may be less likely to abuse children, even when other known risk factors are present. In a case–control study in Buenos Aires, Argentina, for instance, children living in single-parent families were at significantly greater risk for abuse than those in two-parent families. The risk for abuse was lower, though, among those who were better able to gain access to social support (*73*).

Child abuse has also been linked in many studies to substance abuse (*6, 37, 40, 67, 76*), though further research is needed to disentangle the independent effects of substance abuse from the related issues of poverty, overcrowding, mental disorders and health problems associated with this behaviour.

Community factors
Poverty

Numerous studies across many countries have shown a strong association between poverty and child maltreatment (*6, 37, 40, 62, 86–88*). Rates of abuse are higher in communities with high levels of unemployment and concentrated poverty (*89–91*). Such communities are also characterized by high levels of population turnover and overcrowded housing. Research shows that chronic poverty adversely affects children through its impact on parental behaviour and the availability of community resources (*92*). Communities with high levels of poverty tend to have deteriorating physical and social infrastructures and fewer of the resources and amenities found in wealthier communities.

Social capital

Social capital represents the degree of cohesion and solidarity that exists within communities (*85*). Children living in areas with less "social capital" or social investment in the community appear to be at greater risk of abuse and have more psychological or behavioural problems (*85*). On the other hand, social networks and neighbourhood connections have been shown to be protective of children (*4, 58, 93*). This is true even for children with a number of risk factors – such as poverty, violence, substance abuse and parents with low levels of educational achievement – who appear to be protected by high levels of social capital (*85*).

Societal factors

A range of society-level factors are considered to have important influences on the well-being of children and families. These factors – not examined to date in most countries as risk factors for child abuse – include:

- The role of cultural values and economic forces in shaping the choices facing families and shaping their response to these forces.
- Inequalities related to sex and income – factors present in other types of violence and likely to be related to child maltreatment as well.
- Cultural norms surrounding gender roles, parent–child relationships and the privacy of the family.
- Child and family policies – such as those related to parental leave, maternal employment and child care arrangements.
- The nature and extent of preventive health care for infants and children, as an aid in identifying cases of abuse in children.
- The strength of the social welfare system – that is, the sources of support that provide a safety net for children and families.
- The nature and extent of social protection and the responsiveness of the criminal justice system.
- Larger social conflicts and war.

Many of these broader cultural and social factors can affect the ability of parents to care for children – enhancing or lessening the stresses associated with family life and influencing the resources available to families.

The consequences of child abuse
Health burden

Ill health caused by child abuse forms a significant portion of the global burden of disease. While some of the health consequences have been researched (*21, 35, 72, 94–96*), others have only recently been given attention, including psychiatric disorders and suicidal behaviour (*53, 97, 98*). Importantly, there is now evidence that major adult forms of illness – including ischaemic heart disease, cancer, chronic lung disease, irritable bowel syndrome and fibromyalgia – are related to experiences of abuse during childhood (*99–101*). The apparent mechanism to explain these results is the adoption of behavioural risk factors such as smoking, alcohol abuse, poor diet and lack of exercise. Research has also highlighted important

TABLE 3.4
Health consequences of child abuse
Physical
Abdominal/thoracic injuries
Brain injuries
Bruises and welts
Burns and scalds
Central nervous system injuries
Disability
Fractures
Lacerations and abrasions
Ocular damage
Sexual and reproductive
Reproductive health problems
Sexual dysfunction
Sexually transmitted diseases, including HIV/AIDS
Unwanted pregnancy
Psychological and behavioural
Alcohol and drug abuse
Cognitive impairment
Delinquent, violent and other risk-taking behaviours
Depression and anxiety
Developmental delays
Eating and sleep disorders
Feelings of shame and guilt
Hyperactivity
Poor relationships
Poor school performance
Poor self-esteem
Post-traumatic stress disorder
Psychosomatic disorders
Suicidal behaviour and self-harm
Other longer-term health consequences
Cancer
Chronic lung disease
Fibromyalgia
Irritable bowel syndrome
Ischaemic heart disease
Liver disease
Reproductive health problems such as infertility

direct acute and long-term consequences (*21, 23, 99–103*) (see Table 3.4).

Similarly, there are many studies demonstrating short-term and long-term psychological damage (*35, 45, 53, 94, 97*). Some children have a few symptoms that do not reach clinical levels of concern, or else are at clinical levels but not as high as in children generally seen in clinical settings. Other survivors have serious psychiatric symptoms, such as depression, anxiety, substance abuse, aggression, shame or cognitive impairments. Finally, some children meet the full criteria for psychiatric illnesses that include post-traumatic

and alcohol dependence (*96–99, 137*). In addition, victims of child abuse may not be identified as such until later in life and may not have symptoms until long after the abuse has occurred. For these reasons, there has been a recent increase in services for adults who were abused as children, and particularly in referrals to mental health services. Unfortunately, few evaluations have been published on the impact of interventions for adults who were abused during childhood. Most of the studies that have been conducted have focused on girls who were abused by their fathers (*138*).

Legal and related remedies
Mandatory and voluntary reporting

The reporting by health professionals of suspected child abuse and neglect is mandated by law in various countries, including Argentina, Finland, Israel, Kyrgyzstan, the Republic of Korea, Rwanda, Spain, Sri Lanka and the United States. Even so, relatively few countries have mandatory reporting laws for child abuse and neglect. A recent worldwide survey found that, of the 58 countries that responded, 33 had mandatory reporting laws in place and 20 had voluntary reporting laws (*7*).

The reasoning behind the introduction of mandatory reporting laws was that early detection of abuse would help forestall the occurrence of serious injuries, increase the safety of victims by relieving them of the necessity to make reports, and foster coordination between legal, health care and service responses.

In Brazil, there is mandatory reporting to a five-member ''Council of Guardians'' (*8*). Council members, elected to serve a 2-year term, have the duty to protect victims of child abuse and neglect by all social means, including temporary foster care and hospitalization. The legal aspects of child abuse and neglect – such as the prosecution of perpetrators and revoking parental rights – are not handled by the Council.

Mandatory laws are potentially useful for data gathering purposes, but it is not known how effective they are in preventing cases of abuse and neglect. Critics of this approach have raised various concerns, such as whether underfunded social agencies are in a position to benefit the child and his or her family, and whether instead they may do more harm than good by raising false hopes (*139*).

Various types of voluntary reporting systems exist around the world, in countries such as Barbados, Cameroon, Croatia, Japan, Romania and the United Republic of Tanzania (*7*). In the Netherlands, suspected cases of child abuse can be reported voluntarily to one of two separate public agencies – the Child Care and Protection Board and the Confidential Doctor's Office. Both these bodies exist to protect children from abuse and neglect, and both act to investigate suspected reports of maltreatment. Neither agency provides direct services to the child or the family, instead referring children and family members elsewhere for appropriate services (*140*).

Child protection services

Child protection service agencies investigate and try to substantiate reports of suspected child abuse. The initial reports may come from a variety of sources, including health care personnel, police, teachers and neighbours.

If the reports are verified, then staff of the child protection services have to decide on appropriate treatment and referral. Such decisions are often difficult, since a balance has to be found between various potentially competing demands – such as the need to protect the child and the wish to keep a family intact. The services offered to children and families thus vary widely. While some research has been published on the process of decision-making with regard to appropriate treatment, as well as on current shortcomings – such as the need for specific, standard criteria to identify families and children at risk of child abuse – there has been little investigation of the effectiveness of child protection services in reducing rates of abuse.

Child fatality review teams

In the United States, increased awareness of severe violence against children has led to the establishment of teams to review child fatalities in many states (*141*). These multidisciplinary teams review deaths among children, drawing on data and resources of the police, prosecution lawyers, health care professionals, child protection services and coroners or medical examiners. Researchers have found that these specialized review teams are more likely to detect signs of child abuse and neglect than those without relevant training. One of the objectives of this type of intervention, therefore, is to improve the accuracy of classification of child deaths.

Improved accuracy of classification, in turn, may contribute to more successful prosecutions through the collection of better evidence. In an analysis of data gathered from child fatality reviews in the state of Georgia, United States (142), researchers found that child fatality reviews were most sensitive for investigating death from maltreatment and sudden infant death syndrome. After investigation by the child fatality review team, 2% of deaths during the study year not initially classified as related to abuse or neglect were later reclassified as due to maltreatment.

Other review team objectives include preventing future child deaths from maltreatment through the review, analysis and putting in place of corrective actions, and promoting better coordination between the various agencies and disciplines involved.

Arrest and prosecution policies

Criminal justice policies vary markedly, reflecting different views about the role of the justice system with regard to child maltreatment. The decision whether to prosecute alleged perpetrators of abuse depends on a number of factors, including the seriousness of the abuse, the strength of evidence, whether the child would make a competent witness and whether there are any viable alternatives to prosecution (143). One review of the criminal prosecution of child sexual abuse cases (144) found that 72% of 451 allegations filed during a 2-year period were considered probable sexual abuse cases. Formal charges, however, were filed in a little over half of these cases. In another study of allegations of child sexual abuse (145), prosecutors accepted 60% of the cases referred to them.

Mandatory treatment for offenders

Court-mandated treatment for child abuse offenders is an approach recommended in many countries. There is a debate among researchers, though, as to whether treatment mandated through the court system is preferable to voluntary enrolment in treatment programmes. Mandatory treatment follows from the belief that, in the absence of legal repercussions, some offenders will refuse to undergo treatment. Against that, there is the view that enforced treatment imposed by a court could actually create resistance to treatment on the part of the offenders, and that the willing participation of offenders is essential for successful treatment.

Community-based efforts

Community-based interventions often focus on a selected population group or are implemented in a specific setting, such as in schools. They may also be conducted on a wider scale – over a number of population segments, for instance, or even the entire community – with the involvement of many sectors.

School programmes

School-based programmes to prevent child sexual abuse are one of the most widely applied preventive strategies and have been incorporated into the regular school curriculum in several countries. In Ireland, for example, the Stay Safe primary prevention programme is now implemented in almost all primary schools, with the full support of the Department of Education and religious leaders (146).

These programmes are generally designed to teach children how to recognize threatening situations and to provide them with skills to protect themselves against abuse. The concepts underlying the programmes are that children own and can control access to their bodies and that there are different types of physical contact. Children are taught how to tell an adult if they are asked to do something they find uncomfortable. School programmes vary widely in terms of their content and presentation and many also involve parents or caregivers.

Although there is agreement among researchers that children can develop knowledge and acquire skills to protect themselves against abuse, questions have been asked about whether these skills are retained over time and whether they would protect a child in an abusive situation, particularly if the

Gilbert N, ed. *Combatting child abuse: international perspectives and trends.* New York, NY, Oxford University Press, 1997:192–211.

141. Durfee MJ, Gellert GA, Tilton-Durfee D. Origins and clinical relevance of child death review teams. *Journal of the American Medical Association,* 1992, 267:3172–3175.

142. Luallen JJ et al. Child fatality review in Georgia: a young system demonstrates its potential for identifying preventable childhood deaths. *Southern Medical Journal,* 1998, 91:414–419.

143. Myers JEB. *Legal issues in child abuse and neglect practice.* Thousand Oaks, CA, Sage, 1998.

144. Martone M, Jaudes PK, Cavins MK. Criminal prosecution of child sexual abuse cases. *Child Abuse & Neglect,* 1996, 20:457–464.

145. Cross TP, Whitcomb D, DeVos E. Criminal justice outcomes of prosecution of child sexual abuse: a case flow analysis. *Child Abuse & Neglect,* 1995, 19:1431–1442.

146. MacIntyre D, Carr A. Evaluation of the effectiveness of the Stay Safe primary prevention programme for child sexual abuse. *Child Abuse & Neglect,* 1999, 23:1307–1325.

147. Rispens J, Aleman A, Goudena PP. Prevention of child sexual abuse victimization: a meta-analysis of school programs. *Child Abuse & Neglect,* 1997, 21:975–987.

148. Hoefnagels C, Mudde A. Mass media and disclosures of child abuse in the perspective of secondary prevention: putting ideas into practice. *Child Abuse & Neglect,* 2000, 24:1091–1101.

149. Hoefnagels C, Baartman H. On the threshold of disclosure: the effects of a mass media field experiment. *Child Abuse & Neglect,* 1997, 21:557–573.

150. Boocock SS. Early childhood programs in other nations: goals and outcomes. *The Future of Children,* 1995, 5:94–114.

151. Hesketh T, Zhu WX. Health in China. The one-child family policy: the good, the bad, and the ugly. *British Medical Journal,* 1997, 314:1685–1689.

152. Ramiro L, Madrid B, Amarillo M. *The Philippines WorldSAFE Study (Final report).* Manila, International Clinical Epidemiology Network, 2000.

153. Socolar RRS, Runyan DK. Unusual manifestations of child abuse. In: Reece RM, Ludwig S, eds. *Child abuse: medical diagnosis and management,* 2nd ed. Philadelphia, PA, Lippincott Williams & Wilkins, 2001:453–466.

CHAPTER 4

Violence by intimate partners

BOX 4.1

Making data on intimate partner violence more comparable

Various factors affect the quality and comparability of data on intimate partner violence, including:

— inconsistencies in the way violence and abuse are defined;

— variations in the selection criteria for study participants;

— differences resulting from the sources of data;

— the willingness of respondents to talk openly and honestly about experiences with violence.

Because of these factors, most prevalence figures on partner violence from different studies cannot be compared directly. For instance, not all studies separate different kinds of violence, so that it is not always possible to distinguish between acts of physical, sexual and psychological violence. Some studies examine only violent acts from the previous 12 months or 5 years, while others measure lifetime experiences.

There is also considerable variation in the study populations used for research. Many studies on partner violence include all women within a specific age range, while other studies interview only women who are currently married or who have been married. Both age and marital status are associated with a woman's risk of suffering partner abuse. The selection criteria for participants can therefore considerably affect estimates of the prevalence of abuse in a population.

Prevalence estimates are also likely to vary according to the source of data. Several national studies have produced estimates of the prevalence of partner violence — estimates that are generally lower than those obtained from smaller in-depth studies of women's experiences with violence. Smaller in-depth studies tend to concentrate more on the interaction between interviewers and respondents. These studies also tend to cover the subject matter in much greater detail than most national surveys. Prevalence estimates between the two types of studies may also vary because of some of the factors previously mentioned — including differences in the study populations and definitions of violence.

Improving disclosure

All studies on sensitive topics such as violence face the problem of how to achieve openness from people about intimate aspects of their lives. Success will depend partly on the way in which the questions are framed and delivered, as well as on how comfortable interviewees feel during the interview. The latter depends on such factors as the sex of the interviewer, the length of the interview, whether others are present, and how interested and non-judgemental the interviewer appears.

Various strategies can improve disclosure. These include:

■ Giving the interviewee several opportunities during an interview in which to disclose violence.

■ Using behaviourally specific questions, rather than subjective questions such as "Have you ever been abused?".

■ Carefully selecting interviewers and training them to develop a good rapport with the interviewees.

■ Providing support for interviewees, to help avoid retaliation by an abusive partner or family member.

The safety of both respondents and interviewers must always be taken into account in all strategies for improving research into violence.

The World Health Organization has recently published guidelines addressing ethical and safety issues in research into violence against women (*15*). Guidelines for defining and measuring partner violence and sexual assault are being developed to help improve the comparability of data. Some of these guidelines are currently available (*16*) (see also Resources).

with a weapon. Research has shown that behaviourally specific questions such as "Have you ever been forced to have sexual intercourse against your will?" produce greater rates of positive response than questions asking women whether they have been "abused" or "raped" (*17*). Such behaviourally specific questions also allow researchers to gauge the relative severity and frequency of the abuse suffered. Physical acts that are more severe than slapping, pushing or throwing an object at a person are generally defined in studies as "severe violence", though some observers object to defining severity solely according to the act (*18*).

A focus on acts alone can also hide the atmosphere of terror that sometimes permeates violent relationships. In a national survey of violence against women in Canada, for example, one-third of all women who had been physically assaulted by a partner said that they had feared for their lives at some time in the relationship (*19*). Although international studies have concentrated on physical violence because it is more easily conceptualized and measured, qualitative studies suggest that some women find the psychological abuse and degradation even more intolerable than the physical violence (*1, 20, 21*).

Partner violence and murder

Data from a wide range of countries suggest that partner violence accounts for a significant number of deaths by murder among women. Studies from Australia, Canada, Israel, South Africa and the United States of America show that 40–70% of female murder victims were killed by their husbands or boyfriends, frequently in the context of an ongoing abusive relationship (*22–25*). This contrasts starkly with the situation of male murder victims. In the United States, for example, only 4% of men murdered between 1976 and 1996 were killed by their wives, ex-wives or girlfriends (*26*). In Australia between 1989 and 1996, the figure was 8.6% (*27*).

Cultural factors and the availability of weapons define the profiles of murders of intimate partners in different countries. In the United States, more murders of women are committed by guns than by all other types of weapons combined (*28*). In India, guns are rare but beatings and death by fire are common. A frequent ploy is to douse a woman with kerosene and then to claim that she died in a "kitchen accident". Indian public health officials suspect that many actual murders of women are concealed in official statistics as "accidental burns". One study in the mid-1980s found that among women aged 15–44 years in Greater Bombay and other urban areas of Maharashtra state, one out of five deaths were ascribed to "accidental burns" (*29*).

Traditional notions of male honour

In many places, notions of male honour and female chastity put women at risk (see also Chapter 6). For example, in parts of the Eastern Mediterranean, a man's honour is often linked to the perceived sexual "purity" of the women in his family. If a woman is "defiled" sexually – either through rape or by engaging voluntarily in sex outside marriage – she is thought to disgrace the family honour. In some societies, the only way to cleanse the family honour is by killing the "offending" woman or girl. A study of female deaths by murder in Alexandria, Egypt, found that 47% of the women were killed by a relative after they had been raped (*30*).

The dynamics of partner violence

Recent research from industrialized countries suggests that the forms of partner violence that occur are not the same for all couples who experience violent conflict. There would seem to be at least two patterns (*31, 32*):

- A severe and escalating form of violence characterized by multiple forms of abuse, terrorization and threats, and increasingly possessive and controlling behaviour on the part of the abuser.
- A more moderate form of relationship violence, where continuing frustration and anger occasionally erupt into physical aggression.

Researchers hypothesize that community-based surveys are better-suited to detecting the second, more moderate form of violence – also called "common couple violence" – than the severe type of abuse known as battering. This may help explain

TABLE 4.5

Factors associated with a man's risk for abusing his partner

Individual factors	Relationship factors	Community factors	Societal factors
• Young age • Heavy drinking • Depression • Personality disorders • Low academic achievement • Low income • Witnessing or experiencing violence as a child	• Marital conflict • Marital instability • Male dominance in the family • Economic stress • Poor family functioning	• Weak community sanctions against domestic violence • Poverty • Low social capital	• Traditional gender norms • Social norms supportive of violence

(*77*). This study was one of the few that evaluated whether the same risk factors predict aggression by both women and men against a partner.

History of violence in family

Among personal history factors, violence in the family of origin has emerged as an especially powerful risk factor for partner aggression by men. Studies in Brazil, Cambodia, Canada, Chile, Colombia, Costa Rica, El Salvador, Indonesia, Nicaragua, Spain, the United States and Venezuela all found that rates of abuse were higher among women whose husbands had either themselves been beaten as children or had witnessed their mothers being beaten (*12, 57, 76, 78–81*). Although men who physically abuse their wives frequently have violence in their background, not all boys who witness or suffer abuse grow up to become abusive themselves (*82*). An important theoretical question here is: what distinguishes those men who are able to form healthy, non-violent relationships despite childhood adversity from those who become abusive?

Alcohol use by men

Another risk marker for partner violence that appears especially consistent across different settings is alcohol use by men (*81, 83–85*). In the meta-analysis by Black et al. mentioned earlier, every study that examined alcohol use or excessive drinking as a risk factor for partner violence found a significant association, with correlation coefficients ranging from $r = 0.21$ to $r = 0.57$. Population-based surveys from Brazil, Cambodia, Canada, Chile, Colombia, Costa Rica, El Salvador, India,

Indonesia, Nicaragua, South Africa, Spain and Venezuela also found a relationship between a woman's risk of suffering violence and her partner's drinking habits (*9, 19, 79–81, 86, 87*).

There is, however, a considerable debate about the nature of the relationship between alcohol use and violence and whether it is truly causal. Many researchers believe that alcohol operates as a situational factor, increasing the likelihood of violence by reducing inhibitions, clouding judgement and impairing an individual's ability to interpret cues (*88*). Excessive drinking may also increase partner violence by providing ready fodder for arguments between couples. Others argue that the link between violence and alcohol is culturally dependent, and exists only in settings where the collective expectation is that drinking causes or excuses certain behaviours (*89, 90*). In South Africa, for example, men speak of using alcohol in a premeditated way to gain the courage to give their partners the beatings they feel are socially expected of them (*91*).

Despite conflicting opinions about the causal role played by alcohol abuse, the evidence is that women who live with heavy drinkers run a far greater risk of physical partner violence, and that men who have been drinking inflict more serious violence at the time of an assault (*57*). According to the survey of violence against women in Canada, for example, women who lived with heavy drinkers were five times more likely to be assaulted by their partners than those who lived with non-drinkers (*19*).

Personality disorders

A number of studies have attempted to identify whether certain personality factors or disorders are consistently related to partner violence. Studies from Canada and the United States show that men who assault their wives are more likely to be emotionally dependent, insecure and low in self-esteem, and are more likely to find it difficult to control their impulses (*33*). They are also more likely than their non-violent peers to exhibit greater anger and hostility, to be depressed and to score high on certain scales of personality disorder, including antisocial, aggressive and borderline personality disorders (*76*). Although rates of psychopathology generally appear higher among men who abuse their wives, not all physically abusive men show such psychological disorders. The proportion of partner assaults linked to psychopathology is likely to be relatively low in settings where partner violence is common.

Relationship factors

At an interpersonal level, the most consistent marker to emerge for partner violence is marital conflict or discord in the relationship. Marital conflict is moderately to strongly related to partner assault by men in every study reviewed by Black et al. (*76*). Such conflict has also been found to be predictive of partner violence in a population based study of women and men in South Africa (*87*) and a representative sample of married men in Bangkok, Thailand (*92*). In the study in Thailand, verbal marital conflict remained significantly related to physical assault of the wife, even after controlling for socioeconomic status, the husband's stress level and other aspects related to the marriage, such as companionship and stability (*92*).

Community factors

A high socioeconomic status has generally been found to offer some protection against the risk of physical violence against an intimate partner, although exceptions do exist (*39*). Studies from a wide range of settings show that, while physical violence against partners cuts across all socio-economic groups, women living in poverty are disproportionately affected (*12, 19, 49, 78, 79, 81, 92–96*).

It is as yet unclear why poverty increases the risk of violence – whether it is because of low income in itself or because of other factors that accompany poverty, such as overcrowding or hopelessness. For some men, living in poverty is likely to generate stress, frustration and a sense of inadequacy for having failed to live up to their culturally expected role of providers. It may also work by providing ready material for marital disagreements or by making it more difficult for women to leave violent or otherwise unsatisfactory relationships. Whatever the precise mechanisms, it is probable that poverty acts as a "marker" for a variety of social conditions that combine to increase the risk faced by women (*55*).

How a community responds to partner violence may affect the overall levels of abuse in that community. In a comparative study of 16 societies with either high or low rates of partner violence, Counts, Brown & Campbell found that societies with the lowest levels of partner violence were those that had community sanctions against partner violence and those where abused women had access to sanctuary, either in the form of shelters or family support (*73*). The community sanctions, or prohibitions, could take the form either of formal legal sanctions or the moral pressure for neighbours to intervene if a woman was beaten. This "sanctions and sanctuary" framework suggests the hypothesis that intimate partner violence will be highest in societies where the status of women is in a state of transition. Where women have a very low status, violence is not "needed" to enforce male authority. On the other hand, where women have a high status, they will probably have achieved sufficient power collectively to change traditional gender roles. Partner violence is thus usually highest at the point where women begin to assume non-traditional roles or enter the workforce.

Several other community factors have been suggested as possibly affecting the overall incidence of partner violence, but few of these have been tested empirically. An ongoing multi-country study sponsored by the World Health Organization in eight countries (Bangladesh, Brazil, Japan, Namibia, Peru, Samoa, Thailand and the United Republic of Tanzania) is collecting data on a number of community-level factors to examine their possible relationship to partner violence. These factors include:

- Rates of other violent crime.
- Social capital (see Chapter 2).
- Social norms to do with family privacy.
- Community norms related to male authority over women.

The study will shed light on the relative contributions of individual and community-level factors to rates of partner violence.

Societal factors

Research studies across cultures have come up with a number of societal and cultural factors that might give rise to higher levels of violence. Levinson, for example, used statistical analysis of coded ethnographic data from 90 societies to examine the cultural patterns of wife beating – exploring the factors that consistently distinguish societies where wife beating is common from those where the practice is rare or absent (74). Levinson's analysis suggests that wife beating occurs more often in societies in which men have economic and decision-making power in the household, where women do not have easy access to divorce, and where adults routinely resort to violence to resolve their conflicts. The second strongest predictor in this study of the frequency of wife beating was the absence of all-women workgroups. Levinson advances the hypothesis that the presence of female workgroups offers protection from wife beating because they provide women with a stable source of social support as well as economic independence from their husbands and families.

Various researchers have proposed a number of additional factors that might contribute to higher rates of partner violence. It has been argued, for example, that partner violence is more common in places where war or other conflicts or social upheavals are taking place or have recently taken place. Where violence has become commonplace and individuals have easy access to weapons, social relations – including the roles of men and women – are frequently disrupted. During these times of economic and social disruption, women are often more independent and take on greater economic

responsibility, whereas men may be less able to fulfil their culturally expected roles as protectors and providers. Such factors may well increase partner violence, but evidence for this remains largely anecdotal.

Others have suggested that structural inequalities between men and women, rigid gender roles and notions of manhood linked to dominance, male honour and aggression, all serve to increase the risk of partner violence (55). Again, although these hypotheses seem reasonable, they remain to be proved by firm evidence.

The consequences of intimate partner violence

The consequences of abuse are profound, extending beyond the health and happiness of individuals to affect the well-being of entire communities. Living in a violent relationship affects a woman's sense of self-esteem and her ability to participate in the world. Studies have shown that abused women are routinely restricted in the way they can gain access to information and services, take part in public life, and receive emotional support from friends and relatives. Not surprisingly, such women are often unable properly to look after themselves and their children or to pursue jobs and careers.

Impact on health

A growing body of research evidence is revealing that sharing her life with an abusive partner can have a profound impact on a woman's health. Violence has been linked to a host of different health outcomes, both immediate and long-term. Table 4.6 draws on the scientific literature to summarize the consequences that have been associated with intimate partner violence. Although violence can have direct health consequences, such as injury, being a victim of violence also increases a woman's risk of future ill health. As with the consequences of tobacco and alcohol use, being a victim of violence can be regarded as a risk factor for a variety of diseases and conditions.

Studies show that women who have experienced physical or sexual abuse in childhood or

TABLE 4.6

Health consequences of intimate partner violence

Physical

Abdominal/thoracic injuries

Bruises and welts

Chronic pain syndromes

Disability

Fibromyalgia

Fractures

Gastrointestinal disorders

Irritable bowel syndrome

Lacerations and abrasions

Ocular damage

Reduced physical functioning

Sexual and reproductive

Gynaecological disorders

Infertility

Pelvic inflammatory disease

Pregnancy complications/miscarriage

Sexual dysfunction

Sexually transmitted diseases, including HIV/AIDS

Unsafe abortion

Unwanted pregnancy

Psychological and behavioural

Alcohol and drug abuse

Depression and anxiety

Eating and sleep disorders

Feelings of shame and guilt

Phobias and panic disorder

Physical inactivity

Poor self-esteem

Post-traumatic stress disorder

Psychosomatic disorders

Smoking

Suicidal behaviour and self-harm

Unsafe sexual behaviour

Fatal health consequences

AIDS-related mortality

Maternal mortality

Homicide

Suicide

adulthood experience ill-health more frequently than other women – with regard to physical functioning, psychological well-being and the adoption of further risk behaviours, including smoking, physical inactivity, and alcohol and drug abuse (*85, 97–103*). A history of being the target of violence puts women at increased risk of:

— depression;

— suicide attempts;

— chronic pain syndromes;

— psychosomatic disorders;

— physical injury;

— gastrointestinal disorders;

— irritable bowel syndrome;

— a variety of reproductive health consequences (see below).

In general, the following are conclusions emerging from current research about the health consequences of abuse:

• The influence of abuse can persist long after the abuse itself has stopped (*103, 104*).

• The more severe the abuse, the greater its impact on a woman's physical and mental health (*98*).

• The impact over time of different types of abuse and of multiple episodes of abuse appears to be cumulative (*85, 99, 100, 103, 105*).

Reproductive health

Women who live with violent partners have a difficult time protecting themselves from unwanted pregnancy or disease. Violence can lead directly to unwanted pregnancy or sexually transmitted infections, including HIV infection, through coerced sex, or else indirectly by interfering with a woman's ability to use contraceptives, including condoms (*6, 106*). Studies consistently show that domestic violence is more common in families with many children (*5, 47, 49, 50, 78, 93, 107*). Researchers have therefore long assumed that the stress of having many children increases the risk of violence, but recent data from Nicaragua, in fact, suggests that the relationship may be the opposite. In Nicaragua, the onset of violence largely precedes having many children (80% of violence beginning within the first 4 years of marriage), suggesting that violence may be a risk factor for having many children (*9*).

Violence also occurs during pregnancy, with consequences not only for the woman but also for the developing fetus. Population-based studies from Canada, Chile, Egypt and Nicaragua have found that 6–15% of ever-partnered women have been physically or sexually abused during pregnancy, usually by their partners (*9, 48, 49, 57, 78*). In the United States, estimates of abuse during pregnancy range from 3% to 11% among adult women and up to 38% among low-income, teenage mothers (*108–112*).

Violence during pregnancy has been associated with (*6, 110, 113–117*):

— miscarriage;
— late entry into prenatal care;
— stillbirth;
— premature labour and birth;
— fetal injury;
— low birth weight, a major cause of infant death in the developing world.

Intimate partner violence accounts for a substantial but largely unrecognized proportion of maternal mortality. A recent study among 400 villages and seven hospitals in Pune, India, found that 16% of all deaths during pregnancy were the result of partner violence (*118*). The study also showed that some 70% of maternal deaths in this region generally went unrecorded and that 41% of recorded deaths were misclassified. Being killed by a partner has also been identified as an important cause of maternal deaths in Bangladesh (*119*) and in the United States (*120, 121*).

Partner violence also has many links with the growing AIDS epidemic. In six countries in Africa, for instance, fear of ostracism and consequent violence in the home was an important reason for pregnant women refusing an HIV test, or else not returning for their results (*122*). Similarly, in a recent study of HIV transmission between heterosexuals in rural Uganda, women who reported being forced to have sex against their will in the previous year had an eightfold increased risk of becoming infected with HIV (*123*).

Physical health

Obviously, violence can lead to injuries, ranging from cuts and bruises to permanent disability and death. Population-based studies suggest that 40–72% of all women who have been physically abused by a partner are injured at some point in their life (*5, 9, 19, 62, 79, 124*). In Canada, 43% of women injured in this way received medical care and 50% of those injured had to take time off from work (*19*).

Injury, however, is not the most common physical outcome of partner abuse. More common are "functional disorders" – a host of ailments that frequently have no identifiable medical cause, such as irritable bowel syndrome, fibromyalgia, gastro-intestinal disorders and various chronic pain syndromes. Studies consistently link such disorders with a history of physical or sexual abuse (*98, 125–127*). Women who have been abused also experience reduced physical functioning, more physical symptoms and a greater number of days in bed than non-abused women (*97, 98, 101, 124, 125, 128*).

Mental health

Women who are abused by their partners suffer more depression, anxiety and phobias than non-abused women, according to studies in Australia, Nicaragua, Pakistan and the United States (*129–132*). Research similarly suggests that women abused by their partners are at heightened risk for suicide and suicide attempts (*25, 49, 133–136*).

Use of health services

Given the long-term impact of violence on women's health, women who have suffered abuse are more likely to be long-term users of health services, thereby increasing health care costs. Studies in Nicaragua, the United States and Zimbabwe indicate that women who have experienced physical or sexual assault, either in childhood or adulthood, use health services more frequently than their non-abused peers (*98, 100, 137–140*). On average, abuse victims experience more operative surgery, visits by doctors, hospital stays, visits to pharmacies and mental health consultations over their lifetime than non-victims, even after controlling for potential confounding factors.

Economic impact of violence

In addition to its human costs, violence places an enormous economic burden on societies in terms of lost productivity and increased use of social services. Among women in a survey in Nagpur, India, for example, 13% had to forgo paid work because of abuse, missing an average of 7 workdays per incident, and 11% had been unable to perform house-hold chores because of an incident of violence (*141*).

Although partner violence does not consistently affect a woman's overall probability of being employed, it does appear to influence a woman's earnings and her ability to keep a job (*139, 142, 143*). A study in Chicago, IL, United States, found that women with a history of partner violence were more likely to have experienced spells of unem-ployment, to have had a high turnover of jobs, and to have suffered more physical and mental health problems that could affect job performance. They also had lower personal incomes and were significantly more likely to receive welfare assis-tance than women who did not report a history of partner violence (*143*). Similarly, in a study in Managua, Nicaragua, abused women earned 46% less than women who did not report suffering abuse, even after controlling for other factors that could affect earnings (*139*).

Impact on children

Children are often present during domestic alter-cations. In a study in Ireland (*62*), 64% of abused women said that their children routinely witnessed the violence, as did 50% of abused women in Monterrey, Mexico (*11*).

Children who witness marital violence are at a higher risk for a whole range of emotional and behavioural problems, including anxiety, depres-sion, poor school performance, low self-esteem, disobedience, nightmares and physical health complaints (*9, 144–146*). Indeed, studies from North America indicate that children who witness violence between their parents frequently exhibit many of the same behavioural and psychological disturbances as children who are themselves abused (*145, 147*).

Recent evidence suggests that violence may also directly or indirectly affect child mortality (*148, 149*). Researchers in León, Nicaragua, found that after controlling for other possible confounding factors, the children of women who were physically and sexually abused by a partner were six times more likely to die before the age of 5 years than children of women who had not been abused. Partner abuse

accounted for as much as one-third of deaths among children in this region (*149*). Another study in the Indian states of Tamil Nadu and Uttar Pradesh found that women who had been beaten were significantly more likely than non-abused women to have experienced an infant death or pregnancy loss (abortion, miscarriage or stillbirth), even after controlling for well-established predictors of child mortality such as the woman's age, level of education and the number of previous pregnancies that had resulted in a live birth (*148*).

What can be done to prevent intimate partner violence?

The majority of work carried out to date on partner violence has been spearheaded by women's orga-nizations, with occasional funding and assistance from governments. Where governments have become involved – as in Australia, Latin America, North America and parts of Europe – it has generally been in response to demands by civil society for constructive action. The first wave of activity has generally involved elements of legal reform, police training and the establishment of specialized services for victims. Scores of countries have now passed laws on domestic violence, although many officials are either still unaware of the new laws or unwilling to implement them. Those within the system (in the police or the legal system, for instance) frequently share the same prejudices that predominate in society as a whole. Experience has repeatedly shown that without sustained efforts to change institutional culture and practice, most legal and policy reforms have little effect.

Despite over 20 years of activism in the field of violence against women, remarkably few interven-tions have been rigorously evaluated. Indeed, the recent review of programmes to prevent family violence in the United States by the National Research Council found only 34 studies that attempted to evaluate interventions related to partner abuse. Of those, 19 focused on law enforcement, reflecting the strong preference among government officials towards using the criminal justice system to deal with violence (*150*). Research on interventions in developing countries is even more limited. Only a handful of studies exist that attempt critically to examine current interventions. Among these are a review of programmes on violence against women in four states of India. In addition, the United Nations Development Fund for Women has reviewed seven projects across five regions funded by the United Nations Violence Against Women Trust Fund, with the aim of disseminating the lessons learnt from these projects (*151*).

Support for victims

In the developed world, women's crisis centres and battered women's shelters have been the cornerstone of programmes for victims of domestic violence. In 1995, there were approximately 1800 such programmes in the United States, 1200 of which provided emergency shelter in addition to emotional, legal and material support to women and their children (*152*). Such centres generally provide support groups and individual counselling, job training, programmes for children, assistance in dealing with social services and with legal matters, and referrals for treatment for drug and alcohol abuse. Most shelters and crisis centres in Europe and the United States were originally set up by women activists, though many are now run by professionals and receive government funding.

Since the early 1980s, shelters and crisis centres for women have also sprung up in many developing countries. Most countries have at least a few nongovernmental organizations offering specialized services for victims of abuse and campaigning on their behalf. Some countries have hundreds of such organizations. However, maintaining shelters is expensive, and many developing countries have avoided this model, instead setting up telephone hotlines or non-residential crisis centres that provide some of the same services as residential ones.

Where running a formal shelter is not possible, women have often found other ways to deal with emergencies related to domestic abuse. One approach is to set up an informal network of "safe homes", where women in distress can seek temporary shelter in the homes of neighbours. Some communities have designated their local place of worship – a temple or church, for instance – as a sanctuary where women can stay with their children overnight to escape drunken or violent partners.

Legal remedies and judicial reforms
Criminalizing abuse

The 1980s and 1990s saw a wave of legal reforms relating to physical and sexual abuse by an intimate partner (*153, 154*). In the past 10 years, for example, 24 countries in Latin America and the Caribbean have passed specific legislation on domestic violence (*154*). The most common reforms involve criminalizing physical, sexual and psychological abuse by intimate partners, either through new laws on domestic violence or by amending existing penal codes.

The intended message behind such legislation is that partner violence is a crime and will not be tolerated in society. Bringing it into the open is also a way to dispel the idea that violence is a private, family matter. Aside from introducing new laws or extending existing ones, there have been experiments in some developed countries to back up legislation by introducing special domestic violence courts, training police and court officials and prosecution lawyers, and providing special advisers to help women deal with the criminal justice system. Although rigorous evaluation of these measures has so far been sparse, the recent review of family violence interventions by the United States National Academy of Sciences concludes: "Anecdotal evidence suggests that specialized units and comprehensive reforms in police departments, prosecutors' offices and specialized courts have improved the experience of abused children and women" (*150*).

Similar experiments are under way elsewhere. In India, for example, state governments have established legal aid cells, family courts, *lok adalat* (people's courts) and *mahilla lok adalat* (women's courts). A recent evaluation notes that these bodies are primarily conciliatory mechanisms, relying exclusively on mediation and counselling to promote family reconciliation. It has, however, been suggested that these institutions are less than satisfactory even as conciliatory mechanisms, and that the mediators tend to place the well-being of women below the state's interest in keeping families together (*155*).

Laws and policies on arrest

After support services for victims, efforts to reform police practice are the next most common form of intervention against domestic violence. Early on, the focus was on training the police, but when training alone proved largely ineffective in changing police behaviour, efforts shifted to seeking laws requiring mandatory arrest for domestic violence and policies that forced police officers to take a more active stand.

Support for arrest as a means of reducing domestic violence was boosted by a 1984 research experiment in Minneapolis, MN, United States, that suggested that arrest halved the risk of future assaults over a 6-month period, compared with the strategies of separating couples or advising them to seek help (*156*). These results were widely publicized and led to a dramatic shift in police policies toward domestic violence throughout the United States.

Efforts to duplicate the Minneapolis findings in five other areas of the United States, however, failed to confirm the deterrent value of arrest. These new studies found that, on average, arrest was no more effective in reducing violence than other police responses such as issuing warnings or citations, providing counselling to the couples or separating them (*157, 158*). Detailed analysis of these studies also produced some other interesting findings. When the perpetrator of the violence was married, employed or both, arrest reduced repeat assaults, but for unemployed and unattached men, arrest actually led to increased abuse in some cities. The impact of arrest also varied by community. Men living in communities with low unemployment were deterred by arrest regardless of their individual employment status; suspects living in areas of high unemployment, however, were more violent following an arrest than they were after simply receiving a warning (*159*). These findings have led some to question the wisdom of mandatory arrest laws in areas of concentrated poverty (*160*).

Alternative sanctions

As alternatives to arrest, some communities are experimenting with other methods of deterring violent behaviour. One civil law approach is to issue court orders that prohibit a man from contacting or abusing his partner, mandate that he leave the home, order him to pay maintenance or child support, or require him to seek counselling or treatment for substance abuse.

Researchers have found that although victims generally find protection orders useful, the evidence for their effectiveness in deterring violence is mixed (*161, 162*). In a study in the cities of Denver and Boulder, CO, United States, Harrell & Smith (*163*) found that protection orders were effective for at least a year in preventing a reoccurrence of domestic violence, compared with similar situations where there was no protection order. However, studies have shown that arrests for violation of a protection order are rare, which tends to undermine their effectiveness in preventing violence (*164*). Other research shows that protection orders can enhance a woman's self-esteem but have little effect on men with serious criminal records (*165, 166*).

Elsewhere, communities have explored techniques such as public shaming, picketing an abuser's home or workplace, or requiring community service as a punishment for abusive behaviour. Activists in India frequently stage *dharna*, a form of public shaming and protest, in front of the homes or workplaces of abusive men (*155*).

All-women police stations

Some countries have experimented with all-women police stations, an innovation that started in Brazil and has now spread throughout Latin America and parts of Asia (*167, 168*). Although commendable in theory, evaluations show that this initiative has to date experienced many problems (*155, 168–172*). While the presence of a police station staffed entirely by women does increase the number of abused women coming forward, frequently the services that abused women require – such as legal advice and counselling – are not available at the stations. Furthermore, the assumption that female police officers will be more sympathetic to victims has not always proved true, and in some places, the creation of specialized police cells for crimes against women has made it easier for other police units to dismiss women's complaints. A review of all-women police stations in India observes that "women victims are forced to travel great distances to register their complaints with all-women police stations and cannot be assured of speedy neighbourhood police protection." To be viable, the strategy must be accompanied by sensitivity-training for police officers, incentives to encourage such work and the provision of a wider range of services (*155, 168, 170*).

Treatment for abusers

Treatment programmes for perpetrators of partner violence are an innovation that has spread from the United States to Australia, Canada, Europe and a number of developing countries (*173–175*). Most of the programmes use a group format to discuss gender roles and teach skills, including how to cope with stress and anger, take responsibility for one's actions and show feelings for others.

In recent years, there have been efforts to evaluate these programmes, although they have been hindered by methodological difficulties that continue to pose problems in interpreting the results. Research from the United States suggests that the majority of men (53–85%) who complete treatment programmes remain physically non-violent for up to 2 years, with lower rates for longer follow-up periods (*176, 177*). These success rates, however, should be seen in the light of the high drop-out rate that such programmes encounter; overall, between one-third and one-half of all men who enrol in these programmes fail to complete them (*176*) and many who are referred to programmes never formally enrol (*178*). An evaluation of the United Kingdom's flagship Violence Prevention Programme, for example, showed that 65% of men did not show up for the first session, 33% attended fewer than six sessions, and only 33% went on to the second stage (*179*).

A recent evaluation of programmes in four cities in the United States found that most abused women

felt "better off" and "safe" after their partners had entered treatment (*177*). Nevertheless, this study found that after 30 months, nearly half the men had used violence once, and 23% of the men had been repeatedly violent and continued to inflict serious injuries, while 21% of the men were neither physically nor verbally abusive. A total of 60% of couples had split up and 24% were no longer in contact.

According to a recent international review by researchers at the University of North London, England (*179*), evaluations collectively suggest that treatment programmes work best if they:
— continue for longer rather than shorter periods;
— change men's attitudes enough for them to discuss their behaviour;
— sustain participation in the programme;
— work in tandem with a criminal justice system that acts strictly when there are breaches of the conditions of the programme.

In Pittsburgh, PA, United States, for example, the non-attendance rate dropped from 36% to 6% between 1994 and 1997 when the justice system began issuing arrest warrants for men who failed to appear at the programme's initial interview session (*179*).

Health service interventions

In recent years attention has turned towards reforming the response of health care providers to victims of abuse. Most women come into contact with the health system at some point in their lives – when they seek contraception, for instance, or give birth or seek care for their children. This makes the health care setting an important place where women undergoing abuse can be identified, provided with support and referred if necessary to specialized services. Unfortunately, studies show that in most countries, doctors and nurses rarely enquire of women whether they are being abused, or even check for obvious signs of violence (*180–186*).

Existing interventions have focused on sensitizing health care providers, encouraging routine screening for abuse and drawing up protocols for the proper management of abuse. A growing number of countries – including Brazil, Ireland, Malaysia, Mexico, Nicaragua, the Philippines and South Africa – have begun pilot projects training health workers to identify and respond to abuse (*187–189*). Several countries in Latin America have also incorporated guidelines to address domestic violence in their health sector policies (*190*).

Research suggests that making procedural changes in patient care – such as stamping a reminder for the provider on the patient's chart or incorporating questions on abuse in the standard intake forms – have the greatest effect on the behaviour of health care providers (*191, 192*).

Confronting deep-rooted beliefs and attitudes is also important. In South Africa, the Agisanang Domestic Abuse Prevention and Training Project and its partner, the Health Systems Development Unit of the University of Witwatersrand, have developed a reproductive health and gender course for nurses that has a strong domestic violence component. In these courses, popular sayings, wedding songs and role-plays are used in an exercise to dissect commonly held notions on violence and the expected roles of men and women. Following the exercise, there is a discussion on the responsibility of nurses as health professionals. Analysis of a survey completed after one of these courses found that participants no longer believed that beating a woman was justified and that most accepted that a woman could be raped by her husband.

Active screening for abuse – questioning patients about their possible histories of suffering violence by intimate partners – is generally considered good practice in this field. However, while studies repeatedly show that women welcome being queried about violence in a non-judgemental way (*181, 182, 193*), little systematic evaluation has been carried out on whether screening for abuse can improve the safety of women or their health-seeking behaviour – and if it does, under what conditions (*194*).

Community-based efforts

Outreach work

Outreach work has been a major part of the response to partner violence from nongovernmen-

tal organizations. Outreach workers – who are often peer educators – visit victims of violence in their homes and communities. Nongovernmental organizations frequently recruit and train peer workers from the ranks of former clients, themselves earlier victims of partner violence.

Both governmental and nongovernmental projects have been known to employ ''advocates'' – individuals who provide abused women with information and advice, particularly with help in negotiating the intricacies of the legal system and of family welfare and other benefits. These people focus on the rights and entitlements of victims of violence and carry out their work from institutions as diverse as police stations, legal prosecutors' offices and hospitals.

Several outreach schemes have been evaluated. The Domestic Violence Matters project in Islington, London, England, placed civilian advocates in local police stations, with the task of contacting all victims of partner violence within 24 hours of their calling the police. Another initiative in London, the Domestic Violence Intervention project in Hammersmith and Fulham, combined an education programme for violent men with appropriate interventions for their partners. A recent review of these programmes found that the Islington project had reduced the number of repeated calls to the police and – by inference – had reduced the reoccurrence of domestic violence. At the same time, it had increased the use by women of new services, including shelters, legal advice and support groups. The second project had managed to reach greater numbers of women from ethnic minority groups and professional women than other services for victims of domestic violence (*195*).

Coordinated community interventions

Coordinating councils or interagency forums are an increasingly popular means of monitoring and improving responses towards intimate partner violence at the community level (*166*). Their aim is to:

— exchange information;
— identify and address problems in the provision of services;

— promote good practice through training and drawing up guidelines;

— track cases and carry out institutional audits to assess the practice of various agencies;

— promote community awareness and prevention work.

Adapted from the original pilot programmes in California, Massachusetts and Minnesota in the United States, this type of intervention has spread widely throughout the rest of the United States, Canada, the United Kingdom and parts of Latin America.

The Pan American Health Organization (PAHO), for instance, has set up pilot projects in 16 Latin American countries to test this approach in both urban and rural settings. In rural settings, the coordinating councils include individuals such as the local priest, the mayor, community health promoters, magistrates and representatives of women's groups. The PAHO project began with a qualitative research study – known as *La Ruta Crítica* – to examine what happens to women in rural communities when they seek help, and the results are summarized in Box 4.2.

These types of community interventions have seldom been evaluated. One study found a statistically significant increase in the proportion of police calls that resulted in arrests, as well as in the proportion of arrests that resulted in prosecution, after the implementation of a community intervention project (*196*). The study also found a significant increase in the proportion of men sent for mandatory counselling in each of the communities, though it is unclear what impact, if any, these actions had on rates of abuse.

Qualitative evaluations have noted that many of these interventions focus primarily on coordinating refuges and the criminal justice system, at the expense of wider involvement of religious communities, schools, the health system, or other social service agencies. A recent review of interagency forums in the United Kingdom concluded that while coordinating councils can improve the quality of services offered to women and children, interagency work can act as a smokescreen, concealing the fact that little actually changes. The review suggested

that organizations should identify firm criteria for self-evaluation that cover user satisfaction and real changes in policies and practices (*197*).

Prevention campaigns

Women's organizations have long used communication campaigns, small-scale media and other events in an attempt to raise awareness of partner violence and change behaviour. There is evidence that such campaigns reach a large number of people, although only a few campaigns have been evaluated for their effectiveness in changing attitudes or behaviour. During the 1990s, for instance, a network of women's groups in Nicaragua mounted an annual mass media campaign to raise awareness of the impact of violence on women (*198*). Using slogans such as "*Quiero vivir sin violencia*" (I want to live free of violence), the campaigns mobilized communities against abuse. Similarly, the United Nations Development Fund for Women, together with several other United Nations agencies, has been sponsoring a series of regional campaigns against gender violence around the slogan, "A life free of violence: it's our right" (*199*). One communication project that has been evaluated is the multimedia health project known as *Soul City*, in South Africa – a project that combines prime-time television and radio dramas with other educational activities. One component is specifically devoted to domestic violence (see Box 9.1 in Chapter 9). The evaluation found increased knowledge and awareness of domestic violence, changed attitudes and norms, and greater willingness on the part of the project's audience to take appropriate action.

School programmes

Despite a growing number of initiatives aimed at young people on preventing violence, only a small number specifically address the problem of violence in intimate relationships. There is considerable scope, though, to integrate material that explores relationships, gender roles and coercion and control into existing programmes for reducing school violence, bullying, delinquency and other problem behaviours, as well as into reproductive and sexual health programmes.

BOX 4.2

La Ruta Crítica: a study of responses to domestic violence

In 1995, the Pan American Health Organization launched a community study in 10 countries in Latin America (Belize, Bolivia, Costa Rica, Ecuador, El Salvador, Guatemala, Honduras, Nicaragua, Panama and Peru). Its purpose was to record the process that a woman who has suffered domestic violence goes through after making a decision to end her silence and seek assistance. The Spanish name for this process was *La Ruta Crítica* — the critical path — referring to the unfolding series of decisions and actions taken by the woman as she comes to terms with the violent situation and the responses she encounters from others in her search for help. Each action and decision by the woman along the path affects the actions of others, including service providers and members of the community, and what they do, in turn, has an influence on the next step the woman takes.

The questions investigated by the study were therefore concerned with the consequences of a woman deciding to seek help, the sources she approached for assistance, her motivations, and the attitudes and responses, both of institutional service providers and individuals. The qualitative study involved over 500 in-depth interviews with women who had been abused and more than 1000 interviews with service providers, as well as some 50 focus group sessions.

Women who had been victims of violence identified several factors that can act as triggers for action. These included an increase in the severity or frequency of the violence, causing a recognition that the abuser was not going to change. One important factor motivating action was the realization that the life of the woman or those of her children were in danger. As with the factors that precipitated action, the factors inhibiting a woman from seeking help were multiple and interconnected.

The study found that economic considerations seemed to carry more weight than emotional ones. Many women, for instance, expressed concern about their ability to support themselves and their children. The women interviewed also frequently expressed feelings of guilt, self-blame or being abnormal. Corruption and stereotyping by gender in the judicial system and among the police were also mentioned. The greatest inhibiting factor, though, was fear — that the consequences of telling someone or of leaving would be worse than staying in the relationship.

From the *Ruta Crítica* study, it is clear that there are many factors, both internal and external, that have a bearing on an abused woman's decision to take action to stop the violence. The process is often a long one — many years in some cases — involving several attempts at seeking help from a number of sources. Rarely is there just a single event that precipitates action. The evidence indicates that, despite facing formidable obstacles, abused women are often resourceful in seeking help and in finding ways of mitigating the violence inflicted on them.

The programmes for young people that do explicitly address abuse within intimate relationships tend to be independent initiatives sponsored by bodies working to end violence against women (see Box 4.3). Only a handful of these programmes have been evaluated, including one in Canada (*200*) and two in the United States (*201, 202*). Using experimental designs, these evaluations found positive changes in knowledge and attitudes toward relationship violence (see also *203*). One of the programmes in the United States demonstrated a reduction in the perpetration of violence at 1 month. Although its effect on behaviour had vanished after 1 year, its effects on norms of violence within an intimate relationship, on skills for resolving conflict and on knowledge were all maintained (*201*).

Principles of good practice

A growing body of wisdom on partner violence, accumulated over many years by large numbers of service providers, advocates and researchers, suggests a set of principles to help guide "good

BOX 4.3

Promoting non-violence: some examples of primary prevention programmes

The following are a few of the many examples from around the world of innovative programmes to prevent violence between intimate partners.

In Calabar, Nigeria, the Girl's Power Initiative is aimed at young girls. The girls meet weekly over a period of 3 years to discuss frankly a range of issues related to sexuality, women's health and rights, relationships and domestic violence. Specific topics in the programme, designed to build self-esteem and teach skills for self-protection, have included societal attitudes that put women at risk of rape, and distinguishing between love and infatuation.

Education Wife Assault in Toronto, Canada, works with immigrant and refugee women, helping them develop violence prevention campaigns that are culturally appropriate for their communities by means of special "skill shops". Education Wife Assault provides technical assistance, enabling women to conduct their own campaigns. At the same time, it also offers emotional support to the women organizers to help them overcome the discrimination often directed at women campaigning against domestic violence because they are seen as threatening their community's cohesiveness.

In Mexico, the nongovernmental organization Instituto Mexicano de Investigación de Familia y Población has created a workshop for adolescents to help prevent violence in dating and within relationships between friends. Entitled "Faces and Masks of Violence", the project uses participatory techniques to help young people explore expectations and feelings about love, desire and sex, and to understand how traditional gender roles can inhibit behaviour, both in men and women.

In Trinidad and Tobago, the nongovernmental organization SERVOL (Service Volunteered for All) conducts workshops over 14 weeks for adolescents to assist them in developing healthy relationships and learning parenting skills. The project helps these young people understand how their own parenting contributed towards shaping what they are and teaches them how not to repeat the mistakes their parents and other relatives may have made in bringing up their families. As a result, the students discover how to recognize and handle their emotions, and become more sensitive to how early physical and psychological traumas can lead to destructive behaviour later in life.

practice" in this field. These principles include the following:

- Actions to address violence should take place at both national and local level.
- The involvement of women in the development and implementation of projects and the safety of women should guide all decisions relating to interventions.
- Efforts to reform the response of institutions – including the police, health care workers and the judiciary – should extend beyond training to changing institutional cultures.
- Interventions should cover and be coordinated between a range of different sectors.

Action at all levels

An important lesson to emerge from efforts to prevent violence is that actions should take place at both national and local levels. At the national level, priorities include improving the status of women, establishing appropriate norms, policies and laws on abuse, and creating a social environment that is conducive to non-violent relationships.

Many countries, industrialized as well as developing, have found it useful to set up a formal mechanism for developing and implementing national plans of action. Such plans should include clear objectives, lines of responsibility and time schedules, and be backed by adequate resources.

Experience nevertheless suggests that national efforts alone are insufficient to transform the landscape of intimate violence. Even in those industrialized countries where national movements against partner violence have existed for more than 25 years, the options for help available to a woman who has suffered abuse, and the reactions she is likely to meet from institutions such as the police, still vary greatly according to the particular locality. Where there have been efforts in the community to prevent violence, and where there are established groups to conduct training and monitor the activities of formal institutions, victims of abuse fare considerably better than where these are lacking (*204*).

Women's involvement

Interventions should be designed to work with women – who are usually the best judges of their situation – and to respect their decisions. Recent reviews of a range of domestic violence programmes in the Indian states of Gujarat, Karnataka, Madhya Pradesh and Maharashtra, for instance, have consistently shown that the success or failure of projects was determined largely by the attitudes of organizers towards intimate partner violence and their priorities for including the interests of women during the planning and implementation of interventions (*205*).

Women's safety should also be carefully considered when planning and implementing interventions. Those that make women's safety and autonomy a priority have generally proved more successful than those that do not. For example, concern has been raised about laws requiring health care workers to report suspected cases of abuse to the police. These types of interventions take control away from women and have usually proved counterproductive. They may well put a woman's safety at risk and make it less likely that she will come forward for care (*206–208*). Such laws also transform health workers into arms of the judicial system and work against the emotional protection that the environment of the clinic is meant to provide (*150*).

Changing institutional cultures

Little enduring change is usually achieved by short-term efforts to sensitize institutional actors, unless there are also real efforts to engage the whole institution. The nature of the organization's leadership, the way in which performances are evaluated and rewarded, and the embedded cultural biases and beliefs are all of prime importance in this respect (*209, 210*). In the case of reforming health care practice, training alone has seldom been sufficient to change institutional behaviour toward victims of violence (*211, 212*). Although training can improve knowledge and practice in the short term, its impact generally wears off quickly unless accompanied by institutional changes in policies and performance (*211, 213*).

A multisectoral approach

Various sectors such as the police, health services, judiciary and social support services should work together in tackling the problem of intimate partner violence. Historically, the tendency of programmes has been to concentrate on a single sector, which has been shown by experience very often to produce poor results (*155*).

Recommendations

The evidence available shows violence against women by intimate partners to be a serious and widespread problem in all parts of the world. There is also a growing documentation of the damaging impact of violence on the physical and mental health of women and their overall well-being. The following are the main recommendations for action:

- Governments and other donors should be encouraged to invest much more in research on violence by intimate partners over the next decade.

- Programmes should place greater emphasis on enabling families, circles of friends and community groups, including religious communities, to deal with the problem of partner violence.

- Programmes on partner violence should be integrated with other programmes, such as those tackling youth violence, teenage pregnancies, substance abuse and other forms of family violence.

- Programmes should focus more on the primary prevention of intimate partner violence.

Research on intimate partner violence

The lack of a clear theoretical understanding of the causes of intimate partner violence and its relationship to other forms of interpersonal violence has frustrated efforts to build an effective global response. Studies to advance the understanding of violence are needed on a variety of fronts, including:

- Studies that examine the prevalence, consequences and risk and protective factors of violence by intimate partners in different cultural settings, using standardized methodologies.
- Longitudinal research on the trajectory of violent behaviour by intimate partners over time, examining whether and how it differs from the development of other violent behaviours.
- Studies that explore the impact of violence over the course of a person's life, investigating the relative impact of different types of violence on health and well-being, and whether the effects are cumulative.
- Studies that examine the life history of adults who are in healthy, non-violent relationships despite past experiences that are known to increase the risk of partner violence.

In addition, much more research is needed on interventions, both for the purpose of lobbying policy-makers for more investment as well as to improve the design and implementation of programmes. In the next decade, priority should be given to the following:

- Documentation of the various strategies and interventions around the world for combating intimate partner violence.
- Studies assessing the economic costs of intimate partner violence.
- Evaluation of the short-term and long-term effects of programmes to prevent and respond to partner violence – including school education programmes, legal and policy changes, services for victims of violence, programmes that target perpetrators of violence, and

campaigns to change social attitudes and behaviour.

Strengthening informal sources of support

Many women do not seek assistance from the official services or systems that are available to them. Expanding the informal sources of support through neighbourhood networks and networks of friends, religious and other community groups, and workplaces is therefore vital (*6, 61, 183, 214*). How these informal groups and individuals respond will determine whether a victim of partner violence takes action or else retreats into isolation and self-blame (*214*).

There is plenty of room for programmes that can create constructive responses on the part of family and friends. An innovative programme in Iztacalco, Mexico, for instance, used community events, small-scale media (such as posters, pamphlets and audio cassettes) and workshops to help victims of violence discuss the abuse they had undergone and to demonstrate to friends and other family members how best to deal with such situations (*215*).

Making common cause with other social programmes

There is a considerable overlap between the factors that increase the risk of various problem behaviours (*216*). There also appears to be a significant continuity between aggressive behaviour in childhood and a range of problem behaviours in youth and early adulthood (see Chapter 2). The insights gained from research on these types of violence overlap as well. There is an evident need to intervene early with high-risk families and to provide support and other services before dysfunctional patterns of behaviour within the family set in, preparing the stage for abusive behaviour in adolescence or adulthood.

Unfortunately, there is at present little coordination between programmes or research agendas on youth violence, child abuse, substance abuse and partner violence, despite the fact that all these problems regularly coexist in families. If true progress is to be made, attention must be paid to the development of aggressive behaviour patterns – patterns that often begin in childhood. Integrated prevention responses that address the links between different types of violence have the potential to reduce some of these forms of violence.

Investing in primary prevention

The importance of primary prevention of violence by intimate partners is often overshadowed by the importance of the large number of programmes that, understandably, seek to deal with the immediate and numerous consequences of violence.

Both policy-makers and activists in this field must give greater priority to the admittedly immense task of creating a social environment that allows and promotes equitable and non-violent personal relationships. The foundation for such an environment must be the new generation of children, who should come of age with better skills than their parents generally had for managing their relationships and resolving the conflicts within them, with greater opportunities for their future, and with more appropriate notions on how men and women can relate to each other and share power.

Conclusion

Violence by intimate partners is an important public health problem. Resolving it requires the involvement of many sectors working together at community, national and international levels. At each level, responses must include empowering women and girls, reaching out to men, providing for the needs of victims and increasing the penalties for abusers. It is vital that responses should involve children and young people, and focus on changing community and societal norms. The progress made in each of these areas will be the key to achieving global reductions in violence against intimate partners.

References

1. Crowell N, Burgess AW. *Understanding violence against women.* Washington, DC, National Academy Press, 1996.

2. Heise L, Pitanguy J, Germain A. *Violence against women: the hidden health burden.* Washington, DC, World Bank, 1994 (Discussion Paper No. 255).

3. Koss MP et al. *No safe haven: male violence against women at home, at work, and in the community.* Washington, DC, American Psychological Association, 1994.

4. Butchart A, Brown D. Non-fatal injuries due to interpersonal violence in Johannesburg-Soweto: incidence, determinants and consequences. *Forensic Science International,* 1991, 52:35–51.

5. Tjaden P, Thoennes N. *Full report of the prevalence, incidence, and consequences of violence against women: findings from the National Violence Against Women Survey.* Washington, DC, National Institute of Justice, Office of Justice Programs, United States Department of Justice and Centers for Disease Control and Prevention, 2000 (NCJ 183781).

6. Heise LL, Ellsberg M, Gottemoeller M. *Ending violence against women.* Baltimore, MD, Johns Hopkins University School of Public Health, Center for Communications Programs, 1999 (Population Reports, Series L, No. 11).

7. *Violence against women: a priority health issue.* Geneva, World Health Organization, 1997 (document WHO/FRH/WHD/97.8).

8. Yoshihama M, Sorenson SB. Physical, sexual, and emotional abuse by male intimates: experiences of women in Japan. *Violence and Victims,* 1994, 9:63–77.

9. Ellsberg MC et al. Candies in hell: women's experience of violence in Nicaragua. *Social Science and Medicine,* 2000, 51:1595–1610.

10. Leibrich J, Paulin J, Ransom R. *Hitting home: men speak about domestic abuse of women partners.* Wellington, New Zealand Department of Justice and AGB McNair, 1995.

11. Granados Shiroma M. *Salud reproductiva y violencia contra la mujer: un análisis desde la perspectiva de género. [Reproductive health and violence against women: a gender perspective.]* Nuevo León, Asociación Mexicana de Población, Consejo Estatal de Población, 1996.

12. Ellsberg MC et al. Wife abuse among women of childbearing age in Nicaragua. *American Journal of Public Health,* 1999, 89:241–244.

13. Mooney J. *The hidden figure: domestic violence in north London.* London, Middlesex University, 1993.

14. Ellsberg M et al. Researching domestic violence against women: methodological and ethical considerations. *Studies in Family Planning,* 2001, 32:1–16.

15. *Putting women first: ethical and safety recommendations for research on domestic violence against women.* Geneva, World Health Organization, 2001 (document WHO/FCH/GWH/01.01).

16. Saltzman LE et al. *Intimate partner surveillance: uniform definitions and recommended data ele-*

ments, Version 1.0. Atlanta, GA, National Center for Injury Prevention and Control, Centers for Disease Control and Prevention, 1999.

17. Ellsberg M, Heise L, Shrader E. *Researching violence against women: a practical guide for researchers and advocates.* Washington, DC, Center for Health and Gender Equity, 1999.

18. Smith PH, Smith JB, Earp JAL. Beyond the measurement trap: a reconstructed conceptualization and measurement of battering. *Psychology of Women Quarterly,* 1999, 23:177–193.

19. Rodgers K. Wife assault: the findings of a national survey. *Juristat Service Bulletin,* 1994, 14:1–22.

20. Cabaraban M, Morales B. *Social and economic consequences for family planning use in southern Philippines.* Cagayan de Oro, Research Institute for Mindanao Culture, Xavier University, 1998.

21. Cabrejos MEB et al. *Los caminos de las mujeres que rompieron el silencio: un estudio cualitativo sobre la ruta crítica que siguen las mujeres afectadas por la violencia intrafamiliar. [Paths of women who broke the silence: a qualitative study of help-seeking by women affected by family violence.]* Lima, Proyecto Violencia Contra las Mujeres y las Niñas and World Health Organization, 1998.

22. Mouzos J. *Femicide: the killing of women in Australia 1989–1998.* Canberra, Australian Institute of Criminology, 1999.

23. Juristat. *Homicide in Canada.* Ottawa, Statistics Canada, 1998.

24. Gilbert L. Urban violence and health: South Africa 1995. *Social Science and Medicine,* 1996, 43:873–886.

25. Bailey JE et al. Risk factors for violent death of women in the home. *Archives of Internal Medicine,* 1997, 157:777–782.

26. Fox JA, Zawitz MW. *Homicide trends in the United States.* Washington, DC, Bureau of Justice Statistics, United States Department of Justice, 1999.

27. Carcach C, James M. *Homicide between intimate partners in Australia.* Canberra, Australian Institute of Criminology, 1998.

28. *When men murder women: an analysis of 1996 homicide data.* Washington, DC, Violence Policy Center, 2000.

29. Karkal M. How the other half dies in Bombay. *Economic and Political Weekly,* 24 August 1985:1424.

30. Mercy JA et al. Intentional injuries. In: Mashaly AY, Graitcer PL, Youssef ZM, eds. *Injury in Egypt: an analysis of injuries as a health problem.* Cairo, Rose El Youssef New Presses, 1993.

31. Johnson MP. Patriarchal terrorism and common couple violence: two forms of violence against women. *Journal of Marriage and the Family,* 1995, 57:283–294.

32. Johnson MP, Ferraro KJ. Research on domestic violence in the 1990s: making distinctions. *Journal of Marriage and the Family,* 2000, 62:948–963.

33. Kantor GK, Jasinski JL. Dynamics and risk factors in partner violence. In: Jasinski JL, Williams LM, eds. *Partner violence: a comprehensive review of 20 years of research.* Thousand Oaks, CA, Sage, 1998.

34. Morse BJ. Beyond the conflict tactics scale: assessing gender differences in partner violence. *Violence and Victims,* 1995, 10:251–272.

35. Brush LD. Violent acts and injurious outcomes in married couples: methodological issues in the national survey of family and households. *Gender and Society,* 1990, 4:56–67.

36. Canadian Centre for Justice Statistics. *Family violence in Canada: a statistical profile.* Ottawa, Statistics Canada, 2000.

37. Saunders DG. When battered women use violence: husband-abuse or self-defense? *Violence and Victims,* 1986, 1:47–60.

38. DeKeseredy WS et al. The meanings and motives for women's use of violence in Canadian college dating relationships: results from a national survey. *Sociological Spectrum,* 1997, 17:199–222.

39. Schuler SR et al. Credit programs, patriarchy and men's violence against women in rural Bangladesh. *Social Science and Medicine,* 1996, 43:1729–1742.

40. Zimmerman K. *Plates in a basket will rattle: domestic violence in Cambodia. A summary.* Phnom Penh, Project Against Domestic Violence, 1995.

41. Michau L. Community-based research for social change in Mwanza, Tanzania. In: *Third Annual Meeting of the International Research Network on Violence Against Women, Washington, DC, 9–11 January 1998.* Takoma Park, MD, Center for Health and Gender Equity, 1998:4–9.

42. Armstrong A. *Culture and choice: lessons from survivors of gender violence in Zimbabwe.* Harare, Violence Against Women in Zimbabwe Research Project, 1998.

43. Gonzalez Montes S. Domestic violence in Cuetzalan, Mexico: some research questions and results. In: *Third Annual Meeting of the International Research Network on Violence Against Women, Washington, DC, 9–11 January 1998.* Takoma Park, MD, Center for Health and Gender Equity, 1998:36–41.

44. Osakue G, Hilber AM. Women's sexuality and fertility in Nigeria. In: Petchesky R, Judd K, eds. *Negotiating reproductive rights.* London, Zed Books, 1998:180–216.

45. Hassan Y. *The haven becomes hell: a study of domestic violence in Pakistan.* Lahore, Shirkat Gah Women's Resource Centre, 1995.

46. Bradley CS. Attitudes and practices relating to marital violence among the Tolai of East New Britain. In: *Domestic violence in Papua New Guinea.* Boroko, Papua New Guinea Law Reform Commission, 1985:32–71.

47. Jejeebhoy SJ. Wife-beating in rural India: a husband's right? *Economic and Political Weekly*, 1998, 33:855–862.

48. El-Zanaty F et al. *Egypt demographic and health survey 1995.* Calverton, MD, Macro International, 1996.

49. Rosales J et al. *Encuesta Nicaraguense de demografía y salud, 1998. [1998 Nicaraguan demographic and health survey.]* Managua, Instituto Nacional de Estadísticas y Censos, 1999.

50. David F, Chin F. *Economic and psychosocial influences of family planning on the lives of women in Western Visayas.* Iloilo City, Central Philippines University and Family Health International, 1998.

51. Bawah AA et al. Women's fears and men's anxieties: the impact of family planning on gender relations in northern Ghana. *Studies in Family Planning*, 1999, 30:54–66.

52. Wood K, Jewkes R. Violence, rape, and sexual coercion: everyday love in a South African township. *Gender and Development*, 1997, 5:41–46.

53. Khan ME et al. Sexual violence within marriage. *Seminar* (New Delhi), 1996:32–35.

54. Jenkins C for the National Sex and Reproduction Research Team. *National study of sexual and reproductive knowledge and behaviour in Papua New Guinea.* Goroka, Papua New Guinea Institute of Medical Research, 1994.

55. Heise L. Violence against women: an integrated ecological framework. *Violence Against Women* 1998, 4:262–290.

56. Rao V. Wife-beating in rural South India: a qualitative and econometric analysis. *Social Science and Medicine*, 1997, 44:1169–1179.

57. Johnson H. *Dangerous domains: violence against women in Canada.* Ontario, International Thomson Publishing, 1996.

58. Romero M. *Violencia sexual y domestica: informe de la fase cuantitativa realizada en el centro de atencion a adolescentes de San Miguel de Allende. [Sexual and domestic violence: report from the qualitative phase from an adolescent center in San Miguel de Allende.]* Mexico City, Population Council, 1994.

59. Campbell J et al. Voices of strength and resistance: a contextual and longitudinal analysis of women's responses to battering. *Journal of Interpersonal Violence*, 1999, 13:743–762.

60. Dutton MA. Battered women's strategic response to violence: the role of context. In: Edelson JL, Eisikovits ZC, eds. *Future interventions with battered women and their families.* London, Sage, 1996:105–124.

61. Sagot M. *Ruta crítica de las mujeres afectadas por la violencia intrafamiliar en América Latina: estudios de caso de diez países. [The critical path followed by women victims of domestic violence in Latin America: case studies from ten countries.]* Washington, DC, Pan American Health Organization, 2000.

62. O'Conner M. *Making the links: towards an integrated strategy for the elimination of violence against women in intimate relationships with men.* Dublin, Women's Aid, 1995.

63. Short L. Survivor's identification of protective factors and early warning signs in intimate partner violence. In: *Third Annual Meeting of the International Research Network on Violence Against Women, Washington, DC, 9–11 January 1998.* Takoma Park, MD, Center for Health and Gender Equity, 1998:27–31.

64. George A. Differential perspectives of men and women in Mumbai, India on sexual relations and negotiations within marriage. *Reproductive Health Matters*, 1998, 6:87–95.

65. Ellsberg M et al. Women's strategic responses to violence in Nicaragua. *Journal of Epidemiology and Community Health*, 2001, 55:547–555.

66. Bunge VP, Levett A. *Family violence in Canada: a statistical profile.* Ottawa, Statistics Canada, 1998.

67. Campbell JC, Soeken KL. Women's responses to battering: a test of the model. *Research in Nursing and Health*, 1999, 22:49–58.

68. Campbell JC. Abuse during pregnancy: progress, policy, and potential. *American Journal of Public Health*, 1998, 88:185–187.

69. Landenburger KM. The dynamics of leaving and recovering from an abusive relationship. *Journal of Obstetric, Gynecologic, and Neonatal Nursing*, 1998, 27:700–706.

70. Jacobson NS et al. Psychological factors in the longitudinal course of battering: when do the couples split up? When does the abuse decrease? *Violence and Victims*, 1996, 11:371–392.

71. Campbell J. *Assessing dangerousness: violence by sexual offenders, batterers, and child abusers.* Thousand Oaks, CA, Sage, 1995.

72. Wilson M, Daly M. Spousal homicide. *Juristat Service Bulletin*, 1994, 14:1–15.

73. Counts DA, Brown J, Campbell J. *Sanctions and sanctuary: cultural perspectives on the beating of wives.* Boulder, CO, Westview Press, 1992.

74. Levinson D. *Family violence in cross-cultural perspective.* Thousand Oaks, CA, Sage, 1989.

75. Dutton DG. *The domestic assault of women: psychological and criminal justice perspectives.* Vancouver, University of British Colombia Press, 1995.

76. Black DA et al. *Partner, child abuse risk factors literature review.* National Network of Family Resiliency, National Network for Health, 1999 (available on the Internet at http://www.nnh.org/risk).

77. Moffitt TE, Caspi A. *Findings about partner violence from the Dunedin multi-disciplinary health and development study, New Zealand.* Washington, DC, National Institutes of Justice, 1999.

78. Larrain SH. *Violencia puertas adentro: la mujer golpeada. [Violence behind closed doors: the battered women.]* Santiago, Editorial Universitaria, 1994.

79. Nelson E, Zimmerman C. *Household survey on domestic violence in Cambodia.* Phnom Penh, Ministry of Women's Affairs and Project Against Domestic Violence, 1996.

80. Hakimi M et al. *Silence for the sake of harmony: domestic violence and women's health in Central Java, Indonesia.* Yogyakarta, Gadjah Mada University, 2001.

81. Moreno Martín F. La violencia en la pareja. [Intimate partner violence.] *Revista Panamericana de Salud Pública*, 1999, 5:245–258.

82. Caeser P. Exposure to violence in the families of origin among wife abusers and maritally nonviolent men. *Violence and Victims*, 1998, 3:49–63.

83. Parry C et al. Alcohol attributable fractions for trauma in South Africa. *Curationis*, 1996, 19:2–5.

84. Kyriacou DN et al. Emergency department-based study of risk factors for acute injury from domestic violence against women. *Annals of Emergency Medicine*, 1998, 31:502–506.

85. McCauley J et al. The "battering syndrome": prevalence and clinical characteristics of domestic violence in primary health care internal medicine practices. *Annals of Internal Medicine*, 1995, 123:737–746.

86. International Clinical Epidemiologists Network (INCLEN). *Domestic violence in India.* Washington, DC, International Center for Research on Women and Centre for Development and Population Activities, 2000.

87. Jewkes R et al. The prevalence of physical, sexual and emotional violence against women in three South African provinces. *South African Medical Journal*, 2001, 91:421–428.

88. Flanzer JP. Alcohol and other drugs are key causal agents of violence. In: Gelles RJ, Loseke DR, eds. *Current controversies on family violence.* Thousand Oaks, CA, Sage, 1993:171–181.

89. Gelles R. Alcohol and other drugs are associated with violence – they are not its cause. In: Gelles RJ, Loseke DR, eds. *Current controversies on family violence.* Thousand Oaks, CA, Sage, 1993:182–196.

90. MacAndrew D, Edgerton RB. *Drunken comportment: a social explanation.* Chicago, IL, Aldine, 1969.

91. Abrahams N, Jewkes R, Laubsher R. *I do not believe in democracy in the home: men's relationships with and abuse of women.* Tyberberg, Centre for Epidemiological Research in South Africa, Medical Research Council, 1999.

92. Hoffman KL, Demo DH, Edwards JN. Physical wife abuse in a non-Western society: an integrated theoretical approach. *Journal of Marriage and the Family*, 1994, 56:131–146.

93. Martin SL et al. Domestic violence in northern India. *American Journal of Epidemiology*, 1999, 150:417–426.

94. Gonzales de Olarte E, Gavilano Llosa P. Does poverty cause domestic violence? Some answers from Lima. In: Morrison AR, Biehl ML, eds. *Too close to home: domestic violence in the Americas.* Washington, DC, Inter-American Development Bank, 1999:35–49.

95. Straus M et al. Societal change and change in family violence from 1975 to 1985 as revealed by two national surveys. *Journal of Marriage and the Family*, 1986, 48:465–479.

96. Byrne CA et al. The socioeconomic impact of interpersonal violence on women. *Journal of Consulting and Clinical Psychology*, 1999, 67:362–366.

97. Golding JM. Sexual assault history and limitations in physical functioning in two general population samples. *Research in Nursing and Health*, 1996, 19:33–44.

98. Leserman J et al. Sexual and physical abuse history in gastroenterology practice: how types of abuse impact health status. *Psychosomatic Medicine*, 1996, 58:4–15.

99. Koss MP, Koss PG, Woodruff WJ. Deleterious effects of criminal victimization on women's health and medical utilization. *Archives of Internal Medicine*, 1991, 151:342–347.

100. Walker E et al. Adult health status of women HMO members with histories of childhood abuse and

neglect. *American Journal of Medicine*, 1999, 107:332–339.

101. McCauley J et al. Clinical characteristics of women with a history of childhood abuse: unhealed wounds. *Journal of the American Medical Association*, 1997, 277:1362–1368.

102. Dickinson LM et al. Health-related quality of life and symptom profiles of female survivors of sexual abuse. *Archives of Family Medicine*, 1999, 8:35–43.

103. Felitti VJ et al. Relationship of childhood abuse and household dysfunction to many of the leading causes of death in adults: the Adverse Childhood Experiences (ACE) study. *American Journal of Preventive Medicine*, 1998, 14:245–258.

104. Koss MP, Woodruff WJ, Koss PG. Criminal victimization among primary care medical patients: prevalence, incidence, and physician usage. *Behavioral Science and Law*, 1991, 9:85–96.

105. Follette V et al. Cumulative trauma: the impact of child sexual abuse, adult sexual assault, and spouse abuse. *Journal of Traumatic Stress*, 1996, 9:25–35.

106. Heise L, Moore K, Toubia N. *Sexual coercion and women's reproductive health: a focus on research.* New York, NY, Population Council, 1995.

107. Najera TP, Gutierrez M, Bailey P. *Bolivia: follow-up to the 1994 Demographic and Health Survey, and women's economic activities, fertility and contraceptive use.* Research Triangle Park, NC, Family Health International, 1998.

108. Ballard TJ et al. Violence during pregnancy: measurement issues. *American Journal of Public Health*, 1998, 88:274–276.

109. Campbell JC. Addressing battering during pregnancy: reducing low birth weight and ongoing abuse. *Seminars in Perinatology*, 1995, 19:301–306.

110. Curry MA, Perrin N, Wall E. Effects of abuse on maternal complications and birth weight in adult and adolescent women. *Obstetrics and Gynecology*, 1998, 92:530–534.

111. Gazmararian JA et al. Prevalence of violence against pregnant women. *Journal of the American Medical Association*, 1996, 275:1915–1920.

112. Newberger EH et al. Abuse of pregnant women and adverse birth outcome: current knowledge and implications for practice. *Journal of the American Medical Association*, 1992, 267:2370–2372.

113. Bullock LF, McFarlane J. The birth-weight/battering connection. *American Journal of Nursing*, 1989, 89:1153–1155.

114. Murphy C et al. Abuse: a risk factor for low birth weight? A systematic review and meta-analysis. *Canadian Medical Association Journal*, 2001, 164:1567–1572.

115. Parker B, McFarlane J, Soeken K. Abuse during pregnancy: effects on maternal complications and birth weight in adult and teenage women. *Obstetrics and Gynecology*, 1994, 84:323–328.

116. Valdez-Santiago R, Sanin-Aguirre LH. Domestic violence during pregnancy and its relationship with birth weight. *Salud Publica Mexicana*, 1996, 38:352–362.

117. Valladares E et al. *Physical abuse during pregnancy: a risk factor for low birth weight* [Dissertation]. Umeå, Department of Epidemiology and Public Health, Umeå University, 1999.

118. Ganatra BR, Coyaji KJ, Rao VN. Too far, too little, too late: a community-based case–control study of maternal mortality in rural west Maharashtra, India. *Bulletin of the World Health Organization*, 1998, 76:591–598.

119. Fauveau V et al. Causes of maternal mortality in rural Bangladesh, 1976–85. *Bulletin of the World Health Organization*, 1988, 66:643–651.

120. Dannenberg AL et al. Homicide and other injuries as causes of maternal death in New York City, 1987 through 1991. *American Journal of Obstetrics and Gynecology*, 1995, 172:1557–1564.

121. Harper M, Parsons L. Maternal deaths due to homicide and other injuries in North Carolina: 1992–1994. *Obstetrics and Gynecology*, 1997, 90:920–923.

122. Brown D. In Africa, fear makes HIV an inheritance. *Washington Post*, 30 June 1998, Section A:28.

123. Quigley M et al. Case–control study of risk factors for incident HIV infection in rural Uganda. *Journal of Acquired Immune Deficiency Syndrome*, 2000, 5:418–425.

124. Romkens R. Prevalence of wife abuse in the Netherlands: combining quantitative and qualitative methods in survey research. *Journal of Interpersonal Violence*, 1997, 12:99–125.

125. Walker EA et al. Psychosocial factors in fibromyalgia compared with rheumatoid arthritis: II. Sexual, physical, and emotional abuse and neglect. *Psychosomatic Medicine*, 1997, 59:572–577.

126. Walker EA et al. Histories of sexual victimization in patients with irritable bowel syndrome or inflammatory bowel disease. *American Journal of Psychiatry*, 1993, 150:1502–1506.

127. Delvaux M, Denis P, Allemand H. Sexual abuse is more frequently reported by IBS patients than by patients with organic digestive diseases or controls: results of a multicentre inquiry. *European Journal of Gastroenterology and Hepatology*, 1997, 9:345–352.

128. Sutherland C, Bybee D, Sullivan C. The long-term effects of battering on women's health. *Women's Health*, 1998, 4:41–70.

129. Roberts GL et al. How does domestic violence affect women's mental health? *Women's Health*, 1998, 28:117–129.

130. Ellsberg M et al. Domestic violence and emotional distress among Nicaraguan women. *American Psychologist*, 1999, 54:30–36.

131. Fikree FF, Bhatti LI. Domestic violence and health of Pakistani women. *International Journal of Gynaecology and Obstetrics*, 1999, 65:195–201.

132. Danielson KK et al. Comorbidity between abuse of an adult and DSM-III-R mental disorders: evidence from an epidemiological study. *American Journal of Psychiatry*, 1998, 155:131–133.

133. Bergman B et al. Suicide attempts by battered wives. *Acta Psychiatrica Scandinavica*, 1991, 83:380–384.

134. Kaslow NJ et al. Factors that mediate and moderate the link between partner abuse and suicidal behavior in African-American women. *Journal of Consulting and Clinical Psychology*, 1998, 66:533–540.

135. Abbott J et al. Domestic violence against women: incidence and prevalence in an emergency department population. *Journal of the American Medical Association*, 1995, 273:1763–1767.

136. Amaro H et al. Violence during pregnancy and substance use. *American Journal of Public Health*, 1990, 80:575–579.

137. Felitti VJ. Long-term medical consequences of incest, rape, and molestation. *Southern Medical Journal*, 1991, 84:328–331.

138. Koss M. The impact of crime victimization on women's medical use. *Journal of Women's Health*, 1993, 2:67–72.

139. Morrison AR, Orlando MB. Social and economic costs of domestic violence: Chile and Nicaragua. In: Morrison AR, Biehl ML, eds. *Too close to home: domestic violence in the Americas*. Washington, DC, Inter-American Development Bank, 1999:51–80.

140. Sansone RA, Wiederman MW, Sansone LA. Health care utilization and history of trauma among women in a primary care setting. *Violence and Victims*, 1997, 12:165–172.

141. IndiaSAFE Steering Committee. *IndiaSAFE final report*. Washington, DC, International Center for Research on Women, 1999.

142. Browne A, Salomon A, Bassuk SS. The impact of recent partner violence on poor women's capacity to maintain work. *Violence Against Women*, 1999, 5:393–426.

143. Lloyd S, Taluc N. The effects of male violence on female employment. *Violence Against Women*, 1999, 5:370–392.

144. McCloskey LA, Figueredo AJ, Koss MP. The effects of systemic family violence on children's mental health. *Child Development*, 1995, 66:1239–1261.

145. Edleson JL. Children's witnessing of adult domestic violence. *Journal of Interpersonal Violence*, 1999, 14:839–870.

146. Jouriles EN, Murphy CM, O'Leary KD. Interspousal aggression, marital discord, and child problems. *Journal of Consulting and Clinical Psychology*, 1989, 57:453–455.

147. Jaffe PG, Wolfe DA, Wilson SK. *Children of battered women*. Thousand Oaks, CA, Sage, 1990.

148. Jejeebhoy SJ. Associations between wife-beating and fetal and infant death: impressions from a survey in rural India. *Studies in Family Planning*, 1998, 29:300–308.

149. Åsling-Monemi K et al. Violence against women increases the risk of infant and child mortality: a case-referent study in Nicaragua. *Bulletin of the World Health Organization*, in press.

150. Chalk R, King PA. *Violence in families: assessing prevention and treatment programs*. Washington, DC, National Academy Press, 1998.

151. Spindel C, Levy E, Connor M. *With an end in sight: strategies from the UNIFEM trust fund to eliminate violence against women*. New York, NY, United Nations Development Fund for Women, 2000.

152. Plichta SB. Identifying characteristics of programs for battered women. In: Leinman JM et al., eds. *Addressing domestic violence and its consequences: a policy report of the Commonwealth Fund Commission on Women's Health*. New York, NY, The Commonwealth Fund, 1998:45.

153. Ramos-Jimenez P. *Philippine strategies to combat domestic violence against women*. Manila, Task Force on Social Science and Reproductive Health, Social Development Research Center, and De La Salle University, 1996.

154. Mehrotra A. *Gender and legislation in Latin America and the Caribbean*. New York, United Nations Development Programme Regional Bureau for Latin America and the Caribbean, 1998.

155. Mitra N. *Best practices among response to domestic violence: a study of government and non-government response in Madhya Pradesh and Maharashtra [draft]*. Washington, DC, International Center for Research on Women, 1998.

156. Sherman LW, Berk RA. The specific deterrent effects of arrest for domestic assault. *American Sociological Review*, 1984, 49:261–272.

157. Garner J, Fagan J, Maxwell C. Published findings from the spouse assault replication program: a critical review. *Journal of Quantitative Criminology*, 1995, 11:3–28.

158. Fagan J, Browne A. Violence between spouses and intimates: physical aggression between women and men in intimate relationships. In: Reiss AJ, Roth JA, eds. *Understanding and preventing violence: panel on the understanding and control of violent behavior. Vol. 3. Social influences.* Washington, DC, National Academy Press, 1994:115–292.

159. Marciniak E. *Community policing of domestic violence: neighborhood differences in the effect of arrest.* College Park, MD, University of Maryland, 1994.

160. Sherman LW. The influence of criminology on criminal law: evaluating arrests for misdemeanor domestic violence. *Journal of Criminal Law and Criminology*, 1992, 83:1–45.

161. National Institute of Justice and American Bar Association. *Legal interventions in family violence: research findings and policy implications.* Washington, DC, United States Department of Justice, 1998.

162. Grau J, Fagan J, Wexler S. Restraining orders for battered women: issues of access and efficacy. *Women and Politics*, 1984, 4:13–28.

163. Harrell A, Smith B. Effects of restraining orders on domestic violence victims. In: Buzawa ES, Buzawa CG, eds. *Do arrests and restraining orders work?* Thousand Oaks, CA, Sage, 1996.

164. Buzawa ES, Buzawa CG. *Domestic violence: the criminal justice response.* Thousand Oaks, CA, Sage, 1990.

165. Keilitz S et al. *Civil protection orders: victims' views on effectiveness.* Washington, DC, National Institute of Justice, 1998.

166. Littel K et al. *Assessing the justice system response to violence against women: a tool for communities to develop coordinated responses.* Pennsylvania, Pennsylvania Coalition Against Domestic Violence, 1998 (available on the Internet at http://www.vaw.umn.edu/Promise/PP3.htm).

167. Larrain S. Curbing domestic violence: two decades of activism. In: Morrison AR, Biehl ML, eds. *Too close to home: domestic violence in the Americas.* Washington, DC, Inter-American Development Bank, 1999:105–130.

168. Poonacha V, Pandey D. Response to domestic violence in Karnataka and Gujarat. In: Duvvury N, ed. *Domestic violence in India.* Washington, DC, International Center for Research on Women, 1999:28–41.

169. Estremadoyro J. *Violencia en la pareja: comisarías de mujeres en el Perú. [Violence in couples: police stations for women in Peru.]* Lima, Ediciones Flora Tristan, 1993.

170. Hautzinger S. *Machos and policewomen, battered women and anti-victims: combatting violence against women in Brazil.* Baltimore, MD, Johns Hopkins University, 1998.

171. Mesquita da Rocha M. Dealing with crimes against women in Brazil. In: Morrison AR, Biehl L, eds. *Too close to home: domestic violence in the Americas.* Washington, DC, Inter-American Development Bank, 1999:151–154.

172. Thomas DQ. In search of solutions: women's police stations in Brazil. In: Davies M, ed. *Women and violence: realities and responses worldwide.* London, Zed Books, 1994:32–43.

173. Corsi J. Treatment for men who batter women in Latin America. *American Psychologist*, 1999, 54:64.

174. Cervantes Islas F. Helping men overcome violent behavior toward women. In: Morrison AR, Biehl ML, eds. *Too close to home: domestic violence in the Americas.* Washington, DC, Inter-American Development Bank, 1999:143–147.

175. Axelson BL. Violence against women: a male issue. *Choices*, 1997, 26:9–14.

176. Edleson JL. Intervention for men who batter: a review of research. In: Stith SR, Staus MA, eds. *Understanding partner violence: prevalence, causes, consequences and solutions.* Minneapolis, MN, National Council on Family Relations, 1995:262–273.

177. Gondolf E. *A 30-month follow-up of court-mandated batterers in four cities.* Indiana, PA, Mid-Atlantic Addiction Training Institute, Indiana University of Pennsylvania, 1999 (available on the Internet at http://www.iup.edu/maati/publications/30MonthFollowup.shtm).

178. Gondolf EW. Batterer programs: what we know and need to know. *Journal of Interpersonal Violence*, 1997, 12:83–98.

179. Mullender A, Burton S. *Reducing domestic violence: what works? Perpetrator programmes.* London, Policing and Crime Reduction Unit, Home Office, 2000.

180. Sugg NK et al. Domestic violence and primary care: attitudes, practices, and beliefs. *Archives of Family Medicine*, 1999, 8:301–306.

181. Caralis PV, Musialowski R. Women's experiences with domestic violence and their attitudes and expectations regarding medical care of abuse victims. *Southern Medical Journal*, 1997, 90:1075–1080.

182. Friedman LS et al. Inquiry about victimization experiences: a survey of patient preferences and physician practices. *Archives of Internal Medicine*, 1992, 152:1186–1190.

183. *Ruta crítica que siguen las mujeres víctimas de violencia intrafamiliar: análisis y resultados de investigación. [Help-seeking by victims of family violence: analysis and research results.]* Panama City, Pan American Health Organization, 1998.

184. Cohen S, De Vos E, Newberger E. Barriers to physician identification and treatment of family violence: lessons from five communities. *Academic Medicine*, 1997, 72(1 Suppl.):S19–S25.

185. Fawcett G et al. *Detección y manejo de mujeres víctimas de violencia doméstica: desarrollo y evaluación de un programa dirigido al personal de salud. [Detecting and dealing with women victims of domestic violence: the development and evaluation of a programme for health workers.]* Mexico City, Population Council, 1998.

186. Watts C, Ndlovu M. Addressing violence in Zimbabwe: strengthening the health sector response. In: *Violence against women in Zimbabwe: strategies for action.* Harare, Musasa Project, 1997:31–35.

187. d'Oliviera AFL, Schraiber L. Violence against women: a physician's concern? In: *Fifteenth FIGO World Congress of Gynaecology and Obstetrics, Copenhagen, Denmark, 3–8 August 1997.* London, International Federation of Gynaecology and Obstetrics, 1997:157–163.

188. Leye E, Githaniga A, Temmerman M. *Health care strategies for combating violence against women in developing countries.* Ghent, International Centre for Reproductive Health, 1999.

189. *Como atender a las mujeres que viven situationes de violencia doméstica? Orientaciones básicas para el personal de salud. [Care of women living with domestic violence: orientation for health care personnel.]* Managua, Red de Mujeres Contra la Violencia, 1999.

190. *Achievements of project "Toward a comprehensive model approach to domestic violence: expansion and consolidation of interventions coordinated by the state and civil society".* Washington, DC, Pan American Health Organization, 1999.

191. Olson L et al. Increasing emergency physician recognition of domestic violence. *Annals of Emergency Medicine*, 1996, 27:741–746.

192. Freund KM, Bak SM, Blackhall L. Identifying domestic violence in primary care practice. *Journal of General Internal Medicine*, 1996, 11:44–46.

193. Kim J. Health sector initiatives to address domestic violence against women in Africa. In: *Health care strategies for combating violence against women in developing countries.* Ghent, International Centre for Reproductive Health, 1999:101–107.

194. Davison L et al. *Reducing domestic violence: what works? Health services.* London, Policing and Crime Reduction Unit, Home Office, 2000.

195. Kelly L, Humphreys C. *Reducing domestic violence: what works? Outreach and advocacy approaches.* London, Policing and Crime Reduction Unit, Home Office, 2000.

196. Gamache DJ, Edleson JS, Schock MD. Coordinated police, judicial, and social service response to woman battering: a multiple baseline evaluation across three communities. In: Hotaling GT et al., eds. *Coping with family violence: research and policy perspectives.* Thousand Oaks, CA, Sage, 1988:193–209.

197. Hague G. *Reducing domestic violence: what works? Multi-agency fora.* London, Policing and Crime Reduction Unit, Home Office, 2000.

198. Ellsberg M, Liljestrand J, Winkvist A. The Nicaraguan Network of Women Against Violence: using research and action for change. *Reproductive Health Matters*, 1997, 10:82–92.

199. Mehrotra A et al. *A life free of violence: it's our right.* New York, NY, United Nations Development Fund for Women, 2000.

200. Jaffe PG et al. An evaluation of a secondary school primary prevention program on violence in intimate relationships. *Violence and Victims*, 1992, 7:129–146.

201. Foshee VA et al. The Safe Dates program: one-year follow-up results. *American Journal of Public Health*, 2000, 90:1619–1622.

202. Krajewski SS et al. Results of a curriculum intervention with seventh graders regarding violence in relationships. *Journal of Family Violence*, 1996, 11:93–112.

203. Lavoie F et al. Evaluation of a prevention program for violence in teen dating relationships. *Journal of Interpersonal Violence*, 1995, 10:516–524.

204. Heise L. Violence against women: global organizing for change. In: Edleson JL, Eisikovits ZC, eds. *Future interventions with battered women and their families.* Thousand Oaks, CA, Sage, 1996:7–33.

205. *Domestic violence in India.* Washington, DC, International Center for Research on Women, 1999.

206. American College of Obstetricians and Gynecologists. ACOG committee opinion: mandatory reporting of domestic violence. *International Journal of Gynecology and Obstetrics*, 1998, 62:93–95.

207. Hyman A, Schillinger D, Lo B. Laws mandating reporting of domestic violence: do they promote

patient well-being? *Journal of the American Medical Association*, 1995, 273:1781–1787.

208. Jezierski MB, Eickholt T, McGee J. Disadvantages to mandatory reporting of domestic violence. *Journal of Emergency Nursing*, 1999, 25:79–80.

209. Bradley J et al. *Whole-site training: a new approach to the organization of training*. New York, NY, AVSC International, 1998.

210. Cole TB. Case management for domestic violence. *Journal of the American Medical Association*, 1999, 282:513–514.

211. McLeer SV et al. Education is not enough: a systems failure in protecting battered women. *Annals of Emergency Medicine*, 1989, 18:651–653.

212. Tilden VP, Shepherd P. Increasing the rate of identification of battered women in an emergency department: use of a nursing protocol. *Research in Nursing Health*, 1987, 10:209–215.

213. Harwell TS et al. Results of a domestic violence training program offered to the staff of urban community health centers. *American Journal of Preventive Medicine*, 1998, 15:235–242.

214. Kelly L. Tensions and possibilities: enhancing informal responses to domestic violence. In: Edelson JL, Eisidovits ZC, eds. *Future interventions with battered women and their families*. Thousand Oaks, CA, Sage, 1996:67–86.

215. Fawcett GM et al. Changing community responses to wife abuse: a research and demonstration project in Iztacalco, Mexico. *American Psychologist*, 1999, 54:41–49.

216. Carter J. *Domestic violence, child abuse, and youth violence: strategies for prevention and early intervention*. San Francisco, CA, Family Violence Prevention Fund, 2000.

CHAPTER 5

Abuse of the elderly

Background

The abuse of older people by family members dates back to ancient times. Until the advent of initiatives to address child abuse and domestic violence in the last quarter of the 20th century, it remained a private matter, hidden from public view. Initially seen as a social welfare issue and subsequently a problem of ageing, abuse of the elderly, like other forms of family violence, has developed into a public health and criminal justice concern. These two fields – public health and criminal justice – have therefore dictated to a large extent how abuse of the elderly is viewed, how it is analysed, and how it is dealt with. This chapter focuses on abuse of older people by family members or others known to them, either in their homes or in residential or other institutional settings. It does not cover other types of violence that may be directed at older people, such as violence by strangers, street crime, gang warfare or military conflict.

Mistreatment of older people – referred to as "elder abuse" – was first described in British scientific journals in 1975 under the term "granny battering" (*1, 2*). As a social and political issue, though, it was the United States Congress that first seized on the problem, followed later by researchers and practitioners. During the 1980s scientific research and government actions were reported from Australia, Canada, China (Hong Kong SAR), Norway, Sweden and the United States, and in the following decade from Argentina, Brazil, Chile, India, Israel, Japan, South Africa, the United Kingdom and other European countries. Although elder abuse was first identified in developed countries, where most of the existing research has been conducted, anecdotal evidence and other reports from some developing countries have shown that it is a universal phenomenon. That elder abuse is being taken far more seriously now reflects the growing worldwide concern about human rights and gender equality, as well as about domestic violence and population ageing.

Where "older age" begins is not precisely defined, which makes comparisons between studies and between countries difficult. In Western societies, the onset of older age is usually considered to coincide with the age of retirement, at 60 or 65 years of age. In most developing countries, however, this socially constructed concept based on retirement age has little significance. Of more significance in these countries are the roles assigned to people in their lifetime. Old age is thus regarded as that time of life when people, because of physical decline, can no longer carry out their family or work roles.

Concern over the mistreatment of older people has been heightened by the realization that in the coming decades, in both developed and developing countries, there will be a dramatic increase in the population in the older age segment – what in French is termed *"le troisième âge"* (the third age). It is predicted that by the year 2025, the global population of those aged 60 years and older will more than double, from 542 million in 1995 to about 1.2 billion (see Figure 5.1). The total number of older people living in developing countries will also more than double by 2025, reaching 850 million (*3*) – 12% of the overall population of the developing world – though in some countries, including Colombia, Indonesia, Kenya and Thailand, the increase is expected to be more than fourfold. Throughout the world, 1 million people

FIGURE 5.1

Projected growth in the global population aged 60 years and older, 1995–2025

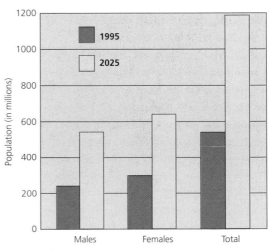

Source: United Nations Population Division, 2002.

reach the age of 60 years every month, 80% of whom are in the developing world.

Women outlive men in nearly all countries of the world, rich and poor (3). This gender gap is, however, considerably narrower in developing countries, mainly because of higher rates of maternal mortality and, in recent years, also because of the AIDS epidemic.

These demographic changes are taking place in developing countries alongside increasing mobility and changing family structures. Industrialization is eroding long-standing patterns of interdependence between the generations of a family, often resulting in material and emotional hardship for the elderly. The family and community networks in many developing countries that had formerly provided support to the older generation have been weakened, and often destroyed, by rapid social and economic change. The AIDS pandemic is also significantly affecting the lives of older people. In many parts of sub-Saharan Africa, for instance, children are being orphaned in large numbers as their parents die from the disease. Older people who had anticipated support from their children in old age are finding themselves to be the main caregivers and without a family to help them in the future.

Only 30% of the world's elderly are covered by pension schemes. In Eastern Europe and the countries of the former Soviet Union, for instance, as a result of the changes from planned to market economies, many older people have been left without a retirement income and the health and welfare services that were provided by the former communist regimes. In the economies of both developed and developing countries, structural inequalities have often been the cause among the general population of low wages, high unemployment, poor health services, lack of educational opportunities and discrimination against women — all of which have tended to make the elderly poorer and more vulnerable.

Older people in developing countries still face a significant risk from communicable diseases. As life expectancy increases in these countries, the elderly will be subject to the same long-term, largely incurable and often disabling diseases associated with old age that are currently most prevalent in developed countries. They will also face environmental dangers and the likelihood of violence in their societies. Nevertheless, advances in medical science and in social welfare will ensure that many older people will enjoy longer periods of disability-free old age. Diseases will be avoided or their impact lessened through better health care strategies. The resulting large number of older people will be a boon for society, constituting a great reservoir of experience and knowledge.

How is elder abuse defined?

It is generally agreed that abuse of older people is either an act of commission or of omission (in which case it is usually described as "neglect"), and that it may be either intentional or unintentional. The abuse may be of a physical nature, it may be psychological (involving emotional or verbal aggression), or it may involve financial or other material maltreatment. Regardless of the type of abuse, it will certainly result in unnecessary suffering, injury or pain, the loss or violation of human rights, and a decreased quality of life for the older person (4). Whether the behaviour is termed abusive, neglectful or exploitative will probably depend on how frequently the mistreatment occurs, its duration, severity and consequences, and above all, the cultural context. Among the Navajo people in the United States, for instance, what had appeared to an outside researcher to be economic exploitation by family members was regarded instead by the tribal elders concerned as their cultural duty, and indeed privilege, to share material belongings with their families (5). Other Indian tribes in the United States viewed elder abuse as a community problem rather than an individual one (6).

The definition developed by Action on Elder Abuse in the United Kingdom (7) and adopted by the International Network for the Prevention of Elder Abuse states that: "Elder abuse is a single or repeated act, or lack of appropriate action, occurring within any relationship where there is an expectation of trust which causes harm or distress to an older person.'' Such abuse is generally divided into the following categories:

- Physical abuse – the infliction of pain or injury, physical coercion, or physical or drug-induced restraint.
- Psychological or emotional abuse – the infliction of mental anguish.
- Financial or material abuse – the illegal or improper exploitation or use of funds or resources of the older person.
- Sexual abuse – non-consensual sexual contact of any kind with the older person.
- Neglect – the refusal or failure to fulfil a caregiving obligation. This may or may not involve a conscious and intentional attempt to inflict physical or emotional distress on the older person.

This definition of elder abuse has been heavily influenced by the work done in Canada, the United Kingdom and the United States. Studies conducted in China (Hong Kong SAR), Finland, Greece, India, Ireland, Israel, Norway, Poland and South Africa have approached the topic in distinctly different ways (8). Norwegian researchers, for instance, identified abuse with a ''triangle of violence'' that includes a victim, a perpetrator and others, who – directly or indirectly – observe the principal players. In countries such as China, that emphasize harmony and respect within society, neglecting the care of an older person is considered an act of elder abuse. If family members fail to fulfil their kinship obligations to provide food and housing, this also constitutes neglect.

Traditional societies

Many traditional societies of the past considered family harmony to be an important factor governing family relationships. This reverence for the family was reinforced by philosophical traditions and public policy. In Chinese society, it was embedded in a value system that stressed ''filial piety''. Mistreatment of older people was unrecognized and certainly unreported. These traditions are still influential today. Studies in the United States of attitudes towards elder abuse revealed that citizens of Korean origin believed in the primacy of family harmony over individual well-being as a yardstick for determining whether a particular behaviour was regarded as abusive or not (9). Similarly, people of Japanese origin considered the ''group'' to be paramount, and that an individual's well-being should be sacrificed for the good of the group (10).

Displacing older people as heads of households and depriving them of their autonomy in the name of affection are cultural norms even in countries where the family is the central institution and the sense of filial obligation is strong (11). Such infantilization and overprotection can leave the older person isolated, depressed and demoralized, and can be considered a form of abuse. In some traditional societies, older widows are abandoned and their property seized. Mourning rites of passage for widows in parts of Africa and India include practices that elsewhere would certainly be considered cruel, for example sexual violence, forced levirate marriages (where a man is obliged by custom to marry the childless widow of his brother) and expulsion from their homes (12). In some places, accusations of witchcraft, often connected with unexplained events in the local community, such as a death or crop failure, are directed at isolated, older women (13). In sub-Saharan Africa, accusations of the practice of witchcraft have driven many older women from their homes and their communities to live in poverty in urban areas. In the United Republic of Tanzania, an estimated 500 older women accused of witchcraft are murdered every year (14). These acts of violence have become firmly entrenched as social customs and may not be considered locally as ''elder abuse'' (see Box 5.1).

A workshop on elder abuse held in South Africa in 1992 drew a distinction between *mistreatment* (such as verbal abuse, passive and active neglect, financial exploitation and overmedication) and *abuse* (including physical, psychological and sexual violence, and theft) (8). Since then, focus groups have been held with older people recruited from three historically ''black'' townships in South Africa to determine the level of knowledge and understanding of elder abuse within these communities. In addition to the typical Western schema that comprises physical, verbal, financial and sexual abuse, and neglect, the participants wished to add to the definition:

— loss of respect for elders, which was equated with neglect;
— accusations of witchcraft;

— abuse by systems (mistreatment at health clinics and by bureaucratic bodies).

The focus groups produced the following definitions (*15*):

• Physical abuse – beating and physical manhandling.

BOX 5.1

Witchcraft: the threat of violence in the United Republic of Tanzania

In the United Republic of Tanzania, some 500 older women are murdered each year following accusations against them of witchcraft. The problem is particularly serious in Sukumaland in the north of the country. Large numbers of older women are driven from their homes and communities in fear of being accused of witchcraft, and end up living destitute in urban areas.

Belief in witchcraft has existed in Sukumaland for centuries, though the violence surrounding it has increased sharply in recent years. This may in part be due to increased poverty caused by too many people living off too little land, as well as an overall lack of education. As poor and uneducated people try to explain the misfortunes that befall them — illness and death, crop failures and dried-up wells — they search for a scapegoat, and witchcraft appears to explain events they cannot otherwise understand or control.

Men are sometimes accused of witchcraft, though the low status of women in society means that women are overwhelmingly the main target. Among some of the particular ways in this region in which women are accused of witchcraft are the following:

■ *Land disputes* are a common underlying cause of violence against widows. According to inheritance laws, widows may continue to live on their husbands' land, without owning the property. When they die, the land becomes the property of their husbands' sons. Accusations of witchcraft are thus used to get rid of widows living on the land as tenants, and blocking the inheritance of others.

■ *Traditional healers* are frequently urged by family members or neighbours to make accusations of witchcraft against women. One young boy killed his mother after a traditional healer told him that she was the cause of his problems.

■ *Myths* about the physical appearance of witches — that they have red eyes, for instance — also often give rise to accusations of witchcraft. The eyes of many older women are red from a lifetime of cooking over smoky stoves, or from medical conditions such as conjunctivitis.

Community leaders in Sukumaland are calling for a strong lead from the Government. One was quoted as saying: "It is a question of educating the people. In other areas of the country where people are better educated, we don't face this problem."

Until recently, the Government was reluctant to acknowledge that belief in witchcraft still existed. Now the subject is being widely discussed and officially condemned. In 1999, the Tanzanian Government made witchcraft the theme for International Women's Day.

A local nongovernmental organization and HelpAge International are also taking measures to improve the security of older women in the United Republic of Tanzania. They aim to change attitudes and beliefs surrounding witchcraft and to address some of the practical matters, such as poverty and poor housing, that have helped to keep such beliefs alive.

Source: reproduced from reference *14* with the permission of the publisher.

- Emotional and verbal abuse – discrimination on the basis of age, insults and hurtful words, denigration, intimidation, false accusations, psychological pain and distress.
- Financial abuse – extortion and control of pension money, theft of property, and exploitation of older people to force them to care for grandchildren.
- Sexual abuse – incest, rape and other types of sexual coercion.
- Neglect – loss of respect for elders, withholding of affection, and lack of interest in the older person's well-being.
- Accusations of witchcraft – stigmatization and ostracization.
- Abuse by systems – the dehumanizing treatment older people are liable to suffer at health clinics and pension offices, and marginalization by the government.

These definitions, produced by the participants and classified by the researchers, were the result of an initial effort in South Africa to obtain information on elder abuse directly from older people. They are also the first attempt to classify elder abuse in a developing country, building on the Western model but bringing in factors that are relevant to the indigenous population.

The extent of the problem
Domestic settings

With most developing nations only recently becoming aware of the problem, information on the frequency of elder abuse has relied on five surveys conducted in the past decade in five developed countries (*16–20*). The results show a rate of abuse of 4–6% among older people if physical, psychological and financial abuse, and neglect are all included. One difficulty in making comparisons between studies is the variation in their time frames. The studies conducted in Canada, the Netherlands and the United States refer to the "preceding year". The study in Finland investigated abuse since the "age of retirement", while the study in Great Britain examined cases from "the past few years". The first set of studies (from

Canada, the Netherlands and the United States) found no significant difference in prevalence rates of abuse by age or by sex, the study in Finland found a higher proportion of female victims (7.0%) than male victims (2.5%), while no breakdown by age or sex was given in the British study. Because of the differences in the methodology used in the five surveys and the relatively small numbers of victims, further comparative analysis is not justified.

A recent survey of family violence in Canada found that 7% of older people had experienced some form of emotional abuse, 1% financial abuse, and 1% physical abuse or sexual assault, at the hands of children, caregivers or partners during the previous 5 years (*21*). Men (9%) were more likely than women (6%) to report suffering emotional or financial abuse. Because of differences in the survey questions and time frame, these findings cannot be compared with the earlier study in Canada which had found a much smaller proportion of emotional abuse (1.4%) and a larger rate of financial abuse (2.5%) (*17*).

Institutional settings

A quarter of a century ago, the proportion of older people living in institutions in developed countries had reached an estimated 9% (*22*). Since that time, there has been a shift in emphasis towards care in the community and the use of less restrictive residential settings. Current rates of use of nursing homes are in the range of 4–7% in countries such as Canada (6.8%), Israel (4.4%), South Africa (4.5%) and the United States (4%). In most African countries, older people can be found in long-stay hospital wards, homes for the destitute and disabled, and – in some sub-Saharan countries – in witches' camps. Social, economic and cultural changes taking place in some of the developing societies will leave families less able to care for their frail relatives and thus portend an increasing demand for institutional care. In China, the expectation of institutional care for older people is becoming the norm. In Taiwan, China, institutional care has rapidly overtaken family care for the elderly (AY Kwan, unpublished data, 2000).

In Latin America, the rates of institutionalization of older people range from 1% to 4%. Institutional care is no longer considered unacceptable for an older person but is seen as an alternative for families. The government-sponsored *asilos*, large institutions resembling the early English work-houses, have been converted into smaller facilities with professional staff from many disciplines. Other homes are operated by religious communities of immigrant origin. Figures for rates of institutionalization are not available in the countries of the former Eastern European bloc, because the authorities at the time did not allow publication of such information.

Despite the fact that a vast literature exists on the quality of care in institutional settings, and that cases of elder abuse have been well documented in reports of governmental inquiries, ethnographic studies and personal histories, there are no national data on the prevalence or incidence of abuse available, but only local data from smaller-scale studies. A survey of nursing-home personnel in one state of the United States disclosed that 36% of the nursing and general staff reported having witnessed at least one incident of physical abuse by other staff members in the preceding year, while 10% admitted having committed at least one act of physical abuse themselves. At least one incident of psychological abuse against a resident had been observed by 81% of the sample in the preceding year, and 40% admitted to having also committed such an act (*23*). The findings suggest that mistreatment of older residents in institutions may be even more extensive than generally believed.

The likely rates of elder abuse both in the community and in institutional settings may be greater than the general statistics collected by countries on violent acts would indicate. Some of the disparity stems from the fact that elder abuse had gone unrecognized until the 1970s. Deaths of older people, both in institutional settings and the community, have often been attributed to natural, accidental or undetermined causes when in fact they were the consequences of abusive or neglectful behaviour.

What are the risk factors for elder abuse?

Most of the early work on abuse of the elderly was limited to domestic settings and carried out in developed countries. In seeking explanations for elder abuse, researchers drew from the literature in the fields of psychology, sociology, gerontology and the study of family violence. To accommodate the complexity of elder abuse and the many factors associated with it, researchers have turned to the ecological model, which was first applied to the study of child abuse and neglect (*24*) and has been applied more recently to elder abuse (*25, 26*). The ecological model can take into account the interactions that take place across a number of systems. As described in Chapter 1, the model consists of a nested hierarchy of four levels of the environment: individual, relationship, community and society.

Individual factors

Early researchers in the field played down individual personality disturbances as causal agents of family violence in favour of social and cultural factors (*27*). More recently, though, research on family violence has shown that abusers who are physically aggressive are more likely to have personality disorders and alcohol-related problems than the general population (*28*). Similarly, studies restricted to violence against older people in domestic settings have found that aggressors are more likely to have mental health and substance abuse problems than family members or caregivers who are not violent or otherwise abusive (*29–31*).

Cognitive and physical impairments of the abused older person were strongly identified in the early studies as risk factors for abuse. However, a later study of a range of cases from a social service agency revealed that the older people who had been mistreated were not more debilitated than their non-abused peers and may even have been less so, particularly in cases of physical and verbal abuse (*32*). In other studies, a comparison of samples of patients with Alzheimer disease showed that the degree of impairment was not a risk factor for being abused (*33, 34*). However, among cases of abuse reported to the authorities, those involving the very old and the most impaired generally constitute a large proportion.

Gender has been proposed by some as a defining factor in elder abuse on the grounds that older women may have been subject to oppression and economically disadvantaged all of their lives (*35*). However, according to community-based prevalence studies, it appears that older men are at risk of abuse by spouses, adult children and other relatives in about the same proportions as women (*16, 17*).

Although the income of the older person was not a significant factor in a study of the prevalence of elder abuse in the United States, financial difficulties on the part of the abuser did appear to be an important risk factor. Sometimes this was related to an adult child's substance abuse problem, leading him or her to extort money, possibly a pension cheque, from the older person. Resentment by family members at having to spend money on the care of the older person may also have played a part in abuse of this nature.

Relationship factors

In the early theoretical models, the level of stress of caregivers was seen as a risk factor that linked elder abuse with care of an elderly relative (*36, 37*). While the popular image of abuse depicts a dependent victim and an overstressed caregiver, there is growing evidence that neither of these factors properly accounts for cases of abuse. Although researchers do not deny the component of stress, they tend now to look at it in a wider context in which the quality of the overall relationship is a causal factor (*30, 34, 38*). Some of the studies involving caregiver stress, Alzheimer disease and elder abuse suggest that the nature of the relationship between the caregiver and the care recipient before abuse begins may be an important predictor of abuse (*34, 39, 40*). Today, therefore, the belief is that stress may be a contributing factor in cases of abuse but does not by itself account for the phenomenon.

Work with patients with dementia has shown that violent acts carried out by a care recipient can act as "triggers" for reciprocal violence by the caregiver (*41*). It may be that the violence is a result of the interplay of several factors, including stress, the relationship between the carer and the care recipient, the existence of disruptive behaviour and aggression by the care recipient, and depression in the caregiver (*42*).

Living arrangements, particularly overcrowded conditions and a lack of privacy, have been associated with conflict within families. Although abuse can occur when the abuser and the older person suffering abuse live apart, the older person is more at risk when living with the caregiver.

The early theories on the subject also sought to associate dependency with increased risk of abuse. At first the emphasis focused on the dependency of the victim on the caregiver or abuser, though later case work identified abusers who were dependent on the older person – usually adult children dependent on elderly parents for housing and financial assistance (*32*). In some of these cases a "web of interdependency" was evident – a strong emotional attachment between the abused and abuser that often hindered efforts at intervention.

Community and societal factors

In almost all studies of risk factors, the community factor of social isolation emerges as a significant one in elder mistreatment (*17, 29, 43, 44*). As with battered women, isolation of older people can be both a cause and a consequence of abuse. Many older people are isolated because of physical or mental infirmities. Furthermore, loss of friends and family members reduces the opportunities for social interaction.

Although there is as yet little solid empirical evidence, societal factors are currently considered important as risk factors for elder abuse in both developing and industrialized countries; in the past the emphasis was generally on individual or interpersonal attributes as potential causal factors for elder abuse. Cultural norms and traditions – such as ageism, sexism and a culture of violence – are also now recognized as playing an important underlying role. Older people are often depicted as being frail, weak and dependent, something that has made them appear less worthy of government investment or even of family care than other groups, and has presented them as ready targets for exploitation.

As regards sub-Saharan Africa in particular, societal and community factors include (*12*):

— the systems of patrilineal and matrilineal inheritance and land rights, affecting the distribution of power;
— the way societies view the role of women;
— the erosion of the close bonds between generations of a family, caused by rural–urban migration and the growth in formal education;
— the loss, through modernization, of the traditional domestic, ritual and family arbitration roles of older people.

According to the focus group study in South Africa mentioned earlier, much of the abuse – and particularly domestic violence – occurred as a result of social disorder, exacerbated by crime, alcohol and drugs. Similar conclusions came from an exercise conducted by seven male community leaders of the Tamaho squatter camp in Katlehong, South Africa (*15*). Drawing a link between poverty and violence, they described how dysfunctional family life, a lack of money for essentials, and a lack of education and job opportunities have all contributed to a life of crime, drug peddling and prostitution by young people. In this society, older people are viewed as targets for abuse and exploitation, their vulnerability being a result of poverty distinguished by a lack of pension support and job opportunities, poor hygiene, disease and malnutrition.

The political transformations within post-communist Eastern Europe have also produced conditions heightening the risk of elder abuse. The factors suggested there as having affected the overall health and psychosocial well-being of people, particularly the elderly, whose vulnerability to mistreatment has thereby increased, include:

— the growing pauperization of significant parts of society;
— high unemployment;
— a lack of stability and social security;

— the outward expression of aggressiveness, especially among the young.

In Chinese societies several reasons have been suggested (*45*) for the mistreatment of older people, including:

— a lack of respect by the younger generation;
— tension between traditional and new family structures;
— restructuring of the basic support networks for the elderly;
— migration of young couples to new towns, leaving elderly parents in deteriorating residential areas within town centres.

Studies on elder abuse have tended to focus on interpersonal and family problems. However, an integrated model encompassing individual, interpersonal, community and societal perspectives is more appropriate, and reduces some of the bias evident in the earlier studies. Such a model takes into account the difficulties faced by older people, especially older women. These people often live in poverty, without the basic necessities of life and without family support – factors that increase their risk of abuse, neglect and exploitation.

The consequences of elder abuse

For older people, the consequences of abuse can be especially serious. Older people are physically weaker and more vulnerable than younger adults, their bones are more brittle and convalescence takes longer. Even a relatively minor injury can cause serious and permanent damage. Many older people survive on limited incomes, so that the loss of even a small sum of money can have a significant impact. They may be isolated, lonely or troubled by illness, in which case they are more vulnerable as targets for fraudulent schemes.

Domestic settings

Very few empirical studies have been conducted to determine the consequences of mistreatment, even though clinical and case study reports about the severe emotional distress experienced by mistreated older people are plentiful. There is some evidence from studies in developed countries to show that a higher proportion of abused elderly people suffer from depression or psychological distress than do their non-abused peers (*31, 46, 47*). Since these studies were cross-sectional in design, it is not possible to tell whether the condition existed before or was a consequence of the mistreatment. Other symptoms that have been proposed as being associated with cases of abuse include feelings of helplessness, alienation, guilt, shame, fear, anxiety, denial and post-traumatic stress (*48, 49*). Emotional effects were also cited by the participants in the focus group study in South Africa, along with health problems and, in the words of one participant, "illness of the heart" (*15*).

In a seminal study in New Haven, CT, United States, data from a comprehensive annual health and welfare study of a representative sample of 2812 older people were merged with the database of the local agency concerned with adult abuse for each year over a 9-year period (*50*). Information for the health survey was recorded by nurses, who saw the older people at a hospital for the first year's data collection and every third year after that. In the intervening years, data were updated by telephone. Information about abuse and neglect was obtained by case workers using existing protocols after investigating claims of mistreatment, usually by a home visit. The merged database allowed the researchers to identify those people from the sample who were confirmed during the 9-year survey as having experienced physical abuse or neglect. Mortality rates were then calculated, beginning with the first year of the survey and for 12 years thereafter, both for those who had been abused or neglected as well as for the non-abused group. When mortality rates for the two groups were compared, 13 years after the study began, 40% of the group where no abuse or neglect had been reported were still alive, compared with 9% of those who had been physically abused or neglected. After controlling for all possible factors that might affect mortality (for example, age, sex, income, functional and cognitive conditions, diagnosis and degree of social support) and finding no significant relationships in these additional factors, the researchers concluded that mistreatment causes extreme interpersonal stress that may confer an additional risk of death.

Institutions

Mistreatment of older people has been identified in facilities for continuing care (such as nursing homes, residential care, hospitals and day care facilities) in almost every country where such institutions exist. Various people may be responsible for the abuse: a paid member of the staff, another resident, a voluntary visitor, or relatives or friends. An abusive or neglectful relationship between the older person and their caregiver at home may not necessarily end once the older person has entered institutional care; the abuse may sometimes continue in a new setting.

A distinction must be made between individual acts of abuse or neglect in institutional settings and institutionalized abuse — where the prevailing regime of the institution itself is abusive or negligent. In practice, though, it is often difficult to say whether the reasons for abuse or neglect found in an institutional setting have been caused by individual acts or through institutional failings, since the two are frequently found together.

The spectrum of abuse and neglect within institutions spans a considerable range (*51*), and may be related to any of the following:

- The provision of care – for example, resistance to changes in geriatric medicine, erosion of individuality in the care, inadequate nutrition and deficient nursing care (such as lack of attention to pressure sores).
- Problems with staffing – for example, work-related stress and staff burnout, poor physical working conditions, insufficient training and psychological problems among staff.
- Difficulties in staff–resident interactions – for example, poor communication, aggressiveness on the part of residents and cultural differences.
- Environment – for example, a lack of basic privacy, dilapidated facilities, the use of restraints, inadequate sensory stimulation, and a proneness to accidents within the institution.

- Organizational policies – for example, those that operate for the benefit of the institution, giving residents few choices over daily living; bureaucratic or unsympathetic attitudes towards residents; staff shortages or high staff turnover; fraud involving residents' possessions or money; and lack of a residents' council or residents' family council.

Anecdotal evidence from India suggests that institutional abuse is often perpetuated by staff through a system of unquestioning regimentation – in the name of discipline or imposed protective care – and exploitation of the dependence of the older people, and is aggravated by a lack of professionally trained management.

With the present state of knowledge, it is impossible to know how pervasive such conditions are. The leading ten deficiencies, cited in broad categories by the United States Government in its 1997 survey of 15 000 nursing homes (*52*), were:

1. Food preparation (21.8%).
2. Comprehensive assessment – a documented assessment of all care needs, including medical, nursing and social care (17.3%).
3. Comprehensive care plans – usually in the form of a document specifying the day-to-day care needs of an individual and stating who is responsible for delivering them, with comments on progress and changes required (17.1%).
4. Accidents (16.6%).
5. Pressure sores (16.1%).
6. Quality of care (14.4%).
7. Physical restraints (13.3%).
8. Housekeeping (13.3%).
9. Lack of dignity (13.2%).
10. Accident prevention (11.9%).

Abuse and neglect can occur in many types of institution, including those that seem to provide high-quality care to patients. A key finding from an examination of inquiries into scandals in residential care suggested that an acceptable or good regime of care could be transformed into an abusive one relatively easily and quickly, with little detectable change in the outward situation (*53*).

What can be done to prevent elder abuse?

The impact that physical and psychological violence have on the health of an older person is exacerbated by the ageing process and diseases of old age. It is more difficult for the elderly to leave an abusive relationship or to make correct decisions because of the physical and cognitive impairments that usually come with old age. In some places, kinship obligations and the use of the extended family network to resolve difficulties may also lessen the ability of older people, particularly women, to escape from dangerous situations. Often, the abuser may be the abused person's only source of companionship. Because of these and other considerations, preventing elder abuse presents a whole host of problems for practitioners. In most cases, the greatest dilemma is how to balance the older person's right to self-determination with the need to take action to end the abuse.

Responses at national level

Efforts to galvanize social action against elder abuse at a national level and to develop legislation and other policy initiatives are at varying stages of development around the world. Some authors (*54, 55*) have used Blumer's model (*56*) of social problems to describe the stages of the process:

— emergence of a problem;

— legitimization of the problem;

— mobilization of action;

— formulation of an official plan;

— implementation of the plan.

The United States is furthest advanced in terms of a national-level response, with a fully developed system for reporting and treating cases of elder abuse. This system operates at the state level, the federal government's involvement being limited to supporting the National Center on Elder Abuse, which gives technical assistance and a small amount of funding to the states for their elder abuse prevention services. A focus at national level is also provided by the National Committee for the Prevention of Elder Abuse, a non-profit organization formed in 1988, and the National Association of State Adult Protective Services Administrators, established in 1989.

In Australia and Canada, some provinces or states have set up systems to deal with cases of elder abuse, but no official federal policy has been announced. New Zealand has established a series of pilot projects throughout the country. All three of these countries have national groups. The New Zealand National Elder Abuse and Neglect Advisory Council was formed in the early 1990s to provide a national perspective on strategies for the care and protection of older people. The Australian Network for the Prevention of Elder Abuse was set up in 1998, as a point of contact and information-sharing for those working with older people in abusive situations. In 1999, the Canadian Network for the Prevention of Elder Abuse was created with similar aims – to find ways to develop policies, programmes and services to eliminate elder abuse.

In the United Kingdom, Action on Elder Abuse, a national nongovernmental organization, has helped focus government attention on the abuse of older people, giving rise to policy documents from the Department of Health and the Social Services Inspectorate. Norway leads among the Scandinavian countries, having obtained parliamentary approval for a service project in Oslo and a resource centre for information and research on violence, the latter largely as a result of action by campaigners against elder abuse. Other European countries – including France, Germany, Italy and Poland – are at the "legitimization" stage of Blumer's model. Activities for the prevention of elder abuse in these countries are limited mainly to individual researchers and to some local programmes.

The Latin American Committee for the Prevention of Elder Abuse has actively campaigned to draw attention to the problem of abuse of the elderly within Latin American and Caribbean countries, and it offers training at regional and national meetings. For some countries – including Cuba, Peru, Uruguay and Venezuela – awareness of the problem is still emerging, and activities consist mainly of meetings of professionals and research studies. Other countries in the region, such as Argentina, Brazil and Chile, have moved on to legitimization and action.

In Buenos Aires, Argentina, the organization "Proteger", dealing exclusively with elder abuse cases, was established in 1998 as one of the programmes of the Department for the Promotion of Social Welfare and Old Age. Professionals and other workers in this programme receive a 6-month training in gerontology, focusing mainly on the prevention of violence and intervention in cases of elder abuse. Proteger also runs a free telephone helpline.

In Brazil, official support for training on elder abuse has been provided by the Ministry of Justice, Health and Welfare. In Chile, as a result of the work of the Interministerial Commission for the Prevention of Intrafamiliar Violence, a law against violence in the family was passed in 1994 (*57*). The law covered all acts of family violence, including those directed at the elderly.

In Asia, studies by researchers in China (Hong Kong SAR), India, Japan and the Republic of Korea have drawn attention to the problem of elder abuse, but no official action, in terms of policies or programme development, has followed so far.

Reports about elder abuse in South Africa first surfaced in 1981. In 1994 a preventive programme on institutional abuse was established jointly by the state and private sector (*58*). Activists working to prevent elder abuse strongly promoted the idea of a national strategy on elder abuse, which the government is now considering, and pushed for the inclusion of elder abuse in the final declaration of the Southern African Development Community Conference on the Prevention of Violence Against Women, held in Maseru, Lesotho, in December 2000. The Nigerian Coalition on Prevention of Elder Abuse brings together all agencies and groups working with and for the elderly. For many other African nations, efforts to deal with elder abuse are overshadowed by other seemingly more pressing concerns – such as conflicts, poverty and debt.

With a rapid expansion of activities worldwide on elder abuse, the International Network for the Prevention of Elder Abuse (INPEA) was formed in 1997, with representation from all six continents.

INPEA's aims are to: increase public awareness; promote education and training; campaign on behalf of abused and neglected older people; and promote research into the causes, consequences, treatment and prevention of elder abuse. During INPEA's early stage of development, workshops have been the main medium of training, and have been conducted at professional meetings in Australia, Brazil, Canada, Cuba, the United Kingdom and the United States. A quarterly newsletter and a web site have been set up. INPEA was also the inspiration for both the Australian and the Canadian networks.

Local responses

Most of the programmes set up to tackle the problem of abuse of the elderly are found in high-income countries. They are generally conducted under the auspices of the social services, health care or legal systems or in conjunction with programmes to combat family violence. Although elder abuse has been proven to exist in several low-income or middle-income countries, few specific programmes have been established. In these countries, cases of elder abuse are generally handled by governmental or nongovernmental social service agencies, even though the staff of such agencies might not always be knowledgeable about the subject. Costa Rica, where there is a strong local programme in place, is an exception (*11*). In some countries, there are no social services or health care systems to deal with elder abuse.

Social services

In general, countries that deliver services to abused, neglected or exploited older people have done so through the existing health and social services network. Such cases frequently involve medical, legal, ethical, psychological, financial, law enforcement and environmental issues. Guidelines and protocols have been developed to help case workers and special training is usually available to them. Care is generally planned by consulting teams drawn from a wide range of disciplines. Typically, these services operate in close collaboration with task forces, usually representing statutory bodies and

voluntary, private and charitable organizations, that offer consultation services, provide training, develop model legislation and identify weak points in the system. Telephone helplines to receive reports of mistreatment are often a feature of such systems (*59, 60*) and are currently operating in the United Kingdom and in local communities in France, Germany and Japan (see Box 5.2). Only the United States and a number of Canadian provinces have created a system solely for handling reports of adult mistreatment. In these adult protection services, as they are known, the case workers investigate and assess cases, develop plans for appropriate care and monitor the cases until they can be handed over to existing social service agencies for the elderly.

There is a growing interest in providing services for victims of elder abuse along the lines of those developed for battered women. Emergency shelters and support groups specifically aimed at older abused people are relatively new. They provide an environment where victims of abuse can share experiences, develop the psychological strength to cope with their fears, self-doubt, stress and anxiety, and raise their self-esteem. One example of how the domestic violence model has been adapted for elder abuse is the programme set up by the Finnish Federation of Mother and Child Homes and Shelters in collaboration with a local nursing home and the Finnish health care system. This project provides emergency shelter beds in the nursing home, a telephone helpline offering advice and an opportunity for older people to talk about their problems, and a biweekly victim support group meeting. Other such emergency shelters exist in Canada, Germany, Japan and the United States.

In low-income countries lacking the social service infrastructure to undertake these types of programmes, local projects can be established to help older people plan programmes and develop their own services, as well as to campaign for change. Such activities will also give the older people strength and self-esteem. In Guatemala, for instance, blind older people who had been ejected from their homes by their families formed their own committee, created a safe house for themselves, and set up local handicraft and other

---

> **BOX 5.2**
>
> ## The Japan Elder Abuse Prevention Centre
>
> In 1993, the Society for the Study of Elder Abuse (SSEA) in Japan, an independent group consisting largely of social workers and academics, carried out a national survey of community care centres. Their study confirmed the existence of elder abuse in Japan. Based on the results, SSEA decided that a telephone counselling service, similar to that run in the United Kingdom by Action on Elder Abuse, was the best way to confront the problem of elder abuse (*60*).
>
> With financial help from a national nongovernmental organization, the Japan Elder Abuse Prevention Centre was set up in 1996 as a non-profit body, offering a volunteer-operated telephone counselling service known simply as *Helpline*. One of the SSEA's members, a director of a nursing home, made a room available in the nursing home for use as an office and provided other help. The counselling service was advertised in newspapers, support centres and other agencies.
>
> *Helpline* now offers a wide range of information as well as legal counselling to anyone — including health care and welfare professionals — with a problem related to elder abuse.
>
> Initially, *Helpline* counsellors were all members of the SSEA, but three outside volunteers were subsequently added to the staff. On any particular day, one or two counsellors are in attendance. Extensive training is given to new counsellors, and all counsellors attend monthly meetings at the SSEA, to exchange information on elder abuse and review their case studies. Outside professionals may be called in, if required, to help deal with special cases.
>
> *Helpline* is exclusively a telephone service. If a caller needs counselling in person, rather than by telephone, their case is handed over to a local home service support centre. Privacy, confidentiality and the anonymity of the callers are key concerns of *Helpline*.

income-generating projects to help fund the safe house (*61*).

Health care

In some Latin American and European countries, as well as in Australia, the medical profession has played a leading role in raising public concern about elder abuse. In other countries, including Canada and the United States, physicians have lagged many years behind the social work and nursing professions. Few intervention programmes for abused older people are housed in hospital settings. Where these do exist, they are usually consultation teams who are on call in the event a suspected case of abuse is reported. Those involved in the provision of health care have an important role to play in programmes that screen for and detect abuse.

While it may be thought that doctors are best placed to notice cases of abuse — partly because of the trust that most elderly people have in them — many doctors do not diagnose abuse because it is not part of their formal or professional training and hence does not feature in their list of differential diagnoses.

In emergency rooms, too, it would seem, scant attention is usually paid to the special needs of elderly people. Health care professionals often feel more comfortable dealing with younger people than they do with elderly ones, and the concerns of older patients are frequently ignored. Most emergency departments do not use protocols to detect and deal with elder abuse, and rarely attempt to address the mental health or behavioural signs of elder abuse, such as depression, attempted suicide, or drug or alcohol abuse (*62*).

There should be an investigation of a patient's condition for possible abuse (*63, 64*) if a doctor or other health care worker notices any of the following signs:

— delays between injuries or illness and seeking medical attention;

— implausible or vague explanations for injuries or ill-health, from either the patient or
his or her caregiver;
— differing case histories from the patient and
the caregiver;
— frequent visits to emergency departments
because a chronic condition has worsened,
despite a care plan and resources to deal with
this in the home;
— functionally impaired older patients who
arrive without their main caregivers;
— laboratory findings that are inconsistent with
the history provided.

When conducting an examination (65), the
doctor or health care worker should:
— interview the patient alone, asking directly
about possible physical violence, restraints or
neglect;
— interview the suspected abuser alone;
— pay close attention to the relationship
between, and the behaviour of, the patient
and his or her suspected abuser;
— conduct a comprehensive geriatric assessment of the patient, including medical,
functional, cognitive and social factors;
— document the patient's social networks, both
formal and informal.

Table 5.1 contains a list of indicators that may
serve as a useful guide if mistreatment is suspected.
The presence of any indicator in this table, though,
should not be taken as proof that abuse has actually
taken place.

Legal action

Despite a growing interest in the problem, most
countries have not introduced specific legislation
on elder abuse. Particular aspects of abuse are
usually covered either by criminal law, or by laws
dealing with civil rights, property rights, family
violence or mental health. Specific and comprehensive legislation on the abuse of older people
would imply a much stronger commitment to
eradicating the problem. However, even where
such laws exist, cases of elder abuse have only rarely
been prosecuted. This is principally because older
people are usually reluctant – or unable – to press
charges against family members, because older
people are often regarded as being unreliable
witnesses, or because of the inherently hidden
nature of elder abuse. As long as elder abuse is
viewed solely as a caregiver issue, legal action is not
likely to be an effective measure.

Only the Atlantic provinces of Canada, Israel,
and a number of states in the United States have
legislation for the mandatory reporting of abuse of
the elderly. In the United States, 43 states require
professionals and others working with older people
to report possible cases of elder abuse to a state-
designated agency, should they have "reason to
believe" that abuse, neglect or exploitation has
taken place. The first of these states passed its
legislation in 1976, and the most recent in 1999.
The Canadian province of Newfoundland passed its
adult protection law as early as 1973, with the last
of the four Atlantic provinces, Prince Edward
Island, following in 1988. Israel's law dates from
1989. As with child abuse reporting laws, all these
laws on elder abuse were introduced to prevent
evidence of abuse from going unnoticed. Mandatory reporting was considered a valuable tool,
particularly in situations where victims were unable
to report and professionals were reluctant to refer
cases. While research on the impact of existing
mandatory reporting does not as yet provide a
conclusive answer, the indications are that whether
a case is reported or not has less to do with legal
requirements than with other organizational,
ethical, cultural and professional factors (66).

Education and public awareness campaigns

Education and public awareness campaigns have
been vital for informing people in industrialized
countries about elder abuse. Education involves not
only teaching new information but also changing
attitudes and behaviour, and is thus a fundamental
preventive strategy. It can be conducted in a wide
variety of ways – for instance, in training sessions,
seminars, continuing educational programmes,
workshops, and scientific meetings and conferences. Those targeted will include not only
practitioners in the various relevant disciplines –
from medicine, mental health and nursing to social

TABLE 5.1

Indicators of elder abuse

Indicators relating to the elderly person				Indicators relating to the caregiver
Physical	Behavioural and emotional	Sexual	Financial	
• Complaints of being physically assaulted	• Change in eating pattern or sleep problems	• Complaints of being sexually assaulted	• Withdrawals of money that are erratic, or not typical of the older person	• Caregiver appears tired or stressed
• Unexplained falls and injuries	• Fear, confusion or air of resignation	• Sexual behaviour that is out of keeping with the older person's usual relationships and previous personality	• Withdrawals of money that are inconsistent with the older person's means	• Caregiver seems excessively concerned or unconcerned
• Burns and bruises in unusual places or of an unusual type	• Passivity, withdrawal or increasing depression	• Unexplained changes in behaviour, such as aggression, withdrawal or self-mutilation	• Changing a will or property title to leave house or assets to "new friends or relatives"	• Caregiver blames the older person for acts such as incontinence
• Cuts, finger marks or other evidence of physical restraint	• Helplessness, hopelessness or anxiety	• Frequent complaints of abdominal pain, or unexplained vaginal or anal bleeding	• Property is missing	• Caregiver behaves aggressively
• Excessive repeat prescriptions or under-usage of medication	• Contradictory statements or other ambivalence not resulting from mental confusion	• Recurrent genital infections, or bruises around the breasts or genital area	• Older person "can't find" jewellery or personal belongings	• Caregiver treats the older person like a child or in a dehumanized way
• Malnourishment or dehydration without an illness-related cause	• Reluctance to talk openly	• Torn, stained or bloody underclothes	• Suspicious activity on credit card account	• Caregiver has a history of substance abuse or abusing others
• Evidence of inadequate care or poor standards of hygiene	• Avoidance of physical, eye or verbal contact with caregiver		• Lack of amenities, when the older person could afford them	• Caregiver does not want the older person to be interviewed alone
• Person seeks medical attention from a variety of doctors or medical centres	• Older person is isolated by others		• Untreated medical or mental health problems	• Caregiver responds defensively when questioned; may be hostile or evasive
			• Level of care is not commensurate with the older person's income or assets	• Caregiver has been providing care to the older person for a long period of time

work, criminal justice and religion – but also researchers, educators, policy-makers and decision-makers. A typical basic syllabus suitable for most disciplines includes an introduction to the topic of elder abuse, consideration of the signs and symptoms of abuse, and details of local organizations that can provide assistance. More specialized training courses will concentrate on developing skills in interviewing, assessment of abuse cases, and planning care programmes. Even more advanced teaching from specialists in the field is needed to cover ethical and legal matters. Courses in

how to work with other professionals and in multidisciplinary teams have also become part of advanced training curricula on elder abuse.

Public education and awareness raising are equally important elements in preventing abuse and neglect. As in public education on child abuse and intimate partner violence, the aim is to inform the general public about the various types of abuse, how to identify the signs and where help can be obtained. People who come into frequent contact with the elderly are a particular target for such education. Apart from family members and friends, they include postal workers, bank tellers, and electricity and gas meter readers. Educational programmes aimed at older people themselves are usually more successful if the information on abuse is woven into wider topics such as successful ageing or health care. Organizations for the elderly, community centres, day-care programmes, schools (see Box 5.3), and self-help and support groups can all help this educational effort.

The media are a powerful tool for raising public awareness. More positive images and a greater prominence for older people in the media can work towards changing attitudes and reducing the stereotyping that exists around the elderly. The participants in the focus group study in South Africa stressed the importance of the media in raising public awareness (*15*), suggesting that awareness of the problem of elder abuse should also be promoted through community workshops with government involvement. In other developing countries with limited resources, local associations can provide basic education along with health care.

To date, few intervention programmes have been evaluated and it is therefore not possible to say which approaches have had the most success. Efforts to assess the effectiveness of various projects have been hindered by a lack of common definitions, a variety of theoretical explanations, a low level of interest on the part of the scientific community and a lack of funding for rigorous studies to be conducted.

A literature review of studies on elder abuse interventions found that 117 such studies had been published, in English, between 1989 and 1998 (G. Bolen, J. Ploeg & B. Hutchinson, unpublished data, 1999). Not one of them, however, included a comparison group or met standard criteria for a valid evaluation study. Based on these findings, the authors of the review felt that there was insufficient evidence in favour of any specific intervention. Six of the studies reviewed were singled out as most closely meeting the necessary criteria, but they too contained serious methodological weaknesses. Among these six studies, the proportion of cases

---

BOX 5.3

A Canadian school curriculum to prevent elder abuse

A nongovernmental organization, Health Canada, has developed a two-part educational project on elder abuse for children and young people. The project is intended to make children aware of and sensitive to old age and what it entails, and to create opportunities for young people to foster relationships across the generations. In so doing, it is hoped that children and young people will develop greater respect for the elderly and will be much less inclined, now and in the future, to mistreat them.

The first part of the project is an interactive story-telling kit for children aged 3–7 years, involving games and stories. While not directly addressing the subject of elder abuse, the kit provides positive images of old age. It has also proved effective with older children with a limited knowledge of English.

A formal school curriculum is at the core of the second part of the project, developed after extensive consultations with a range of people — including teachers, youth workers, religious leaders, health care providers, young people, those working with the elderly and older people themselves. The curriculum — appropriate mainly for adolescents — aims to change the deeply-rooted negative attitudes in society about older people and ageing, and to reduce the level of elder abuse.

Also in Canada, schools in Ontario have included the topic of conflict resolution in their curricula, and teachers there have found that a discussion of elder abuse can easily be introduced in this subject.

successfully resolved following a particular intervention ranged from 22% to 75%.

Recommendations

Although abuse of the elderly by family members, caregivers and others is better understood today than it was 25 years ago, a firmer base of knowledge is needed for policy, planning and programming purposes. Many aspects of the problem remain unknown, including its causes and consequences, and even the extent to which it occurs. Research on the effectiveness of interventions has to date yielded almost no useful or reliable results.

Perhaps the most insidious form of abuse against the elderly lies in the negative attitudes towards, and stereotypes of, older people and the process of ageing itself, attitudes that are reflected in the frequent glorification of youth. As long as older people are devalued and marginalized by society, they will suffer from loss of self-identity and remain highly susceptible to discrimination and all forms of abuse.

Among the priorities for confronting and eradicating the problem of elder abuse are:
— greater knowledge about the problem;
— stronger laws and policies;
— more effective prevention strategies.

Greater knowledge

Better knowledge about elder abuse is a top priority worldwide. In 1990 the Council of Europe convened a broad-ranging conference on the subject that looked at definitions, statistics, laws and policies, prevention and treatment, as well as the available sources of information on elder abuse (67). A global working group on elder abuse should be set up to deal with all these subjects. Among other things, such a body could bring together and standardize global statistics, and work out the requirements for a common data-reporting form. The precise role of different cultures in elder abuse should also be researched and better explained.

Research leading to effective interventions is urgently needed. Studies should be conducted to ascertain how older people can play a greater part in designing and participating in prevention pro-grammes, something that has already been started in Canada. This could be particularly relevant in developing countries, where involving older people in the design and implementation of programmes can help raise awareness about their rights, address the problems related to social exclusion and help to empower them (3).

More rigorous standards are needed in scientific research on elder abuse. Too much past research has involved small samples and weak methodology, sometimes producing conflicting results. Some studies have shown that the mental state of the abuser and substance abuse are risk factors, but exactly how these factors contribute to abuse or neglect in some cases but not in others has not been investigated. Further work is also needed to resolve the currently contradictory data about cognitive and physical impairment in older people as risk factors for abuse.

Causes of abuse

More research is needed on the role of stress among caregivers, originally considered a primary cause of elder abuse. With the increasing prevalence of Alzheimer disease worldwide and the greater level of abusive behaviour found in families where a family member suffers from the disease, more attention should be given to the relationship between the caregiver and the care recipient. While it may be obvious that social isolation or lack of support can contribute to abuse or neglect, the sufferers of abuse in these situations are generally unwilling to join programmes that encourage social interaction, such as centres for the elderly or day-care activities. Research on who these victims are and on their situations might produce better solutions.

The role of ageism — discrimination against and stigmatization of older people — as a possible cause of elder abuse has yet to be properly investigated, although some specialists in the field have suggested that the marginalization of the elderly is a contributory factor. Cross-cultural studies would probably be helpful in understanding this effect.

Clearly there are certain social and cultural factors in some developing countries that are directly linked to abuse, such as a belief in witchcraft and the abandonment of widows. Other practices, which are also often quoted as being important causal factors, need to be examined, since there has been no research to confirm the claims.

Other cultural and socioeconomic factors, such as poverty, modernization and inheritance systems, may be indirect causes of abuse. The use of the ecological model to explain elder abuse is still new and more research is needed on the factors operating at different levels of the model.

Impact of abuse

The aspect of elder abuse that has perhaps received least attention is the impact on the older person. Longitudinal studies that track both abused and non-abused people over a long period of time should therefore form part of the research agenda. In particular, few studies have looked at the psychological impact on an abused person. Except for depression, little is known about the emotional damage caused to the victims.

Evaluation of interventions

A variety of interventions have been developed, including interventions related to mandatory reporting, protective service units, social service protocols, emergency shelters, support and self-help groups, and consultation teams. Very few of these, however, have been evaluated using an experimental or quasi-experimental research design, and evaluative research of a high standard is urgently required. Unfortunately, the topic of elder abuse has not attracted the attention of many established researchers, whose expertise is nonetheless much needed. A greater investment of resources in studies on elder abuse would encourage such research.

Stronger laws

Basic rights

The human rights of older people must be guaranteed worldwide. To this end:

- Existing laws on domestic or intrafamily violence should be extended to include older people as a group.
- Relevant existing criminal and civil laws should explicitly cover the abuse, neglect and exploitation of older people.
- Governments should introduce new laws specifically to protect older people.

Abusive traditions

Many existing traditions are abusive towards older women, including belief in witchcraft and the practice of abandoning widows. Ending these customs will require a high degree of collaboration among many groups, probably over a long period of time. To help this process:

- Advocacy groups, consisting of older people as well as younger people, should be formed at local, provincial and national levels to campaign for change.
- Governmental health and welfare programmes should actively seek to mitigate the negative impact that many modernization processes and the consequent changes in family structure have on older people.
- National governments should establish an adequate pension system, in all countries where it does not exist.

More effective prevention strategies

At the most basic level, greater importance must be attached to primary prevention. This requires building a society in which older people are allowed to live out their lives in dignity, adequately provided with the necessities of life and with genuine opportunities for self-fulfilment. For those societies overwhelmed by poverty, the challenge is enormous.

Prevention starts with awareness. One important way to raise awareness – both among the public and concerned professionals – is through education and training. Those providing health care and social services at all levels, both in the community and in institutional settings, should receive basic training on the detection of elder abuse. The media are a second powerful tool for raising awareness of the problem and its possible solutions, among the general public as well as the authorities.

Programmes, in which older people themselves play a leading role, for preventing abuse of the elderly in their homes include:

— recruiting and training older people to serve as visitors or companions to other older people who are isolated;
— creating support groups for victims of elder abuse;
— setting up community programmes to stimulate social interaction and participation among the elderly;
— building social networks of older people in villages, neighbourhoods or housing units;
— working with older people to create "self-help" programmes that enable them to be productive.

Preventing elder abuse by helping abusers, particularly adult children, to resolve their own problems is a difficult task. Measures that may be useful include:

— offering services for the treatment of mental health problems and substance abuse;
— making jobs and education available;
— finding new ways of resolving conflict, especially where the traditional role of older people in conflict resolution has been eroded.

Much can also be done to prevent abuse of the elderly in institutional settings. Measures that may be useful include:

— the development and implementation of comprehensive care plans;
— training for staff;
— policies and programmes to address work-related stress among staff;
— the development of policies and programmes to improve the physical and social environment of the institution.

Conclusion

The problem of elder abuse cannot be properly solved if the essential needs of older people — for food, shelter, security and access to health care — are not met. The nations of the world must create an environment in which ageing is accepted as a natural part of the life cycle, where anti-ageing attitudes are discouraged, where older people are given the right to live in dignity — free of abuse and exploitation — and are given opportunities to participate fully in educational, cultural, spiritual and economic activities (*3*).

References

1. Baker AA. Granny-battering. *Modern Geriatrics,* 1975, 5:20–24.
2. Burston GR. "Granny battering". *British Medical Journal,* 1975, 3:592.
3. Randal J, German T. *The ageing and development report: poverty, independence, and the world's people.* London, HelpAge International, 1999.
4. Hudson MF. Elder mistreatment: a taxonomy with definitions by Delphi. *Journal of Elder Abuse and Neglect,*1991, 3:1–20.
5. Brown AS. A survey on elder abuse in one Native American tribe. *Journal of Elder Abuse and Neglect,*1989, 1.17–37.
6. Maxwell EK, Maxwell RJ. Insults to the body civil: mistreatment of elderly in two Plains Indian tribes. *Journal of Cross-Cultural Gerontology,* 1992, 7:3–22.
7. What is elder abuse? *Action on Elder Abuse Bulletin,* 1995, 11 (May–June).
8. Kosberg JI, Garcia JL. Common and unique themes on elder abuse from a worldwide perspective. In: Kosberg JI, Garcia JL, eds. *Elder abuse: international and cross-cultural perspectives.* Binghamton, NY, Haworth Press, 1995:183–198.
9. Moon A, Williams O. Perceptions of elder abuse and help-seeking patterns among African-American, Caucasian American, and Korean-American elderly women. *The Gerontologist,* 1993, 33:386–395.
10. Tomita SK. Exploration of elder mistreatment among the Japanese. In: Tatara T, ed. *Understanding elder abuse in minority populations.* Philadelphia, PA, Francis & Taylor, 1999:119–139.
11. Gilliland N, Picado LE. Elder abuse in Costa Rica. *Journal of Elder Abuse and Neglect,* 2000, 12:73–87.
12. Owen M. *A world of widows.* London, Zed Books, 1996.
13. Gorman M, Petersen T. *Violence against older people and its health consequences: experience from Africa and Asia.* London, HelpAge International, 1999.
14. Witchcraft: a violent threat. *Ageing and Development,* 2000, 6:9.

15. Keikelame J, Ferreira M. *Mpathekombi, ya bantu abadala: elder abuse in black townships on the Cape Flats.* Cape Town, Human Sciences Research Council and University of Cape Town Centre for Gerontology, 2000.

16. Pillemer K, Finkelhor D. Prevalence of elder abuse: a random sample survey. *The Gerontologist,* 1988, 28:51–57.

17. Podnieks E. National survey on abuse of the elderly in Canada. *Journal of Elder Abuse and Neglect,* 1992, 4:5–58.

18. Kivelä SL et al. Abuse in old age: epidemiological data from Finland. *Journal of Elder Abuse and Neglect,* 1992, 4:1–18.

19. Ogg J, Bennett GCJ. Elder abuse in Britain. *British Medical Journal,* 1992, 305:998–999.

20. Comijs HC et al. Elder abuse in the community: prevalence and consequences. *Journal of the American Geriatrics Society,* 1998, 46:885–888.

21. Canadian Centre for Justice Statistics. *Family violence in Canada: a statistical profile 2000.* Ottawa, Health Canada, 2000.

22. Kane RL, Kane RA. *Long-term care in six countries: implications for the United States.* Washington, DC, United States Department of Health, Education and Welfare, 1976.

23. Pillemer KA, Moore D. Highlights from a study of abuse of patients in nursing homes. *Journal of Elder Abuse and Neglect,* 1990, 2:5–30.

24. Garbarino J, Crouter A. Defining the community context for parent–child relations: the correlates of child maltreatment. *Child Development,* 1978, 49:604–616.

25. Schiamberg LB, Gans D. An ecological framework for contextual risk factors in elder abuse by adult children. *Journal of Elder Abuse and Neglect,* 1999, 11:79–103.

26. Carp RM. *Elder abuse in the family: an interdisciplinary model for research.* New York, NY, Springer, 2000.

27. Gelles RJ. Through a sociological lens: social structure and family violence. In: Gelles RJ, Loeske DR, eds. *Current controversies on family violence.* Thousand Oaks, CA, Sage, 1993:31–46.

28. O'Leary KD. Through a psychological lens: personality traits, personality disorders, and levels of violence. In: Gelles RJ, Loeske DR, eds. *Current controversies on family violence.* Thousand Oaks, CA, Sage, 1993:7–30.

29. Wolf RS, Pillemer KA. *Helping elderly victims: the reality of elder abuse.* New York, NY, Columbia University Press, 1989.

30. Homer AC, Gilleard C. Abuse of elderly people by their carers. *British Medical Journal,* 1990, 301:1359–1362.

31. Bristowe E, Collins JB. Family mediated abuse of non-institutionalised elder men and women living in British Columbia. *Journal of Elder Abuse and Neglect,* 1989, 1:45–54.

32. Pillemer KA. Risk factors in elder abuse: results from a case–control study. In: Pillemer KA, Wolf RS, eds. *Elder abuse: conflict in the family.* Dover, MA, Auburn House, 1989:239–264.

33. Paveza GJ et al. Severe family violence and Alzheimer's disease: prevalence and risk factors. *The Gerontologist,* 1992, 32:493–497.

34. Cooney C, Mortimer A. Elder abuse and dementia: a pilot study. *International Journal of Social Psychiatry,* 1995, 41:276–283.

35. Aitken L, Griffin G. *Gender issues in elder abuse.* London, Sage, 1996.

36. Steinmetz SK. *Duty bound: elder abuse and family care.* Thousand Oaks, CA, Sage, 1988.

37. Eastman M. *Old age abuse: a new perspective,* 2nd ed. San Diego, CA, Singular Publishing Group, Inc., 1994.

38. Reis M, Nahamish D. Validation of the indicators of abuse (IOA) screen. *The Gerontologist,* 1998, 38:471–480.

39. Hamel M et al. Predictors and consequences of aggressive behavior by community-based dementia patients. *The Gerontologist,* 1990, 30:206–211.

40. Nolan MR, Grant G, Keady J. *Understanding family care: a multidimensional model of caring and coping.* Buckingham, Open University Press, 1996.

41. Pillemer KA, Suitor JJ. Violence and violent feelings: what causes them among family caregivers? *Journal of Gerontology,* 1992, 47:S165–S172.

42. O'Loughlin A, Duggan J. *Abuse, neglect and mistreatment of older people: an exploratory study.* Dublin, National Council on Ageing and Older People, 1998 (Report No. 52).

43. Phillips LR. Theoretical explanations of elder abuse. In: Pillemer KA, Wolf RS, eds. *Elder abuse: conflict in the family.* Dover, MA, Auburn House, 1989:197–217.

44. Grafstrom M, Nordberg A, Winblad B. Abuse is in the eye of the beholder. *Scandinavian Journal of Social Medicine,* 1994, 21:247–255.

45. Kwan AY. Elder abuse in Hong Kong: a new family problem for the east? In: Kosberg JI, Garcia JL, eds. *Elder abuse: international and cross-cultural perspectives.* Binghamton, NY, Haworth Press, 1995:65–80.

46. Phillips LR. Abuse and neglect of the frail elderly at home: an exploration of theoretical relationships. *Advanced Nursing,* 1983, 8:379–382.

47. Pillemer KA, Prescott D. Psychological effects of elder abuse: a research note. *Journal of Elder Abuse and Neglect*, 1989, 1:65–74.

48. Booth BK, Bruno AA, Marin R. Psychological therapy with abused and neglected patients. In: Baumhover LA, Beall SC, eds. *Abuse, neglect, and exploitation of older persons: strategies for assessment and intervention.* Baltimore, MD, Health Professions Press, 1996:185–206.

49. Goldstein M. Elder mistreatment and PTSD. In: Ruskin PE, Talbott JA, eds. *Aging and post-traumatic stress disorder.* Washington, DC, American Psychiatric Association, 1996:126–135.

50. Lachs MS et al. The mortality of elder mistreatment. *Journal of the American Medical Association*, 1998, 20:428–432.

51. Bennett G, Kingston P, Penhale B. *The dimensions of elder abuse: perspectives for practitioners.* London, Macmillan, 1997.

52. Harrington CH et al. *Nursing facilities, staffing, residents, and facility deficiencies, 1991–1997.* San Francisco, CA, Department of Social and Behavioral Sciences, University of California, 2000.

53. Clough R. Scandalous care: interpreting public inquiry reports of scandals in residential care. In: Glendenning F, Kingston P, eds. *Elder abuse and neglect in residential settings: different national backgrounds and similar responses.* Binghamton, NY, Haworth Press, 1999:13–28.

54. Leroux TG, Petrunik M. The construction of elder abuse as a social problem: a Canadian perspective. *International Journal of Health Services*, 1990, 20:651–663.

55. Bennett G, Kingston P. *Elder abuse: concepts, theories and interventions.* London, Chapman & Hall, 1993.

56. Blumer H. Social problems as collective behaviour. *Social Problems*, 1971, 18:298–306.

57. Mehrotra A. *Situation of gender-based violence against women in Latin America and the Caribbean: national report for Chile.* New York, United Nations Development Programme, 1999.

58. Eckley SCA, Vilakas PAC. Elder abuse in South Africa. In: Kosberg JI, Garcia JL, eds. *Elder abuse: international and cross-cultural perspectives.* Binghamton, NY, Haworth Press, 1995:171–182.

59. *Hearing the despair: the reality of elder abuse.* London, Action on Elder Abuse, 1997.

60. Yamada Y. A telephone counseling program for elder abuse in Japan. *Journal of Elder Abuse and Neglect*, 1999, 11:105–112.

61. Checkoway B. Empowering the elderly: gerontological health promotion in Latin America. *Ageing and Society*, 1994, 14:75–95.

62. Sanders AB. Care of the elderly in emergency departments: conclusions and recommendations. *Annals of Emergency Medicine*, 1992, 21:79–83.

63. Lachs MS, Pillemer KA. Abuse and neglect of elderly persons. *New England Journal of Medicine*, 1995, 332:437–443.

64. Jones JS. Geriatric abuse and neglect. In: Bosker G et al., eds. *Geriatric emergency medicine.* St Louis, MO, CV Mosby, 1990:533–542.

65. *Elder mistreatment guidelines: detection, assessment and intervention.* New York, NY, Mount Sinai/Victim Services Agency Elder Abuse Project, 1988.

66. Wolf RS. Elder abuse: mandatory reporting revisited. In: Cebik LE, Graber GC, Marsh FH, eds. *Violence, neglect, and the elderly.* Greenwich, CT, JAI Press, 1996:155–170.

67. *Violence against elderly people.* Strasbourg, Council of Europe, Steering Committee on Social Policy, 1991.

CHAPTER 6

Sexual violence

Background

Sexual violence occurs throughout the world. Although in most countries there has been little research conducted on the problem, available data suggest that in some countries nearly one in four women may experience sexual violence by an intimate partner (*1–3*), and up to one-third of adolescent girls report their first sexual experience as being forced (*4–6*).

Sexual violence has a profound impact on physical and mental health. As well as causing physical injury, it is associated with an increased risk of a range of sexual and reproductive health problems, with both immediate and long-term consequences (*4, 7–16*). Its impact on mental health can be as serious as its physical impact, and may be equally long lasting (*17–24*). Deaths following sexual violence may be as a result of suicide, HIV infection (*25*) or murder – the latter occurring either during a sexual assault or subsequently, as a murder of "honour" (*26*). Sexual violence can also profoundly affect the social well-being of victims; individuals may be stigmatized and ostracized by their families and others as a consequence (*27, 28*).

Coerced sex may result in sexual gratification on the part of the perpetrator, though its underlying purpose is frequently the expression of power and dominance over the person assaulted. Often, men who coerce a spouse into a sexual act believe their actions are legitimate because they are married to the woman.

Rape of women and of men is often used as a weapon of war, as a form of attack on the enemy, typifying the conquest and degradation of its women or captured male fighters (*29*). It may also be used to punish women for transgressing social or moral codes, for instance, those prohibiting adultery or drunkenness in public. Women and men may also be raped when in police custody or in prison.

While sexual violence can be directed against both men and women, the main focus of this chapter will be on the various forms of sexual violence against women, as well as those directed against young girls by people other than caregivers.

How is sexual violence defined?

Sexual violence is defined as:

> any sexual act, attempt to obtain a sexual act, unwanted sexual comments or advances, or acts to traffic, or otherwise directed, against a person's sexuality using coercion, by any person regardless of their relationship to the victim, in any setting, including but not limited to home and work.

Coercion can cover a whole spectrum of degrees of force. Apart from physical force, it may involve psychological intimidation, blackmail or other threats – for instance, the threat of physical harm, of being dismissed from a job or of not obtaining a job that is sought. It may also occur when the person aggressed is unable to give consent – for instance, while drunk, drugged, asleep or mentally incapable of understanding the situation.

Sexual violence includes *rape*, defined as physically forced or otherwise coerced penetration – even if slight – of the vulva or anus, using a penis, other body parts or an object. The attempt to do so is known as *attempted rape*. Rape of a person by two or more perpetrators is known as *gang rape*.

Sexual violence can include other forms of assault involving a sexual organ, including coerced contact between the mouth and penis, vulva or anus.

Forms and contexts of sexual violence

A wide range of sexually violent acts can take place in different circumstances and settings. These include, for example:

— rape within marriage or dating relationships;
— rape by strangers;
— systematic rape during armed conflict;
— unwanted sexual advances or sexual harassment, including demanding sex in return for favours;
— sexual abuse of mentally or physically disabled people;
— sexual abuse of children;
— forced marriage or cohabitation, including the marriage of children;
— denial of the right to use contraception or to adopt other measures to protect against sexually transmitted diseases;
— forced abortion;

— violent acts against the sexual integrity of women, including female genital mutilation and obligatory inspections for virginity;

— forced prostitution and trafficking of people for the purpose of sexual exploitation.

There is no universally accepted definition of trafficking for sexual exploitation. The term encompasses the organized movement of people, usually women, between countries and within countries for sex work. Such trafficking also includes coercing a migrant into a sexual act as a condition of allowing or arranging the migration.

Sexual trafficking uses physical coercion, deception and bondage incurred through forced debt. Trafficked women and children, for instance, are often promised work in the domestic or service industry, but instead are usually taken to brothels where their passports and other identification papers are confiscated. They may be beaten or locked up and promised their freedom only after earning – through prostitution – their purchase price, as well as their travel and visa costs (*30–33*).

The extent of the problem
Sources of data
Data on sexual violence typically come from police, clinical settings, nongovernmental organizations and survey research. The relationship between these sources and the global magnitude of the problem of sexual violence may be viewed as corresponding to an iceberg floating in water (*34*) (see Figure 6.1). The small visible tip represents cases reported to police. A

larger section may be elucidated through survey research and the work of nongovernmental organizations. But beneath the surface remains a substantial although unquantified component of the problem.

In general, sexual violence has been a neglected area of research. The available data are scanty and fragmented. Police data, for instance, are often incomplete and limited. Many women do not report sexual violence to police because they are ashamed, or fear being blamed, not believed or otherwise mistreated. Data from medico-legal clinics, on the other hand, may be biased towards the more violent incidents of sexual abuse. The proportion of women who seek medical services for immediate problems related to sexual violence is also relatively small.

Although there have been considerable advances over the past decade in measuring the phenomenon through survey research, the definitions used have varied considerably across studies. There are also significant differences across cultures in the willingness to disclose sexual violence to researchers. Caution is therefore needed when making global comparisons of the prevalence of sexual violence.

Estimates of sexual violence
Surveys of victims of crime have been undertaken in many cities and countries, using a common methodology to aid comparability, and have generally included questions on sexual violence. Table 6.1 summarizes data from some of these surveys on the prevalence of sexual assault over the preceding 5 years (*35, 36*). According to these

FIGURE 6.1

Magnitude of the problem of sexual violence

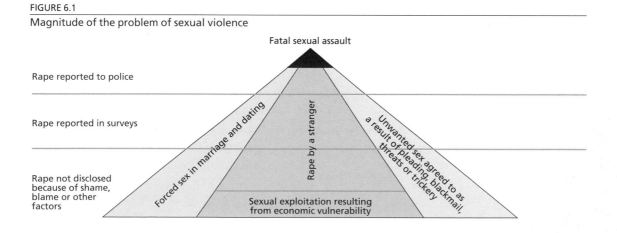

TABLE 6.1

Percentage of women aged 16 years and older who report having been sexually assaulted in the previous 5 years, selected cities, 1992–1997

Country	Study population	Year	Sample size	Percentage of women (aged 16 years and older) sexually assaulted in the previous 5 years (%)
Africa				
Botswana	Gaborone	1997	644	0.8
Egypt	Cairo	1992	1000	3.1
South Africa	Johannesburg	1996	1006	2.3
Tunisia	Grand-Tunis	1993	1087	1.9
Uganda	Kampala	1996	1197	4.5
Zimbabwe	Harare	1996	1006	2.2
Latin America				
Argentina	Buenos Aires	1996	1000	5.8
Bolivia	La Paz	1996	999	1.4
Brazil	Rio de Janiero	1996	1000	8.0
Colombia	Bogotá	1997	1000	5.0
Costa Rica	San José	1996	1000	4.3
Paraguay	Asunción	1996	587	2.7
Asia				
China	Beijing	1994	2000	1.6
India	Bombay	1996	1200	1.9
Indonesia	Jakarta and Surabaya	1996	1400	2.7
Philippines	Manila	1996	1500	0.3
Eastern Europe				
Albania	Tirana	1996	1200	6.0
Hungary	Budapest	1996	756	2.0
Lithuania	Điauliai, Kaunas, Klaipêda, Panevêžys, Vilnius	1997	1000	4.8
Mongolia	Ulaanbaatar, Zuunmod	1996	1201	3.1

Source: references *35* and *36*.

studies, the percentage of women reporting having been a victim of sexual assault ranges from less than 2% in places such as La Paz, Bolivia (1.4%), Gaborone, Botswana (0.8%), Beijing, China (1.6%), and Manila, Philippines (0.3%), to 5% or more in Tirana, Albania (6.0%), Buenos Aires, Argentina (5.8%), Rio de Janeiro, Brazil (8.0%), and Bogotá, Colombia (5.0%). It is important to note that no distinction has been made in these figures between rape by strangers and that by intimate partners. Surveys that fail to make this distinction or those that only examine rape by strangers usually underestimate substantially the prevalence of sexual violence (*34*).

Apart from crime surveys, there have been a small number of surveys, with representative samples, that have asked women about sexual violence. For instance, in a national survey conducted in the United States of America, 14.8% of women over 17 years of age reported having been raped in their lifetime (with an additional 2.8% having experienced attempted rape) and 0.3% of the sample reported having been raped in the previous year (*37*). A survey of a representative sample of women aged 18–49 years in three provinces of South Africa found that in the previous year 1.3% of women had been forced, physically or by means of verbal threats, to have non-consensual sex (*34*). In a survey of a representative sample of the general population over 15 years of age in the Czech Republic (*38*), 11.6% of women reported forced sexual contact in their lifetime, 3.4% reporting that this had occurred more than once. The most common form of contact was forced vaginal intercourse.

Sexual violence by intimate partners

In many countries a substantial proportion of women experiencing physical violence also experience sexual abuse. In Mexico and the United States, studies estimate that 40–52% of women experiencing physical violence by an intimate partner have also been sexually coerced by that partner (*39, 40*). Sometimes, sexual violence occurs without physical violence (*1*). In the Indian state of Uttar Pradesh, in a representative sample of over 6000 men, 7% reported having sexually and physically abused their wives, 22% reported using sexual violence without physical violence and 17% reported that they had used physical violence alone (*41*).

Table 6.2 summarizes some of the available data on the prevalence of sexual coercion by intimate partners (*1–3, 37, 42–53*). Findings from these

TABLE 6.2

Percentage of adult women reporting sexual victimization by an intimate partner, selected population-based surveys, 1989–2000

Country	Study population	Year	Sample size	Percentage assaulted in past 12 months	Percentage ever assaulted	
				Attempted or completed forced sex (%)	Attempted or completed forced sex (%)	Completed forced sex (%)
Brazil[a]	Sao Paulo	2000	941[a]	2.8	10.1	
	Pernambuco	2000	1 188[a]	5.6	14.3	
Canada	National	1993	12 300		8.0	
	Toronto	1991–1992	420		15.3[b]	
Chile	Santiago	1997	310	9.1		
Finland	National	1997–1998	7 051	2.5	5.9	
Japan[a]	Yokohama	2000	1 287[a]	1.3	6.2	
Indonesia	Central Java	1999–2000	765	13.0		22.0
Mexico	Durango	1996	384		42.0	
	Guadalajara	1996	650	15.0	23.0	
Nicaragua	León	1993	360		21.7	
	Managua	1997	378	17.7		
Peru[a]	Lima	2000	1 086[a]	7.1	22.5	
	Cusco	2000	1 534[a]	22.9	46.7	
Puerto Rico	National	1993–1996	7 079			5.7[b]
Sweden	Teg, Umeå	1991	251		7.5[c]	
Switzerland	National	1994–1995	1 500		11.6	
Thailand[a]	Bangkok	2000	1 051[a]	17.1	29.9	
	Nakornsawan	2000	1 027[a]	15.6	28.9	
Turkey	East and south-east Anatolia	1998	599			51.9[b]
United Kingdom	England, Scotland and Wales	1989	1 007			14.2[d]
	North London, England	1993	430	6.0[b]	23.0[b]	
United States	National	1995–1996	8 000	0.2[b]	7.7[b]	
West Bank and Gaza Strip	Palestinians	1995	2 410	27.0		
Zimbabwe	Midlands Province	1996	966		25.0	

Sources: references *1–3, 37, 42–53.*

[a] Preliminary results from the *WHO multi-country study on women's health and domestic violence.* Geneva, World Health Organization, 2000 (unpublished). Sample size reported is the denominator for the prevalence rate and not the total sample size of the study.

[b] Sample group included women who had never been in a relationship and therefore were not at risk of being assaulted by an intimate partner.

[c] Offenders reported to be husbands, boyfriends and acquaintances.

[d] Weighted estimate; unweighted prevalence rate was 13.9%.

studies show that sexual assault by an intimate partner is neither rare nor unique to any particular region of the world. For instance, 23% of women in North London, England, reported having been the victim of either an attempted or completed rape by a partner in their lifetime. Similar figures have been reported for Guadalajara, Mexico (23.0%), León, Nicaragua (21.7%), Lima, Peru (22.5%), and for the Midlands Province in Zimbabwe (25.0%). The prevalence of women sexually assaulted by an intimate partner in their lifetime (including attempted assaults) has also been estimated in a few national surveys (for example, Canada 8.0%, England, Wales and Scotland (combined) 14.2%, Finland 5.9%, Switzerland 11.6% and the United States 7.7%).

Forced sexual initiation

A growing number of studies, particularly from sub-Saharan Africa, indicate that the first sexual experience of girls is often unwanted and forced. In a case–control study, for example, of 191 adolescent girls (mean age 16.3 years) attending an antenatal clinic in Cape Town, South Africa, and 353 non-pregnant adolescents matched for age and neighbourhood or school, 31.9% of the study cases and 18.1% of the controls reported that force was used during their sexual initiation. When asked about the consequences of refusing sex, 77.9% of the study cases and 72.1% of the controls said that they feared being beaten if they refused to have sex (*4*).

Forced sexual initiation and coercion during adolescence have been reported in many studies of young women and men (see Table 6.3 and Box 6.1). Where studies have included both men and women in the sample, the prevalence of reported rape or sexual coercion has been higher among the women than the men (*5, 6, 54–60*). For example, nearly half of the sexually active adolescent women in a multi-country study in the Caribbean reported that their first sexual inter course was forced, compared with one-third of the adolescent men (*60*). In Lima, Peru, the percentage of young women reporting forced sexual initiation was almost four times that reported by the young men (40% against 11%, respectively) (*56*).

Gang rape

Rape involving at least two or more perpetrators is widely reported to occur in many parts of the world. Systematic information on the extent of the problem, however, is scant. In Johannesburg, South Africa, surveillance studies of women attending medico-legal clinics following a rape found that one-third of the cases had been gang rapes (*61*). National data on rape and sexual assault in the United States reveal that about 1 out of 10 sexual assaults involve multiple perpetrators. Most of these assaults are committed by people unknown to their victims (*62*). This pattern, though, differs from that in South Africa where boyfriends are often involved in gang rapes.

Sexual trafficking

Each year hundreds of thousands of women and girls throughout the world are bought and sold into prostitution or sexual slavery (*30–32, 63, 64*). Research in Kyrgyzstan has estimated that around 4000 people were trafficked from the country in 1999, with the principal destinations being China, Germany, Kazakhstan, the Russian Federation, Turkey and the United Arab Emirates. Of those trafficked, 62% reported being forced to work without pay, while over 50% reported being physically abused or tortured by their employers (*31*). A World Organization against Torture (OMCT) report suggested that more than 200 000 Bangladeshi women had been trafficked between 1990 and 1997 (*65*). Some 5000–7000 Nepali

TABLE 6.3

Percentage of adolescents reporting forced sexual initiation, selected population-based surveys, 1993–1999

Country or area	Study population	Year	Sample		Percentage reporting first sexual intercourse as forced (%)	
			Size[a]	Age group (years)	Females	Males
Cameroon	Bamenda	1995	646	12–25	37.3	29.9
Caribbean	Nine countries[b]	1997–1998	15 695	10–18	47.6[c]	31.9[c]
Ghana	Three urban towns	1996	750	12–24	21.0	5.0
Mozambique	Maputo	1999	1 659	13–18	18.8	6.7
New Zealand	Dunedin	1993–1994	935	Birth cohort[d]	7.0	0.2
Peru	Lima	1995	611	16–17	40.0	11.0
South Africa	Transkei	1994–1995	1 975	15–18	28.4	6.4
United Republic of Tanzania	Mwanza	1996	892	12–19	29.1	6.9
United States	National	1995	2 042	15–24	9.1	—

Source: references *5, 6* and *54–60*.

[a] Total number of adolescents in the study. Rates are based on those who have had sexual intercourse.

[b] Antigua, Bahamas, Barbados, British Virgin Islands, Dominica, Grenada, Guyana, Jamaica and Saint Lucia.

[c] Percentage of adolescents responding that their first intercourse was forced or "somewhat" forced.

[d] Longitudinal study of a cohort born in 1972–1973. Subjects were questioned at 18 years of age and again at 21 years of age about their current and previous sexual behaviour.

BOX 6.1

Sexual violence against men and boys

Sexual violence against men and boys is a significant problem. With the exception of childhood sexual abuse, though, it is one that has largely been neglected in research. Rape and other forms of sexual coercion directed against men and boys take place in a variety of settings, including in the home, the workplace, schools, on the streets, in the military and during war, as well as in prisons and police custody.

In prisons, forced sex can occur among inmates to establish hierarchies of respect and discipline. Sexual violence by prison officials, police and soldiers is also widely reported in many countries. Such violence may take the form of prisoners being forced to have sex with others as a form of "entertainment", or to provide sex for the officers or officials in command. Elsewhere, men who have sex with other men may be "punished", by rape, for their behaviour which is perceived to transgress social norms.

The extent of the problem

Studies conducted mostly in developed countries indicate that 5–10% of men report a history of childhood sexual abuse. In a few population-based studies conducted with adolescents in developing countries, the percentage of males reporting ever having been the victim of a sexual assault ranges from 3.6% in Namibia and 13.4% in the United Republic of Tanzania to 20% in Peru. Studies from both industrialized and developing countries also reveal that forced first intercourse is not rare. Unfortunately, there are few reliable statistics on the number of boys and men raped in settings such as schools, prisons and refugee camps.

Most experts believe that official statistics vastly under-represent the number of male rape victims. The evidence available suggests that males may be even less likely than female victims to report an assault to the authorities. There are a variety of reasons why male rape is under-reported, including shame, guilt and fear of not being believed or of being denounced for what has occurred. Myths and strong prejudices surrounding male sexuality also prevent men from coming forward.

Consequences of sexual violence

As is the case with female victims of sexual assault, research suggests that male victims are likely to suffer from a range of psychological consequences, both in the immediate period after the assault and over the longer term. These include guilt, anger, anxiety, depression, post-traumatic stress disorder, sexual dysfunction, somatic complaints, sleep disturbances, withdrawal from relationships and attempted suicide. In addition to these reactions, studies of adolescent males have also found an association between suffering rape and substance abuse, violent behaviour, stealing and absenteeism from school.

Prevention and policy responses

Prevention and policy responses to sexual violence against men need to be based on an understanding of the problem, its causes and the circumstances in which it occurs. In many countries the phenomenon is not adequately addressed in legislation. In addition, male rape is frequently not treated as an equal offence with rape of women.

Many of the considerations relating to support for women who have been raped — including an understanding of the healing process, the most urgent needs following an assault and the effectiveness of support services — are also relevant for men. Some countries have progressed in their response to male sexual assault, providing special telephone hotlines, counselling, support

> **BOX 6.1 (continued)**
> groups and other services for male victims. In many places, though, such services are either not available or else are very limited — for instance, focusing primarily on women, with few, if any, counsellors on hand who are experienced in discussing problems with male victims.
>
> In most countries, there is much to be done before the issue of sexual violence against men and boys can be properly acknowledged and discussed, free of denial or shame. Such a necessary development, though, will enable more comprehensive prevention measures and better support for the victims to be implemented.

women and girls are illegally traded to India each year and trafficking of Thai women to Japan has also been reported (*32*). Trafficking of women also takes place internally within some countries, often from rural areas to cities.

North America is also an important destination for international trafficking. A study undertaken under the auspices of the United States Central Intelligence Agency, estimated that 45 000–50 000 women and children are trafficked annually to the United States (*63*). Over 150 cases of trafficking were prosecuted between 1996 and 1999 by the United States Department of Justice (*63*). The problem also exists in Europe. A study conducted by the International Organization for Migration estimated that 10–15% of 2000 known foreign prostitutes in Belgium had been forcibly sold from abroad (*30*). In Italy, a study of some 19 000–25 000 foreign prostitutes estimated that 2000 of them had been trafficked (*66*). Most of these women were under 25 years of age, many of them between 15 and 18 years (*30, 66*). Their origin was mainly central and eastern Europe, particularly Albania, as well as Colombia, Nigeria and Peru (*66*).

Sexual violence against sex workers

Whether trafficked or not, sex workers are at high risk for both physical and sexual violence, particularly where sex work is illegal (*67*). A survey of female sex workers in Leeds, England, and Glasgow and Edinburgh, Scotland, revealed that 30% had been slapped, punched or kicked by a client while working, 13% had been beaten, 11% had been raped and 22% had experienced an attempted rape (*68*). Only 34% of those who had suffered violence at the hands of a client reported it to police. A survey

of sex workers in Bangladesh revealed that 49% of the women had been raped and 59% beaten by police in the previous year; the men reported much lower levels of violence (*69*). In Ethiopia, a study of sex workers also found high rates of physical and sexual violence from clients, especially against the child sex workers (*70*).

Sexual violence in schools, health care settings, armed conflicts and refugee settings

Schools

For many young women, the most common place where sexual coercion and harassment are experienced is in school. In an extreme case of violence in 1991, 71 teenage girls were raped by their classmates and 19 others were killed at a boarding school in Meru, Kenya (*71*). While much of the research in this field comes from Africa, it is not clear whether this reflects a particularly high prevalence of the problem or simply the fact that the problem has had a greater visibility there than in other parts of the world.

Harassment of girls by boys is in all likelihood a global problem. In Canada, for example, 23% of girls had experienced sexual harassment while attending school (*72*). The research done in Africa, however, has highlighted the role of teachers there in facilitating or perpetrating sexual coercion. A report by Africa Rights (*28*) found cases of schoolteachers attempting to gain sex, in return for good grades or for not failing pupils, in the Democratic Republic of the Congo, Ghana, Nigeria, Somalia, South Africa, Sudan, Zambia and Zimbabwe. A recent national survey in South Africa that included questions about experience of rape before the age of 15 years found that schoolteachers were responsible for 32% of disclosed child rapes (*34*). In Zimbabwe, a retrospective study of reported cases of child sexual abuse over an 8-year period (1990–1997) found high rates of sexual abuse committed by teachers in rural primary schools. Many of the victims were girls between 11 and 13 years of age and penetrative sex was the most prevalent type of sexual abuse (*73*).

Health care settings

Sexual violence against patients in health facilities has been reported in many places (*74–79*). A study of physicians disciplined for sexual offences in the United States, for instance, found that the number of cases had increased from 42 in 1989 to 147 in 1996, with the proportion of all disciplinary action that was sex-related rising from 2.1% to 4.4% over the same period (*76*). This increase, though, could reflect a greater readiness to lodge complaints.

Other documented forms of sexual violence against female patients include the involvement of medical staff in the practice of clitoridectomy in Egypt (*80*), forced gynaecological examinations and the threat of forced abortions in China (*81*), and inspections of virginity in Turkey (*82*). Sexual violence is part of the broader problem of violence against women patients perpetrated by health workers that has been reported in a large number of countries and until recently has been much neglected (*83–87*). Sexual harassment of female nurses by male doctors has also been reported (*88, 89*).

Armed conflicts and refugee settings

Rape has been used as a strategy in many conflicts, including in Korea during the Second World War and in Bangladesh during the war of independence, as well as in a range of armed conflicts such as those in Algeria (*90*), India (Kashmir) (*91*), Indonesia (*92*), Liberia (*29*), Rwanda and Uganda (*93*). In some armed conflicts – for example, the ones in Rwanda and the states of the former Yugoslavia – rape has been used as a deliberate strategy to subvert community bonds and thus the perceived enemy, and furthermore as a tool of "ethnic cleansing". In East Timor, there were reports of extensive sexual violence against women by the Indonesian military (*94*).

A study in Monrovia, Liberia, found that women under 25 years were more likely than those aged 25 years and over to report experiencing attempted rape and sexual coercion during the conflict (18% compared with 4%) (*29*). Women who were forced to cook for a warring faction were at significantly higher risk.

Another inevitable consequence of armed conflicts is the ensuing economic and social disruption which can force large numbers of people into prostitution (*94*), an observation that applies equally to the situation of refugees, whether they are fleeing armed conflicts or natural disasters such as floods, earthquakes or powerful storms.

Refugees fleeing conflicts and other threatening conditions are often at risk of rape in their new setting. Data from the Office of the United Nations High Commissioner for Refugees, for instance, indicated that among the "boat people" who fled Viet Nam in the late 1970s and early 1980s, 39% of the women were abducted or raped by pirates while at sea – a figure that is likely to be an underestimate (*27*). In many refugee camps as well, including those in Kenya and the United Republic of Tanzania, rape has been found to be a major problem (*95, 96*).

"Customary" forms of sexual violence
Child marriage

Marriage is often used to legitimize a range of forms of sexual violence against women. The custom of marrying off young children, particularly girls, is found in many parts of the world. This practice – legal in many countries – is a form of sexual violence, since the children involved are unable to give or withhold their consent. The majority of them know little or nothing about sex before they are married. They therefore frequently fear it (*97*) and their first sexual encounters are often forced (*98*).

Early marriage is most common in Africa and South Asia, though it also occurs in the Middle East and parts of Latin America and Eastern Europe (*99, 100*). In Ethiopia and parts of West Africa, for instance, marriage at the age of 7 or 8 years is not uncommon. In Nigeria, the mean age at first marriage is 17 years, but in the Kebbi State of northern Nigeria, the average age at first marriage is just over 11 years (*100*). High rates of child marriage have also been reported in the Democratic Republic of the Congo, Mali, Niger and Uganda (*99, 100*).

In South Asia, child marriage is especially common in rural areas, but exists also in urban areas (*100–102*). In Nepal, the average age at first marriage is 19 years. Seven per cent of girls, though, are married before the age of 10 years, and 40% by the age of 15 years (*100*). In India, the median age at first marriage for women is 16.4 years. A survey of 5000 women in the Indian state of Rajasthan found that 56% of the women had married before the age of 15 years, and of these, 17% were married before they were 10 years old. Another survey, conducted in the state of Madhya Pradesh, found that 14% of girls were married between the ages of 10 and 14 years (*100*).

Elsewhere, in Latin America for instance, early age at first marriage has been reported in Cuba, Guatemala, Honduras, Mexico and Paraguay (*99, 100*). In North America and Western Europe, less than 5% of marriages involve girls younger than 19 years of age (for example, 1% in Canada, Switzerland and the United Kingdom, 2% in Belgium and Germany, 3% in Spain, and 4% in the United States) (*103*).

Other customs leading to violence

In many places, there are customs other than child marriage that result in sexual violence towards women. In Zimbabwe, for instance, there is the custom of *ngozi*, whereby a girl can be given to a family as compensation for a death of a man caused by a member of the girl's family. On reaching puberty the girl is expected to have sexual intercourse with the brother or father of the deceased person, so as to produce a son to replace the one who died. Another custom is *chimutsa mapfiwa* – wife inheritance – according to which, when a married woman dies, her sister is obliged to replace her in the matrimonial home.

What are the risk factors for sexual violence?

Explaining sexual violence against women is complicated by the multiple forms it takes and contexts in which it occurs. There is considerable overlap between forms of sexual violence and intimate partner violence; many of the causes are similar to those already discussed in Chapter 4. There are factors increasing the risk of someone being coerced into sex, factors increasing the risk of an individual man forcing sex on another person, and factors within the social environment – including peers and family – influencing the likelihood of rape and the reaction to it. Research suggests that the various factors have an additive effect, so that the more factors present, the greater the likelihood of sexual violence. In addition, a particular factor may vary in importance according to the life stage.

Factors increasing women's vulnerability

One of the most common forms of sexual violence around the world is that which is perpetrated by an intimate partner, leading to the conclusion that one of the most important risk factors for women – in terms of their vulnerability to sexual assault – is being married or cohabiting with a partner. Other factors influencing the risk of sexual violence include:

— being young;
— consuming alcohol or drugs;
— having previously been raped or sexually abused;
— having many sexual partners;
— involvement in sex work;
— becoming more educated and economically empowered, at least where sexual violence perpetrated by an intimate partner is concerned;
— poverty.

Age

Young women are usually found to be more at risk of rape than older women (*24, 62, 104*). According to data from justice systems and rape crisis centres in Chile, Malaysia, Mexico, Papua New Guinea, Peru and the United States, between one-third and two-thirds of all victims of sexual assault are aged 15 years or less (*62, 104*). Certain forms of sexual violence, for instance, are very closely associated with a young age, in particular violence taking place in schools and colleges, and trafficking in women for sexual exploitation.

Alcohol and drug consumption

Increased vulnerability to sexual violence also stems from the use of alcohol and other drugs. Consuming alcohol or drugs makes it more difficult for women to protect themselves by interpreting and effectively acting on warning signs. Drinking alcohol may also place women in settings where their chances of encountering a potential offender are greater (*105*).

Having previously been raped or sexually abused

There is some evidence linking experiences of sexual abuse in childhood or adolescence with patterns of victimization during adulthood (*24, 37, 105–108*). A national study of violence against women in the United States found that women who were raped before the age of 18 years were twice as likely to be raped as adults, compared with those who were not raped as children or adolescents (18.3% and 8.7%, respectively) (*37*). The effects of early sexual abuse may also extend to other forms of victimization and problems in adulthood. For instance, a case–control study in Australia on the long-term impact of abuse reported significant associations between child sexual abuse and experiencing rape, sexual and mental health problems, domestic violence and other problems in intimate relationships – even after accounting for various family background characteristics (*108*). Those who had experienced abuse involving intercourse had more negative outcomes than those suffering other types of coercion.

Having many sexual partners

Young women who have many sexual partners are at increased risk of sexual violence (*105, 107, 109*). It is not clear, though, if having more sexual partners is a cause or consequence of abuse, including childhood sexual abuse. For example,

findings from a representative sample of men and women in León, Nicaragua, found that women who had experienced attempted or completed rape during childhood or adolescence were more likely to have a higher number of sexual partners in adulthood, compared with non-abused or moderately abused women (*110*). Similar findings have been reported in longitudinal studies of young women in New Zealand and Norway (*107, 109*).

Educational level

Women are at increased risk of sexual violence, as they are of physical violence by an intimate partner, when they become more educated and thus more empowered. Women with no education were found in a national survey in South Africa to be much less likely to experience sexual violence than those with higher levels of education (*34*). In Zimbabwe, women who were working were much more likely to report forced sex by a spouse than those who were not (*42*). The likely explanation is that greater empowerment brings with it more resistance from women to patriarchal norms (*111*), so that men may resort to violence in an attempt to regain control. The relationship between empowerment and physical violence is an inverted U-shape – with greater empowerment conferring greater risk up to a certain level, beyond which it starts to become protective (*105, 112*). It is not known, though, whether this is also the case for sexual violence.

Poverty

Poor women and girls may be more at risk of rape in the course of their daily tasks than those who are better off, for example when they walk home on their own from work late at night, or work in the fields or collect firewood alone. Children of poor women may have less parental supervision when not in school, since their mothers may be at work and unable to afford child care. The children themselves may, in fact, be working and thus vulnerable to sexual exploitation.

Poverty forces many women and girls into occupations that carry a relatively high risk of sexual violence (*113*), particularly sex work (*114*). It also creates enormous pressures for them to find

TABLE 6.4
Factors increasing men's risk of committing rape

Individual factors	Relationship factors	Community factors	Societal factors
• Alcohol and drug use • Coercive sexual fantasies and other attitudes and beliefs supportive of sexual violence • Impulsive and antisocial tendencies • Preference for impersonal sex • Hostility towards women • History of sexual abuse as a child • Witnessed family violence as a child	• Associate with sexually aggressive and delinquent peers • Family environment characterized by physical violence and few resources • Strongly patriarchal relationship or family environment • Emotionally unsupportive family environment • Family honour considered more important than the health and safety of the victim	• Poverty, mediated through forms of crisis of male identity • Lack of employment opportunities • Lack of institutional support from police and judicial system • General tolerance of sexual assault within the community • Weak community sanctions against perpetrators of sexual violence	• Societal norms supportive of sexual violence • Societal norms supportive of male superiority and sexual entitlement • Weak laws and policies related to sexual violence • Weak laws and policies related to gender equality • High levels of crime and other forms of violence

or maintain jobs, to pursue trading activities and, if studying, to obtain good grades – all of which render them vulnerable to sexual coercion from those who can promise these things (*28*). Poorer women are also more at risk of intimate partner violence, of which sexual violence is often a manifestation (*41, 115*).

Factors increasing men's risk of committing rape

Data on sexually violent men are somewhat limited and heavily biased towards apprehended rapists, except in the United States, where research has also been conducted on male college students. Despite the limited amount of information on sexually violent men, it appears that sexual violence is found in almost all countries (though with differences in prevalence), in all socioeconomic classes and in all age groups from childhood onwards. Data on sexually violent men also show that most direct their acts at women whom they already know (*116, 117*). Among the factors increasing the risk of a man committing rape are those related to attitudes and beliefs, as well as behaviour arising from situations and social conditions that provide opportunities and support for abuse (see Table 6.4).

Alcohol and drug consumption

Alcohol has been shown to play a disinhibiting role in certain types of sexual assault (*118*), as have some drugs, notably cocaine (*119*). Alcohol has a psychopharmacological effect of reducing inhibitions, clouding judgements and impairing the ability to interpret cues (*120*). The biological links between alcohol and violence are, however, complex (*118*). Research on the social anthropology of alcohol consumption suggests that connections between violence, drinking and drunkenness are socially learnt rather than universal (*121*). Some researchers have noted that alcohol may act as a cultural "break time", providing the opportunity for antisocial behaviour. Thus men are more likely to act violently when drunk because they do not consider that they will be held accountable for their behaviour. Some forms of group sexual violence are also associated with drinking. In these settings, consuming alcohol is an act of group bonding, where inhibitions are collectively reduced and individual judgement ceded in favour of that of the group.

Psychological factors

There has been considerable research in recent times on the role of cognitive variables among the set of factors that can lead to rape. Sexually violent men have been shown to be more likely to consider victims responsible for the rape and are less knowledgeable about the impact of rape on victims (*122*). Such men may misread cues given out by women in social situations and may lack the inhibitions that act to suppress associations between sex and aggression (*122, 123*). They have coercive sexual fantasies (*122, 123*), generally encouraged by access to pornography (*124*), and overall are more hostile towards women than men who are not sexually violent (*106, 125, 126*). In addition to these factors, sexually violent men are believed to differ from other men in terms of impulsivity and antisocial tendencies (*105*). They also tend to have an exaggerated sense of masculinity.

Sexual violence is also associated with a preference for impersonal sexual relationships as opposed to emotional bonding, with having many sexual partners and with the inclination to assert personal interests at the expense of others (*125, 127*). A further association is with adversarial attitudes on gender, that hold that women are opponents to be challenged and conquered (*128*).

Peer and family factors

Gang rape

Some forms of sexual violence, such as gang rape, are predominantly committed by young men (*129*). Sexual aggression is often a defining characteristic of manhood in the group and is significantly related to the wish to be held in high esteem (*130*). Sexually aggressive behaviour among young men has been linked with gang membership and having delinquent peers (*126, 131*). Research also suggests that men with sexually aggressive peers are also much more likely to report coercive or enforced intercourse outside the gang context than men lacking sexually aggressive peers (*132*).

Gang rape is often viewed by the men involved, and sometimes by others too, as legitimate, in that it is seen to discourage or punish perceived "immoral" behaviour among woman – such as wearing short skirts or frequenting bars. For this reason, it may not be equated by the perpetrators with the idea of a crime. In several areas in Papua New Guinea, women can be punished by public gang rape, often sanctioned by elders (*133*).

Early childhood environments

There is evidence to suggest that sexual violence is also a learnt behaviour in some men, particularly as regards child sexual abuse. Studies on sexually abused boys have shown that around one in five continue in later life to molest children themselves (*134*). Such experiences may lead to a pattern of behaviour where the man regularly justifies being violent, denies doing wrong, and has false and unhealthy notions about sexuality.

Childhood environments that are physically violent, emotionally unsupportive and characterized by competition for scarce resources have been associated with sexual violence (*105, 126, 131, 135*). Sexually aggressive behaviour in young men, for instance, has been linked to witnessing family violence, and having emotionally distant and uncaring fathers (*126, 131*). Men raised in families with strongly patriarchal structures are also more likely to become violent, to rape and use sexual coercion against women, as well as to abuse their intimate partners, than men raised in homes that are more egalitarian (*105*).

Family honour and sexual purity

Another factor involving social relationships is a family response to sexual violence that blames women without punishing men, concentrating instead on restoring "lost" family honour. Such a response creates an environment in which rape can occur with impunity.

While families will often try to protect their women from rape and may also put their daughters on contraception to prevent visible signs should it occur (*136*), there is rarely much social pressure to control young men or persuade them that coercing sex is wrong. Instead, in some countries, there is frequently support for family members to do whatever is necessary – including murder – to alleviate the "shame" associated with a rape or other sexual transgression. In a review of all crimes of honour occurring in Jordan in 1995 (*137*), researchers found that in over 60% of the cases, the victim died from multiple gunshot wounds – mostly at the hands of a brother. In cases where the victim was a single pregnant female, the offender was either acquitted of murder or received a reduced sentence.

Even though poverty is often the driving force behind child marriage, factors such as maintaining the sexual purity of a young girl and protecting her from premarital sex, HIV infection and unwelcome sexual advances are also reasons commonly given by families to justify such marriages (*100*).

Community factors

Poverty

Poverty is linked to both the perpetration of sexual violence and the risk of being a victim of it. Several authors have argued that the relationship between poverty and perpetration of sexual violence is mediated through forms of crisis of masculine identity (*95, 112, 138–140*). Bourgois, writing about life in East Harlem, New York, United States (*138*), described how young men felt pressured by models of "successful" masculinity and family structure passed down from their parents' and grandparents' generations, together with modern-day ideals of manhood that also place an emphasis on material consumption. Trapped in their slums, with little or no available employment, they are unlikely to attain either of these models or expectations of masculine "success". In these circumstances, ideals of masculinity are reshaped to emphasize misogyny, substance abuse and participation in crime (*138*) – and often also xenophobia and racism. Gang rape and sexual conquest are normalized, as men turn their aggression against women they can no longer control patriarchally or support economically.

Physical and social environment

While fear of rape is typically associated with being outside the home (*141, 142*), the great majority of sexual violence actually occurs in the home of the victim or the abuser. Nonetheless, abduction by a stranger is quite often the prelude to a rape and the opportunities for such an abduction are influenced by the physical environment.

The social environment within a community is, however, usually more important than the physical surrounding. How deeply entrenched in a community beliefs in male superiority and male entitlement to sex are will greatly affect the likelihood of sexual violence taking place, as will the general tolerance in the community of sexual

assault and the strength of sanctions, if any, against perpetrators (*116, 143*). For instance, in some places, rape can even occur in public, with passers-by refusing to intervene (*133*). Complaints of rape may also be treated leniently by the police, particularly if the assault is committed during a date or by the victim's husband. Where police investigations and court cases do proceed, the procedures may well be either extremely lax or else corrupt – for instance, with legal papers being "lost" in return for a bribe.

Societal factors

Factors operating at a societal level that influence sexual violence include laws and national policies relating to gender equality in general and to sexual violence more specifically, as well as norms relating to the use of violence. While the various factors operate largely at local level, within families, schools, workplaces and communities, there are also influences from the laws and norms working at national and even international level.

Laws and policies

There are considerable variations between countries in their approach to sexual violence. Some countries have far-reaching legislation and legal procedures, with a broad definition of rape that includes marital rape, and with heavy penalties for those convicted and a strong response in supporting victims. Commitment to preventing or controlling sexual violence is also reflected in an emphasis on police training and an appropriate allocation of police resources to the problem, in the priority given to investigating cases of sexual assault, and in the resources made available to support victims and provide medico-legal services. At the other end of the scale, there are countries with much weaker approaches to the issue – where conviction of an alleged perpetrator on the evidence of the women alone is not allowed, where certain forms or settings of sexual violence are specifically excluded from the legal definition, and where rape victims are strongly deterred from bringing the matter to court through the fear of being punished for filing an "unproven" rape suit.

Social norms

Sexual violence committed by men is to a large extent rooted in ideologies of male sexual entitlement. These belief systems grant women extremely few legitimate options to refuse sexual advances (*139, 144, 145*). Many men thus simply exclude the possibility that their sexual advances towards a woman might be rejected or that a woman has the right to make an autonomous decision about participating in sex. In many cultures women, as well as men, regard marriage as entailing the obligation on women to be sexually available virtually without limit (*34, 146*), though sex may be culturally proscribed at certain times, such as after childbirth or during menstruation (*147*).

Societal norms around the use of violence as a means to achieve objectives have been strongly associated with the prevalence of rape. In societies where the ideology of male superiority is strong – emphasizing dominance, physical strength and male honour – rape is more common (*148*). Countries with a culture of violence, or where violent conflict is taking place, experience an increase in almost all forms of violence, including sexual violence (*148–151*).

Global trends and economic factors

Many of the factors operating at a national level have an international dimension. Global trends, for instance towards free trade, have been accompanied by an increase in the movement around the world of women and girls for labour, including for sex work (*152*). Economic structural adjustment programmes, drawn up by international agencies, have accentuated poverty and unemployment in a number of countries, thereby increasing the likelihood of sexual trafficking and sexual violence (*153*) – something particularly noted in Central America, the Caribbean (*114*) and parts of Africa (*113*).

The consequences of sexual violence

Physical force is not necessarily used in rape, and physical injuries are not always a consequence. Deaths associated with rape are known to occur, though the prevalence of fatalities varies consider-ably across the world. Among the more common consequences of sexual violence are those related to reproductive, mental health and social well-being.

Pregnancy and gynaecological complications

Pregnancy may result from rape, though the rate varies between settings and depends particularly on the extent to which non-barrier contraceptives are being used. A study of adolescents in Ethiopia found that among those who reported being raped, 17% became pregnant after the rape (*154*), a figure which is similar to the 15–18% reported by rape crisis centres in Mexico (*155, 156*). A longitudinal study in the United States of over 4000 women followed for 3 years found that the national rape-related pregnancy rate was 5.0% per rape among victims aged 12–45 years, producing over 32 000 pregnancies nationally among women from rape each year (*7*). In many countries, women who have been raped are forced to bear the child or else put their lives at risk with back-street abortions.

Experience of coerced sex at an early age reduces a woman's ability to see her sexuality as something over which she has control. As a result, it is less likely that an adolescent girl who has been forced into sex will use condoms or other forms of contraception, increasing the likelihood of her becoming pregnant (*4, 16, 157, 158*). A study of factors associated with teenage pregnancy in Cape Town, South Africa, found that forced sexual initiation was the third most strongly related factor, after frequency of intercourse and use of modern contraceptives (*4*). Forced sex can also result in unintended pregnancy among adult women. In India, a study of married men revealed that men who admitted forcing sex on their wives were 2.6 times more likely to have caused an unintended pregnancy than those who did not admit to such behaviour (*41*).

Gynaecological complications have been con-sistently found to be related to forced sex. These include vaginal bleeding or infection, fibroids, decreased sexual desire, genital irritation, pain during intercourse, chronic pelvic pain and urinary tract infections (*8–15*). Women who experience both physical and sexual abuse from intimate partners are at higher risk of health problems generally than those experiencing physical violence alone (*8, 14*).

Sexually transmitted diseases

HIV infection and other sexually transmitted diseases are recognized consequences of rape (*159*). Research on women in shelters has shown that women who experience both sexual and physical abuse from intimate partners are significantly more likely to have had sexually transmitted diseases (*160*). For women who have been trafficked into sex work, the risks of HIV and other sexually transmitted diseases are likely to be particularly high. The links between HIV and sexual violence, and the relevant prevention strategies, are discussed in Box 6.2.

Mental health

Sexual violence has been associated with a number of mental health and behavioural problems in adolescence and adulthood (*17–20, 22, 23, 161*). In one population-based study, the prevalence of symptoms or signs suggestive of a psychiatric disorder was 33% in women with a history of sexual abuse as adults, 15% in women with a history of physical violence by an intimate partner and 6% in non-abused women (*162*). Sexual violence by an intimate partner aggravates the effects of physical violence on mental health.

Abused women reporting experiences of forced sex are at significantly greater risk of depression and post-traumatic stress disorder than non-abused women (*14, 18, 22, 23*). Post-traumatic stress disorder after rape is more likely if there is injury during the rape, or a history of depression or alcohol abuse (*24*). A study of adolescents in France also found a relationship between having been raped and current sleep difficulties, depressive symptoms, somatic complaints, tobacco consumption and behavioural problems (such as aggressive behaviour, theft and truancy) (*163*). In the absence of trauma counselling, negative psychological effects have been known to persist for at least a year following a rape, while physical

health problems and symptoms tend to decrease over such a period (*164*). Even with counselling, up to 50% of women retain symptoms of stress (*165–167*).

Suicidal behaviour

Women who experience sexual assault in childhood or adulthood are more likely to attempt or commit suicide than other women (*21, 168 173*). The association remains, even after controlling for sex, age, education, symptoms of post-traumatic stress disorder and the presence of psychiatric disorders (*168, 174*). The experience of being raped or sexually assaulted can lead to suicidal behaviour as early as adolescence. In Ethiopia, 6% of raped schoolgirls reported having attempted suicide (*154*). A study of adolescents in Brazil found prior sexual abuse to be a leading factor predicting several health risk behaviours, including suicidal thoughts and attempts (*161*).

Experiences of severe sexual harassment can also result in emotional disturbances and suicidal behaviour. A study of female adolescents in Canada found that 15% of those experiencing frequent, unwanted sexual contact had exhibited suicidal behaviour in the previous 6 months, compared with 2% of those who had not had such harassment (*72*).

Social ostracization

In many cultural settings it is held that men are unable to control their sexual urges and that women are responsible for provoking sexual desire in men (*144*). How families and communities react to acts of rape in such settings is governed by prevailing ideas about sexuality and the status of women.

In some societies, the cultural "solution" to rape is that the woman should marry the rapist, thereby preserving the integrity of the woman and her family by legitimizing the union (*175*). Such a "solution" is reflected in the laws of some countries, which allow a man who commits rape to be excused his crime if he marries the victim (*100*). Apart from marriage, families may put pressure on the woman not to report or pursue a case or else to concentrate on

> **BOX 6.2**
>
> ## Sexual violence and HIV/AIDS
>
> Violent or forced sex can increase the risk of transmitting HIV. In forced vaginal penetration, abrasions and cuts commonly occur, thus facilitating the entry of the virus — when it is present — through the vaginal mucosa. Adolescent girls are particularly susceptible to HIV infection through forced sex, and even through unforced sex, because their vaginal mucous membrane has not yet acquired the cellular density providing an effective barrier that develops in the later teenage years. Those who suffer anal rape — boys and men, as well as girls and women — are also considerably more susceptible to HIV than would be the case if the sex were not forced, since anal tissues can be easily damaged, again allowing the virus an easier entry into the body.
>
> Being a victim of sexual violence and being susceptible to HIV share a number of risk behaviours. Forced sex in childhood or adolescence, for instance, increases the likelihood of engaging in unprotected sex, having multiple partners, participating in sex work, and substance abuse. People who experience forced sex in intimate relationships often find it difficult to negotiate condom use — either because using a condom could be interpreted as mistrust of their partner or as an admission of promiscuity, or else because they fear experiencing violence from their partner. Sexual coercion among adolescents and adults is also associated with low self-esteem and depression — factors that are associated with many of the risk behaviours for HIV infection.
>
> Being infected with HIV or having an HIV-positive family member can also increase the risk of suffering sexual violence, particularly for women. Because of the stigma attached to HIV and AIDS in many countries, an infected woman may be evicted from her home. In addition, an AIDS-related illness or death in a poor household may make the economic situation desperate. Women may be forced into sex work and consequently be at increased risk for both HIV/AIDS and sexual violence. Children orphaned by AIDS, impoverished and with no one to care for them, may be forced to live on the streets, at considerable risk of sexual abuse.
>
> Among the various ways of reducing the incidence of both sexual violence and HIV infection, education is perhaps the foremost. For young people, above all, there must be comprehensive interventions in schools and other educational institutes, youth groups and workplaces. School curricula should cover relevant aspects of sexual and reproductive health, relationships and violence. They should also teach life skills, including how to avoid risky or threatening situations — related to such things as violence, sex or drugs — and how to negotiate safe sexual behaviour.
>
> For the adult population in general there should be full and accessible information on sexual health and the consequences of specific sexual practices, as well as interventions to change harmful patterns of behaviour and social norms that hinder communication on sexual matters.
>
> It is important that health care workers and other service providers receive integrated training on gender and reproductive health, including gender-based violence and sexually transmitted diseases such as HIV infection.
>
> For rape victims, there should be screening and referral for HIV infection. Also, the use of postexposure prophylaxis for HIV — given soon after the assault, together with counselling — may be considered. Similarly, women with HIV should be screened for a possible history of sexual violence. Voluntary counselling programmes for HIV should consider incorporating violence prevention strategies.

obtaining financial "damages" from the rapist's family (*42, 176*). Men may reject their wives if they have been raped (*27*) and in some countries, as mentioned previously, restoring lost honour calls for the woman to be cast out – or in extreme cases, murdered (*26*).

What can be done to prevent sexual violence?

The number of initiatives addressing sexual violence is limited and few have been evaluated. Most interventions have been developed and implemented in industrialized countries. How relevant they may be in other settings is not well known. The interventions that have been developed can be categorized as follows.

Individual approaches

Psychological care and support

Counselling, therapy and support group initiatives have been found to be helpful following sexual assaults, especially where there may be complicating factors related to the violence itself or the process of recovery. There is some evidence that a brief cognitive-behavioural programme administered shortly after assault can hasten the rate of improvement of psychological damage arising from trauma (*177, 178*). As already mentioned, victims of sexual violence sometimes blame themselves for the incident, and addressing this in psychological therapy has also been shown to be important for recovery (*179*). Short-term counselling and treatment programmes after acts of sexual violence, though, require considerable further evaluation.

Formal psychological support for those experiencing sexual violence has been provided largely by the nongovernmental sector, particularly rape crisis centres and various women's organizations. Inevitably, the number of victims of sexual violence with access to these services is small. One solution to extend access is through establishing telephone helplines, ideally ones that are free of charge. A "Stop Woman Abuse" helpline in South Africa, for example, answered 150 000 calls in the first 5 months of operation (*180*).

Programmes for perpetrators

The few programmes targeting perpetrators of sexual violence have generally been aimed at men convicted of assault. They are found mainly in industrialized countries and have only recently begun to be evaluated (see Chapter 4 for a discussion of such programmes). A common response of men who commit sexual violence is to deny both that they are responsible and that what they are doing is violent (*146, 181*). To be effective, programmes working with perpetrators need to make them admit responsibility and to be publicly seen as responsible for their actions (*182*). One way of achieving this is for programmes that target male perpetrators of sexual violence to collaborate with support services for victims as well as with campaigns against sexual violence.

Life-skills and other educational programmes

In recent years, several programmes for sexual and reproductive health promotion, particularly those promoting HIV prevention, have begun to introduce gender issues and to address the problem of sexual and physical violence against women. Two notable examples – developed for Africa but used in many parts of the developing world – are "Stepping Stones" and "Men As Partners" (*183, 184*). These programmes have been designed for use in peer groups of men and women and are delivered over several workshop sessions using participatory learning approaches. Their comprehensive approach helps men, who might otherwise be reluctant to attend programmes solely concerned with violence against women, participate and discuss a range of issues concerning violence. Furthermore, even if the men are perpetrators of sexual violence, the programmes are careful to avoid labelling them as such.

A review of the effect of the Stepping Stones programme in Africa and Asia found that the workshops helped the men participating take greater responsibility for their actions, relate better to others, have greater respect for women and communicate more effectively. As a result of the programme, reductions in violence against women have been reported in communities in Cambodia, the Gambia, South Africa, Uganda and the United Republic of Tanzania. The evaluations to date, though, have generally used qualitative methods and further research is needed to adequately test the effectiveness of this programme (*185*).

Developmental approaches

Research has stressed the importance of encouraging nurturing, with better and more gender-balanced parenting, to prevent sexual violence (124, 125). At the same time, Schwartz (186) has developed a prevention model that adopts a developmental approach, with interventions before birth, during childhood and in adolescence and young adulthood. In this model, the prenatal element would include discussions of parenting skills, the stereotyping of gender roles, stress, conflict and violence. In the early years of childhood, health providers would pursue these issues and introduce child sexual abuse and exposure to violence in the media to the list of discussion topics, as well as promoting the use of non-sexist educational materials. In later childhood, health promotion would include modelling behaviours and attitudes that avoid stereotyping, encouraging children to distinguish between "good" and "bad" touching, and enhancing their ability and confidence to take control over their own bodies. This intervention would allow room for talking about sexual aggression. During adolescence and young adulthood, discussions would cover myths about rape, how to set boundaries for sexual activity, and breaking the links between sex, violence and coercion. While Schwartz's model was designed for use in industrialized countries, some of the principles involved could be applicable to developing countries.

Health care responses

Medico-legal services

In many countries, where sexual violence is reported the health sector has the duty to collect medical and legal evidence to corroborate the accounts of the victims or to help in identifying the perpetrator. Research in Canada suggests that medico-legal documentation can increase the chance of a perpetrator being arrested, charged or convicted (187, 188). For instance, one study found that documented physical injury, particularly of the moderate to severe type, was associated with charges being filed – irrespective of the patient's income level or whether the patient knew the assailant,

either as an acquaintance or an intimate partner (188). However, a study of women attending a hospital in Nairobi, Kenya, following a rape, has highlighted the fact that in many countries rape victims are not examined by a gynaecologist or an experienced police examiner and that no standard protocols or guidelines exist on this matter (189).

The use of standard protocols and guidelines can significantly improve the quality of treatment and psychological support of victims, as well as the evidence that is collected (190). Comprehensive protocols and guidelines for female victims of assault should include:

— recording a full description of the incident, listing all the assembled evidence;
— listing the gynaecological and contraceptive history of the victim;
— documenting in a standard way the results of a full physical examination;
— assessment of the risk of pregnancy;
— testing for and treating sexually transmitted diseases, including, where appropriate, testing for HIV;
— providing emergency contraception and, where legal, counselling on abortion;
— providing psychological support and referral.

In some countries, the protocol forms part of the procedure of a "sexual assault evidence kit" that includes instructions and containers for collecting evidence, appropriate legal forms and documents for recording histories (191). Examinations of rape victims are by their nature extremely stressful. The use of a video to explain the procedure before an examination has been shown significantly to reduce the stress involved (192).

Training for health care professionals

Issues concerning sexual violence need to be addressed in the training of all health service staff, including psychiatrists and counsellors, in basic training as well as in specialized postgraduate courses. Such training should, in the first place, give health care workers greater knowledge and awareness of sexual violence and make them more able to detect and handle cases of abuse in a sensitive but effective way. It should also help reduce instances of sexual abuse within the health sector, something that can be a significant, though generally unacknowledged, problem.

In the Philippines, the Task Force on Social Science and Reproductive Health, a body that includes doctors, nurses and social scientists and is supported by the Department of Health, has produced training modules for nursing and medical students on gender-based violence. The aims of this programme are (*193*):

- To understand the roots of violence in the context of culture, gender and other social aspects.
- To identify situations, within families or homes that are at a high risk for violence, where it would be appropriate to undertake:
  - primary interventions, in particular in collaboration with other professionals;
  - secondary interventions, including identifying victims of violence, understanding basic legal procedures and how to present evidence, referring and following up patients, and helping victims reintegrate into society.

These training modules are built into the curricula for both nursing and medical students. For the nursing curriculum, the eleven modules are spread over the 4 years of formal instruction, and for medical students over their final 3 years of practical training.

Prophylaxis for HIV infection

The possibility of transmission of HIV during rape is a major cause for concern, especially in countries with a high prevalence of HIV infection (*194*). The use of antiretroviral drugs following exposure to HIV is known in certain contexts to be reasonably effective. For instance, the administration of the antiretroviral drug zidovudine (AZT) to health workers following an occupational needle-stick exposure (puncturing the skin with a contaminated needle) has been shown to reduce the subsequent risk of developing HIV infection by 81% (*195*).

The average risk of HIV infection from a single act of unprotected vaginal sex with an infected partner is relatively low (approximately 1–2 per 1000, from male to female, and around 0.5–1 per 1000 from female to male). This risk, in fact, is of a similar order to that from a needle-stick injury (around 3 per 1000), for which postexposure prophylaxis is now routine treatment (*196*). The average risk of HIV infection from unprotected anal sex is considerably higher, though, at around 5–30 per 1000. However, during rape, because of the force used, it is very much more likely that there will be macroscopic or microscopic tears to the vaginal mucosa, something that will greatly increase the probability of HIV transmission (*194*).

There is no information about the feasibility or cost-effectiveness in resource-poor settings of routinely offering rape victims prophylaxis for HIV. Testing for HIV infection after rape is difficult in any case. In the immediate aftermath of an incident, many women are not in a position fully to comprehend complicated information about HIV testing and risks. Ensuring proper follow-up is also difficult as many victims will not attend further scheduled visits for reasons that probably relate to their psychological coping following the assault. The side-effects of antiretroviral treatment may also be significant, causing people to drop out from a course (*195, 197*), though those who perceive themselves as being at high risk are much more likely to be compliant (*197*).

Despite the lack of knowledge about the effectiveness of HIV prophylaxis following rape, many organizations have recommended its use. For instance, medical aid schemes in high-income countries are increasingly including it in their care packages. Research is urgently needed in middle-income and low-income countries on the effectiveness of antiretroviral treatment after rape and how it could be included in patient care.

Centres providing comprehensive care to victims of sexual assault

Because of the shortage of doctors in many countries, specially trained nurses have been used in some places to assist victims of sexual assault (*187*). In Canada, nurses, known as "sexual assault nurse examiners", are trained to provide comprehensive care to victims of sexual violence. These nurses refer clients to a physician when medical intervention is needed. In the province of Ontario, Canada, the first sexual assault care centre opened in 1984 and since then 26 others have been established. These centres provide or coordinate a wide range of services, including emergency medical care and medical follow-up, counselling, collecting forensic evidence of assault, legal support, and community consultation and education (*198*). Centres that provide a range of services for victims of sexual assault, often located in places such as a hospital or police station, are being developed in many countries (see Box 6.3). Specialized centres such as these have the advantage of providing appropriately trained and experienced staff. In some places, on the other hand, integrated centres exist providing services for victims of different forms of violence.

Community-based efforts
Prevention campaigns

Attempts to change public attitudes towards sexual violence using the media have included advertising on hoardings ("billboards") and in public transport, and on radio and television. Television has been used effectively in South Africa and Zimbabwe. The South African prime-time television series *Soul City* is described in Box 9.1 of Chapter 9. In Zimbabwe, the nongovernmental organization Musasa has produced awareness-raising initiatives using theatre, public meetings and debates, as well as a television series where survivors of violence described their experiences (*199*).

Other initiatives, besides media campaigns, have been used in many countries. The Sisterhood Is Global Institute in Montreal, Canada, for instance, has developed a manual suitable for Muslim communities aimed at raising awareness and

---

BOX 6.3

Integrated services for rape victims in Malaysian hospitals

In 1993, the first "One-Stop Crisis Centre" for battered women was established in the accident and emergency department of Kuala Lumpur Hospital in Malaysia. Its aim was to provide a coordinated interagency response to violence against women, in such a way as to enable victims of assault to address their medical, legal, psychological and social problems at a single location. Initially, the centre dealt exclusively with domestic violence, but has since extended its scope to cover rape, with specific procedures for victims of rape.

At Kuala Lumpur Hospital, a crisis intervention team handles around 30 rape cases and 70 cases of domestic violence each month. This team brings in expertise from the hospital itself and from various women's groups, the police, the department of medical social workers, the legal aid office and the Islamic Religious Bureau.

In 1996, the Malaysian Ministry of Health decided to extend this innovative health care strategy and to establish similar centres in every public hospital of the country. Within 3 years, 34 such centres had been set up. In these centres, psychiatrists, counsellors and medical social workers carry out counselling on rape, and some of the clients become outpatients in the hospital's psychiatric department. Trained social workers need to be on call 24 hours a day.

As the "One-Stop Crisis Centre" programme developed, various problems came to light. One was the need for hospital staff to be better trained in handling issues of sexual violence with sensitivity. Some hospital workers were seen to blame victims of rape for the violence they had suffered, while others regarded the victims with voyeuristic curiosity instead of concentrating on providing support. There was also a lack of forensic medical officers and of sufficient sheltered accommodation for rape victims. Identifying these problems was an important first step towards improving the programme and providing a higher quality of service for rape victims.

stimulating debate on issues related to gender equality and violence against women and girls (*200*). The manual has been pilot-tested in Egypt, Jordan and Lebanon and – in an adaptation for non-Muslim settings – used in Zimbabwe.

A United Nations interagency initiative to combat gender-based violence is being conducted in 16 countries of Latin America and the Caribbean (*201*). The campaign is designed:

— to raise awareness about the human, social and economic costs of violence against women and girls;

— to build capacity at the governmental level to develop and implement legislation against gender violence;

— to strengthen networks of public and private organizations and carry out programmes to prevent violence against women and girls.

Community activism by men

An important element in preventing sexual and physical violence against women is a collective initiative by men. Men's groups against domestic violence and rape can be found in Australia, Africa, Latin America and the Caribbean and Asia, and in many parts of North America and Europe. The underlying starting point for this type of initiative is that men as individuals should take measures to reduce their use of violence (*202*). Typical activities include group discussions, education campaigns and rallies, work with violent men, and workshops in schools, prisons and workplaces. Actions are frequently conducted in collaboration with women's organizations that are involved in preventing violence and providing services to abused women.

In the United States alone, there are over 100 such men's groups, many of which focus specifically on sexual violence. The "Men Can Stop Rape" group in Washington, DC, for instance, seeks to promote alternative forms of masculinity that foster non-violence and gender equality. Its recent activities have included conducting presentations in secondary schools, designing posters, producing a handbook for teachers and publishing a youth magazine (*202*).

School-based programmes

Action in schools is vital for reducing sexual and other forms of violence. In many countries a sexual relation between a teacher and a pupil is not a serious disciplinary offence and policies on sexual harassment in schools either do not exist or are not implemented. In recent years, though, some countries have introduced laws prohibiting sexual relations between teachers and pupils. Such measures are important in helping eradicate sexual harassment in schools. At the same time, a wider range of actions is also needed, including changes to teacher training and recruitment and reforms of curricula, so as to transform gender relations in schools.

Legal and policy responses
Reporting and handling cases of sexual violence

Many countries have a system to encourage people to report incidents of sexual violence to the police and to improve the speed and sensitivity of the processing of cases by the courts. The specific mechanisms include dedicated domestic violence units, sexual crime units, gender training for the police and court officials, women-only police stations and courts for rape offences. Some of these mechanisms are discussed in Chapter 4.

Problems are sometimes created by the unwillingness of medical experts to attend court. The reason for this is frequently that the court schedules are unpredictable, with cases often postponed at short notice and long waits for witnesses who are to give short testimonies. In South Africa, to counter this, the Directorate of Public Prosecutions has been training magistrates to interrupt proceedings in sexual violence cases when the medical expert arrives so that testimonies can be taken and witnesses cross-examined without delay.

Legal reform

Legal interventions that have been adopted in many places have included:

— broadening the definition of rape;

— reforming the rules on sentencing and on admissibility of evidence;

— removing the requirements for victims' accounts to be corroborated.

In 1983, the Canadian laws on rape were reformed, in particular removing the requirement that accounts of rape be corroborated. Nonetheless, an evaluation has found that the prosecutors have tended to ignore this easing of the requirement for corroboration and that few cases go to court without forensic evidence (*203*).

Several countries in Asia, including the Philippines, have recently enacted legislation radically redefining rape and mandating state assistance to victims. The result has been a substantial increase in the number of reported cases. Campaigns to inform the general public of their legal rights must also take place if the reformed legislation is to be fully effective.

To ensure that irrelevant information was not admitted in court, the International Criminal Tribunal for the Former Yugoslavia drew up certain rules, which could serve as a useful model for effective laws and procedures elsewhere. Rule 96 of the Tribunal specifies that in cases of sexual assault there is no need for corroboration of the victim's testimony and that the earlier sexual history of the victim is not to be disclosed as evidence. The rule also deals with the possible claim by the accused that there was consent to the act, stating that consent as a defence shall not be allowed if the victim has been subjected to or threatened with physical or psychological violence, or detention, or has had reason to fear such violence or detention. Furthermore, consent shall not be allowed under the rule if the victim had good reason to believe that if he or she did not submit, another person might be so subjected, threatened or put in fear. Even where the claim of consent is allowed to proceed, the accused has to satisfy the court that the evidence for such a claim is relevant and credible, before this evidence can be presented.

In many countries, judges hand out particularly short sentences for sexual violence (*204, 205*). One way of overcoming this has been to introduce minimum sentencing for convictions for rape, unless there are extenuating circumstances.

International treaties

International treaties are important as they set standards for national legislation and provide a lever for local groups to campaign for legal reforms.

Among the relevant treaties that impinge on sexual violence and its prevention include:

— the Convention on the Elimination of All Forms of Discrimination Against Women (1979);
— the Convention on the Rights of the Child (1989) and its Optional Protocol on the Sale of Children, Child Prostitution and Child Pornography (2000);
— the Convention Against Transnational Organized Crime (2000) and its supplemental Protocol to Prevent, Suppress and Punish Trafficking in Persons, Especially Women and Children (2000);
— the Convention Against Torture and Other Cruel, Inhuman or Degrading Treatment or Punishment (1984).

A number of other international agreements set norms and limits of behaviour, including behaviour in conflicts, that necessitate provisions in national legislation. The Rome Statute of the International Criminal Court (1998), for instance, covers a broad spectrum of gender-specific crimes, including rape, sexual slavery, enforced prostitution, forced pregnancy and forced sterilization. It also includes certain forms of sexual violence that constitute a breach or serious violation of the 1949 Geneva Conventions, as well as other forms of sexual violence that are comparable in gravity to crimes against humanity. The inclusion of gender crimes in the definitions of the statute is an important historical development in international law (*206*).

Actions to prevent other forms of sexual violence

Sexual trafficking

Initiatives to prevent the trafficking of people for sexual purposes have generally aimed to:

— create economic programmes in certain countries for women at risk of being trafficked;
— provide information and raise awareness so that women at potential risk are aware of the danger of trafficking.

In addition, several government programmes and nongovernmental organizations are developing services for the victims of trafficking (*207*). In Cyprus, the Aliens and Immigration Department approaches women entering the country to work in the entertainment or domestic service sectors. The Department advises the women on their rights and obligations and on available forms of protection against abuse, exploitation and procurement into prostitution. In the European Union and the United States, victims of trafficking willing to cooperate with the judicial system in prosecuting traffickers can receive temporary residence permits. In Belgium and Italy, shelters have been set up for victims of trafficking. In Mumbai, India, an anti-trafficking centre has been set up to facilitate the arrest and prosecution of offenders, and to provide assistance and information to trafficked women.

Female genital mutilation

Addressing cultural practices that are sexually violent requires an understanding of their social, cultural and economic context. Khafagi has argued (*208*) that such practices – which include female genital mutilation – should be understood from the perspective of those who perform them and that such knowledge can be used to design culturally appropriate interventions to prevent the practices. In the Kapchorwa district of Uganda, the REACH programme has been successful in reducing rates of female genital mutilation. The programme, led by the Sabiny Elders' Association, sought to enlist the support of elders in the community in detaching the practice of female genital mutilation from the cultural values it purported to serve. In its place, alternative activities were substituted, that upheld the original cultural tradition (*209*). Box 6.4 describes another programme, in Egypt, to prevent female genital mutilation.

Child marriage

Child marriage has a cultural basis and is often legal, so the task of achieving change is considerable. Simply outlawing early marriages will not, of itself, usually be sufficient to prevent the practice. In many countries the process of registering births is so irregular that age at first marriage may not be known (*100*). Approaches that address poverty –

an important factor underlying many such marriages – and those that stress educational goals, the health consequences of early childbirth and the rights of children are more likely to achieve results.

Rape during armed conflicts

The issue of sexual violence in armed conflicts has recently again been brought to the fore by organizations such as the Association of the Widows of the Genocide (AVEGA) and the Forum for African Women Educationalists. The former has supported war widows and rape victims in Rwanda and the latter has provided medical care and counselling to victims in Sierra Leone (*210*).

In 1995, the Office of the United Nations High Commissioner for Refugees released guidelines on the prevention of and response to sexual violence among refugee populations (*211*). These guidelines include provisions for:

— the design and planning of camps, to reduce susceptibility to violence;

— documenting cases;

— educating and training staff to identify, respond to and prevent sexual violence;

— medical care and other support services, including procedures to avoid further trauma to victims.

The guidelines also cover public awareness campaigns, educational activities and the setting up of women's groups to report and respond to violence.

Based on work in Guinea (*212*) and the United Republic of Tanzania (*96*), the International Rescue Committee has developed a programme to combat sexual violence in refugee communities. It includes the use of participatory methods to assess the prevalence of sexual and gender-based violence in refugee populations, the training and deployment of community workers to identify cases and set up appropriate prevention systems, and measures for community leaders and other officials to prosecute perpetrators. The programme has been used in many places against sexual and gender-based violence, including Bosnia and Herzegovina, the Democratic Republic of the Congo, East Timor, Kenya, Sierra Leone and The former Yugoslav Republic of Macedonia.

BOX 6.4

Putting an end to female genital mutilation: the case of Egypt

Female genital mutilation is extremely common among married women in Egypt. The 1995 Demographic and Health Survey found that the age group in which the practice was most frequently used was 9–13 years. Nearly half of those performing female circumcisions were doctors and 32% were midwives or nurses. Sociological research has found that the main reasons given for practising female circumcision were to uphold tradition, to control the sexual desires of women, to make women "clean and pure" and, most importantly, to make them eligible for marriage.

Largely stemming from the public awareness created by the International Conference on Population and Development held in Cairo in 1994, a movement against female genital mutilation, spanning a broad range of sectors, was built up.

In terms of the response from health officials and professionals, a joint statement in 1998 from the Egyptian Society of Gynaecology and Obstetrics and the Egyptian Fertility Care Society declared that female genital mutilation was both useless and harmful, and constituted unethical practice for a doctor. The Egyptian Minister of Health and Population also issued a decree banning anyone from performing female genital mutilation.

Religious leaders in the Muslim world also voiced their opposition to the practice. The Grand Mufti put out a statement pointing out that there was no mention of female circumcision in the Koran and that sayings (*hadith*) attributed to the Prophet Muhammad on the subject were not definitively confirmed by evidence. Furthermore, in 1998, the Conference on Population and Reproductive Health in the Muslim World adopted a recommendation calling on Islamic countries to move to end all forms of violence against women, with a reminder that under Islamic law (*sharia*) no obligation existed to circumcise girls.

Egyptian nongovernmental organizations have mobilized on the issue, disseminating information on female genital mutilation and including it in community development, health awareness and other programmes. A task force of some 60 nongovernmental organizations has been set up to combat the practice.

Several nongovernmental organizations — often working through male community leaders — are now actively involving men, educating them about the dangers of female genital mutilation. In this process, young men are being encouraged to declare that they will marry uncircumcised women.

In Upper Egypt there is a programme aimed at various social groups — including community leaders, religious leaders and professional people — to train them as campaigners against female genital mutilation. Counselling is also offered to families who are considering not circumcising their daughters and discussions are conducted with health workers to dissuade them from performing the practice.

Recommendations

Sexual violence has generally been a neglected area of research in most parts of the world, yet the evidence suggests that it is a public health problem of substantial proportions. Much more needs to be done both to understand the phenomenon and to prevent it.

More research

The lack of an agreed definition of sexual violence and the paucity of data describing the nature and extent of the problem worldwide have contributed to its lack of visibility on the agendas of policy-makers and donors. There is a need for substantial further research on almost every aspect of sexual violence, including:

— the incidence and prevalence of sexual violence in a range of settings, using a standard research tool for measuring sexual coercion;

— the risk factors for being a victim or a perpetrator of sexual violence;

— the health and social consequences of different forms of sexual violence;

— the factors influencing recovery of health following a sexual assault;

— the social contexts of different forms of sexual violence, including sexual trafficking, and the relationships between sexual violence and other forms of violence.

Determining effective responses

Interventions must also be studied to produce a better understanding of what is effective in different settings for preventing sexual violence and for treating and supporting victims. The following areas should be given priority:

- Documenting and evaluating services and interventions that support survivors or work with perpetrators of sexual violence.
- Determining the most appropriate health sector responses to sexual violence, including the role of prophylactic antiretroviral therapy for HIV prevention after rape – with different basic packages of services being recommended for different settings, depending on the level of resources.
- Determining what constitutes appropriate psychological support for different settings and circumstances.
- Evaluating programmes aimed at preventing sexual violence, including community-based interventions – particularly those focusing on men – and school-based programmes.
- Studying the impact of legal reforms and criminal sanctions.

Greater attention to primary prevention

Primary prevention of sexual violence is often marginalized in favour of providing services for survivors. Policy-makers, researchers, donors and nongovernmental organizations should therefore give much greater attention to this important area.

Priority should be given to the following:

— the primary prevention of all forms of sexual violence through programmes in communities, schools and refugee settings;

— support for culturally sensitive and participatory approaches to changing attitudes and behaviour;

— support for programmes addressing the prevention of sexual violence in the broader context of promoting gender equality;

— programmes that address some of the underlying socioeconomic causes of violence, including poverty and lack of education, for example by providing job opportunities for young people;

— programmes to improve child rearing, reduce the vulnerability of women and promote more gender-equitable notions of masculinity.

Addressing sexual abuse within the health sector

Sexual violence against patients in the health sector exists in many places, but is not usually acknowledged as a problem. Various steps need to be taken to overcome this denial and to confront the problem, including the following (*83, 85*):

— incorporating topics pertaining to gender and sexual violence, including ethical considerations relevant to the medical profession, in the curricula for basic and postgraduate training of physicians, nurses and other health workers;

— actively seeking ways to identify and investigate possible cases of abuse of patients within health institutions;

— utilizing international bodies of the medical and nursing professions, and nongovernmental organizations (including women's organizations) to monitor and compile evidence of abuse and campaign for action on the part of governments and health services;

— establishing proper codes of practice and complaints procedures, and strict disciplinary procedures for health workers who abuse patients in health care settings.

Conclusion

Sexual violence is a common and serious public health problem affecting millions of people each year throughout the world. It is driven by many factors operating in a range of social, cultural and economic contexts. At the heart of sexual violence directed against women is gender inequality.

In many countries, data on most aspects of sexual violence are lacking, and there is a great need everywhere for research on all aspects of sexual violence. Of equal importance are interventions. These are of various types, but the essential ones concern the primary prevention of sexual violence, targeting both women and men, interventions supporting the victims of sexual assault, measures to make it more likely that perpetrators of rape will be caught and punished, and strategies for changing social norms and raising the status of women. It is vital to develop interventions for resource-poor settings and rigorously to evaluate programmes in both industrialized and developing countries.

Health professionals have a large role to play in supporting the victims of sexual assault – medically and psychologically – and collecting evidence to assist prosecutions. The health sector is considerably more effective in countries where there are protocols and guidelines for managing cases and collecting evidence, where staff are well-trained and where there is good collaboration with the judicial system. Ultimately, the strong commitment and involvement of governments and civil society, along with a coordinated response across a range of sectors, are required to end sexual violence.

References

1. Hakimi M et al. *Silence for the sake of harmony: domestic violence and women's health in central Java.* Yogyakarta, Gadjah Mada University, 2001.

2. Ellsberg MC. *Candies in hell: domestic violence against women in Nicaragua.* Umeå, Umeå University, 1997.

3. Mooney J. *The hidden figure: domestic violence in north London.* London, Middlesex University, 1993.

4. Jewkes R et al. Relationship dynamics and adolescent pregnancy in South Africa. *Social Science and Medicine*, 2001, 5:733–744.

5. Matasha E et al. Sexual and reproductive health among primary and secondary school pupils in Mwanza, Tanzania: need for intervention. *AIDS Care*, 1998, 10:571–582.

6. Buga GA, Amoko DH, Ncayiyana DJ. Sexual behaviour, contraceptive practice and reproductive health among school adolescents in rural Transkei. *South African Medical Journal*, 1996, 86:523–527.

7. Holmes MM et al. Rape-related pregnancy: estimates and descriptive characteristics from a national sample of women. *American Journal of Obstetrics and Gynecology*, 1996, 175:320–324.

8. Eby K et al. Health effects of experiences of sexual violence for women with abusive partners. *Health Care for Women International*, 1995, 16:563–576.

9. Leserman J et al. Selected symptoms associated with sexual and physical abuse among female patients with gastrointestinal disorders: the impact on subsequent health care visits. *Psychological Medicine*, 1998, 28:417–425.

10. McCauley J et al. The "battering syndrome": prevalence and clinical characteristics of domestic violence in primary care internal medicine practices. *Annals of Internal Medicine*, 1995, 123:737–746.

11. Coker AL et al. Physical health consequences of physical and psychological intimate partner violence. *Archives of Family Medicine*, 2000, 9:451–457.

12. Letourneau EJ, Holmes M, Chasendunn-Roark J. Gynecologic health consequences to victims of interpersonal violence. *Women's Health Issues*, 1999, 9:115–120.

13. Plichta SB, Abraham C. Violence and gynecologic health in women less than 50 years old. *American Journal of Obstetrics and Gynecology*, 1996, 174:903–907.

14. Campbell JC, Soeken K. Forced sex and intimate partner violence: effects on women's health. *Violence Against Women*, 1999, 5:1017–1035.

15. Collett BJ et al. A comparative study of women with chronic pelvic pain, chronic nonpelvic pain and those with no history of pain attending general practitioners. *British Journal of Obstetrics and Gynaecology*, 1998, 105:87–92.

16. Boyer D, Fine D. Sexual abuse as a factor in adolescent pregnancy. *Family Planning Perspectives*, 1992, 24:4–11.

17. Briggs L, Joyce PR. What determines post-traumatic stress disorder symptomatology for survivors of childhood sexual abuse? *Child Abuse & Neglect*, 1997, 21:575–582.

18. Creamer M, Burgess P, McFarlane AC. Post-traumatic stress disorder: findings from the Australian National Survey of Mental Health and Well-being. *Psychological Medicine*, 2001, 31:1237–1247.

19. Cheasty M, Clare AW, Collins C. Relation between sexual abuse in childhood and adult depression: case–control study. *British Medical Journal*, 1998, 316:198–201.

20. Darves-Bornoz JM. Rape-related psychotraumatic syndromes. *European Journal of Obstetrics, Gynecology and Reproductive Biology*, 1997, 71:59–65.

21. Felitti VJ et al. Relationship of childhood abuse and household dysfunction to many of the leading causes of death in adults: the Adverse Childhood Experiences (ACE) study. *American Journal of Preventive Medicine*, 1998, 14:245–258.

22. Fergusson DM, Horwood LJ, Lynskey MT. Childhood sexual abuse and psychiatric disorder in young adulthood: II. Psychiatric outcomes of childhood sexual abuse. *Journal of the American Academy of Child and Adolescent Psychiatry*, 1996, 35:1365–1374.

23. Levitan RD et al. Major depression in individuals with a history of childhood physical or sexual abuse: relationship of neurovegetative features, mania, and gender. *American Journal of Psychiatry*, 1998, 155:1746–1752.

24. Acierno R et al. Risk factors for rape, physical assault, and post-traumatic stress disorder in women: examination of differential multivariate relationships. *Journal of Anxiety Disorders*, 1999, 13:541–563.

25. Miller M. A model to explain the relationship between sexual abuse and HIV risk among women. *AIDS Care*, 1999, 11:3–20.

26. Mercy JA et al. Intentional injuries. In: Mashaly AY, Graitcer PH, Youssef ZM, eds. *Injury in Egypt: an analysis of injuries as a health problem*. Cairo, Rose El Youssef New Presses, 1993:65–84.

27. Mollica RF, Son L. Cultural dimensions in the evaluation and treatment of sexual trauma: an overview. *Psychiatric Clinics of North America*, 1989, 12:363–379.

28. Omaar R, de Waal A. Crimes without punishment: sexual harassment and violence against female students in schools and universities in Africa. *African Rights*, July 1994 (Discussion Paper No. 4).

29. Swiss S et al. Violence against women during the Liberian civil conflict. *Journal of the American Medical Association*, 1998, 279:625–629.

30. Migration Information Programme. *Trafficking and prostitution: the growing exploitation of migrant women from central and eastern Europe*. Geneva, International Organization for Migration, 1995.

31. Chauzy JP. *Kyrgyz Republic: trafficking*. Geneva, International Organization for Migration, 20 January 2001 (Press briefing notes).

32. Dinan K. *Owed justice: Thai women trafficked into debt bondage in Japan*. New York, NY, Human Rights Watch, 2000.

33. *The economics of sex*. Geneva, International Labour Organization, 1998 (World of Work, No. 26).

34. Jewkes R, Abrahams N. The epidemiology of rape and sexual coercion in South Africa: an overview. *Social Science and Medicine* (in press).

35. *The international crime victim survey in countries in transition: national reports*. Rome, United Nations Interregional Crime and Justice Research Institute, 1998.

36. *Victims of crime in the developing world*. Rome, United Nations Interregional Crime and Justice Research Institute, 1998.

37. Tjaden P, Thoennes N. *Full report of the prevalence, incidence and consequences of violence against women: findings from the National Violence Against Women Survey*. Washington, DC, National Institute of Justice, Office of Justice Programs, United States Department of Justice and Centers for Disease Control and Prevention, 2000 (NCJ 183781).

38. Weiss P, Zverina J. Experiences with sexual aggression within the general population in the Czech Republic. *Archives of Sexual Behavior*, 1999, 28:265–269.

39. Campbell JC, Soeken KL. Forced sex and intimate partner violence: effects on women's risk and women's health. *Violence Against Women*, 1999, 5:1017–1035.

40. Granados Shiroma M. *Salud reproductiva y violencia contra la mujer: un análisis desde la perspectiva de género. [Reproductive health and violence against women: an analysis from the gender perspective.]* Nuevo León, Asociación Mexicana de Población, Colegio de México, 1996.

41. Martin SL et al. Sexual behaviour and reproductive health outcomes: associations with wife abuse in India. *Journal of the American Medical Association*, 1999, 282:1967–1972.

42. Watts C et al. Withholding sex and forced sex: dimensions of violence against Zimbabwean women. *Reproductive Health Matters*, 1998, 6:57–65.

43. Gillioz L, DePuy J, Ducret V. *Domination et violences envers la femme dans le couple. [Domination and violence against women in the couple.]* Lausanne, Payot-Editions, 1997.

44. Rodgers K. Wife assault: the findings of a national survey. *Juristat Service Bulletin*, 1994, 14:1–22.

45. Randall M et al. Sexual violence in women's lives: findings from the women's safety project, a community-based survey. *Violence Against Women*, 1995, 1:6–31.

46. Morrison A et al. *The socio-economic impact of domestic violence against women in Chile and Nicaragua.* Washington, DC, Inter-American Development Bank, 1997.

47. Painter K, Farrington DP. Marital violence in Great Britain and its relationship to marital and nonmarital rape. *International Review of Victimology*, 1998, 5:257–276.

48. *Puerto Rico: encuesto de salud reproductiva 1995– 1996. [Puerto Rico: reproductive health survey 1995–1996.]* San Juan, University of Puerto Rico and Centers for Disease Control and Prevention, 1998.

49. Risberg G, Lundgren E, Westman G. Prevalence of sexualized violence among women: a population-based study in a primary healthcare district. *Scandinavian Journal of Public Health*, 1999, 27:247–253.

50. Heiskanen M, Piispa M. *Faith, hope and battering: a survey of men's violence against women in Finland.* Helsinki, Statistics Finland, 1998.

51. Haj Yahia MM. *The incidence of wife abuse and battering and some demographic correlates revealed in two national surveys in Palestinian society.* Ramallah, Besir Centre for Research and Development, 1998.

52. Ilkkaracan P et al. Exploring the context of women's sexuality in Eastern Turkey. *Reproductive Health Matters*, 1998, 6:66–75.

53. Heise LL, Ellsberg M, Gottemoeller M. *Ending violence against women.* Baltimore, MD, Johns Hopkins University School of Public Health, Center for Communications Programs, 1999 (Population Reports, Series L, No.11).

54. Rwenge M. Sexual risk behaviours among young people in Bamenda, Cameroon. *International Family Planning Perspectives*, 2000, 26:118–123.

55. *Estudo CAP nas escolas: conhecimento, attitudas, practicas e comportamento em saude sexual e reproductiva em uma era de SIDA. [A KAP study in schools: knowledge, attitudes, practices and behaviour regarding sexual and reproductive health during an AIDS era.]* Maputo, Geração Biz and Ministry of Youth and Sport, 1999.

56. Caceres CF, Vanoss M, Sid Hudes E. Sexual coercion among youth and young adolescents in Lima, Peru. *Journal of Adolescent Health*, 2000, 27:361–367.

57. Abma J, Driscoll A, Moore K. Young women's degree of control over first intercourse: an exploratory analysis. *Family Planning Perspectives*, 1998, 30:12–18.

58. Dickson N et al. First sexual intercourse: age, coercion, and later regrets reported by a birth cohort. *British Medical Journal*, 1998, 316:29–33.

59. *Adolescents.* (Programme brief on the findings from the Operations research and technical assistance, Africa Project II.) Nairobi, The Population Council, 1998.

60. Halcón L, Beuhring T, Blum R. *A portrait of adolescent health in the Caribbean, 2000.* Minneapolis, MN, University of Minnesota and Pan American Health Organization, 2000.

61. Swart L et al. Rape surveillance through district surgeons' offices in Johannesburg, 1996–1998: findings, evaluation and prevention implications. *South African Journal of Psychology*, 2000, 30:1–10.

62. Greenfeld LA. *Sex offenses and offenders: an analysis of data on rape and sexual assault.* Washington, DC, United States Department of Justice, Office of Justice Programs, Bureau of Justice Statistics (NCJ 163392).

63. Richard AO. *International trafficking in women to the United States: a contemporary manifestation of slavery and organized crime.* Washington, DC, Center for the Study of Intelligence, 1999.

64. Brown L. *Sex slaves: the trafficking of women in Asia.* London, Virago Press, 2001.

65. Benninger-Budel C et al. *Violence against women: a report.* Geneva, World Organization Against Torture, 1999.

66. Migration Information Programme. *Trafficking in women to Italy for sexual exploitation.* Geneva, International Organization for Migration, 1996.

67. Barnard M. Violence and vulnerability: conditions of work for streetworking prostitutes. *Sociology of Health and Illness*, 1993, 15:683–705.

68. Church S et al. Violence by clients towards female prostitutes in different work settings: questionnaire survey. *British Medical Journal*, 2001, 322:524–525.

69. Jenkins C. Street sex workers in Dhaka: their clients and enemies. In: *The Proceedings of the International Conference on Violence Against Women and Children, Dhaka, Bangladesh, June 1998.* Dhaka, 1998.

70. Ayalew T, Berhane Y. Child prostitution: magnitude and related problems. *Ethiopian Medical Journal*, 2000, 38:153–163.

71. Perlez J. For the oppressed sex: brave words to live by. *New York Times*, 6 June 1990.

72. Bagley C, Bolitho F, Bertrand L. Sexual assault in school, mental health and suicidal behaviors in adolescent women in Canada. *Adolescence*, 1997, 32:361–366.

73. Nhundu TJ, Shumba A. The nature and frequency of reported cases of teacher perpetrated child sexual abuse in rural primary schools in Zimbabwe. *Child Abuse & Neglect*, 2001, 25:1517–1534.

74. *Silencio y complicidad: violencia contra las mujeres en los servicios públicos en el Perú. [Silence and complicity: violence against women in public services in Peru.]* Lima, Committee of Latin America and the Caribbean for the Defense of the Rights of the Woman, and Center for Reproductive Law and Policy, 1998.

75. McPhedran M. Sexual abuse in the health professions: who's counting? *World Health Statistics Quarterly*, 1996, 49:154–157.

76. Dehlendorf CE, Wolfe SM. Physicians disciplined for sex-related offenses. *Journal of the American Medical Association*, 1998, 279:1883–1888.

77. Thomasson GO. Educating physicians to prevent sex-related contact with patients. *Journal of the American Medical Association*, 1999, 281:419–420.

78. Lamont JA, Woodward C. Patient–physician sexual involvement: a Canadian survey of obstetrician-gynecologists. *Canadian Medical Association Journal*, 1994, 150:1433–1439.

79. Fary T, Fisher N. Sexual contact between doctors and patients: almost always harmful. *British Medical Journal*, 1992, 304:1519–1520.

80. Fayad M. *Female genital mutilation (female circumcision)*. Cairo, Star Press, 2000.

81. *Human rights are women's rights*. London, Amnesty International, 1999.

82. Frank MW et al. Virginity examinations in Turkey: role for forensic physicians in controlling female sexuality. *Journal of the American Medical Association*, 1999, 282:485–490.

83. d'Oliveira AF, Diniz SG, Schraiber LB. Violence against women in health-care institutions: an emerging problem. *Lancet*, 2002, 359:1681–1685.

84. Sargent C, Rawlins J. Transformations in maternity services in Jamaica. *Social Science and Medicine*, 1992, 35:1225–1232.

85. Jewkes R, Abrahams N, Mvo Z. Why do nurses abuse patients? Reflections from South African obstetric services. *Social Science and Medicine*, 1998, 47:1781–1795.

86. Gilson L, Alilio M, Heggenhougen K. Community satisfaction with primary health care services: an evaluation undertaken in the Morogoro region of Tanzania. *Social Science and Medicine*, 1994, 39:767–780.

87. Jaffre Y, Prual AM. Midwives in Niger: an uncomfortable position between social behaviours and health care constraints. *Social Science and Medicine*, 1994, 38:1069–1073.

88. Shaikh MA. Sexual harassment in medical profession: perspectives from Pakistan. *Journal of the Pakistan Medical Association*, 2000, 50:130–131.

89. Kisa A, Dziegielewski SF. Sexual harassment of female nurses in a hospital in Turkey. *Health Services Management Research*, 1996, 9:243–253.

90. Chelala C. Algerian abortion controversy highlights rape of war victims. *Lancet*, 1998, 351:1413.

91. Asia Watch. *Rape in Kashmir: a crime of war*. New York, NY, Human Rights Watch, 1993.

92. Xiau W. Silent consent: Indonesian abuse of women. *Harvard International Review*, 1999, 21:16–17.

93. Swiss S, Giller JE. Rape as a crime of war: a medical perspective. *Journal of the American Medical Association*, 1993, 270:612–615.

94. Pacific Women Against Violence. Violence against East Timor women. *Pacific Women's Network Against Violence Against Women*, 2000, 5:1–3.

95. Morrell R, ed. *Changing men in Southern Africa*. Pietermaritzburg, University of Natal Press, 2001.

96. Nduna S, Goodyear L. *Pain too deep for tears: assessing the prevalence of sexual and gender violence among Burundian refugees in Tanzania*. Kibondo, International Rescue Committee, 1997.

97. George A. *Sexual behavior and sexual negotiation among poor women and men in Mumbai: an exploratory study*. Baroda, Sahaj Society for Health Alternatives, 1997.

98. Sharma V, Sujay R, Sharma A. Can married women say no to sex? Repercussions of the denial of the sexual act. *Journal of Family Welfare*, 1998, 44:1–8.

99. *Early marriage: whose right to choose?* London, Forum on Marriage and the Rights of Women and Girls, 2000.

100. UNICEF Innocenti Research Center. Early marriage: child spouses. *Innocenti Digest*, 2001, No. 7.

101. Kumari R, Singh R, Dubey A. *Growing up in rural India: problems and needs of adolescent girls*. New Delhi, Radiant Publishers, 1990.

102. Ahmed EM. *Violence against women: the legal system and institutional responses*. Lahore, AGHS Legal Aid Cell, 1998.

103. Indicators on marriage and marital status. In: *1997 Demographic yearbook*, 49th ed. New York, NY, United Nations Statistics Division, 1999.

104. Heise L, Pitanguy J, Germain A. *Violence against women: the hidden health burden*. Washington, DC, World Bank, 1994 (Discussion Paper No. 255).

105. Crowell NA, Burgess AW, eds. *Understanding violence against women*. Washington, DC, National Academy Press, 1996.

106. Koss M, Dinero TE. Discriminant analysis of risk factors for sexual victimisation among a national sample of college women. *Journal of Consulting and Clinical Psychology*, 1989, 57:242–250.

107. Fergusson DM, Horwood LJ, Lynskey MT. Childhood sexual abuse, adolescent sexual behaviours and sexual revictimization. *Child Abuse & Neglect*, 1997, 21:789–803.

108. Fleming J et al. The long-term impact of childhood sexual abuse in Australian women. *Child Abuse & Neglect*, 1999, 23:145–159.

109. Pederson W, Skrondal A. Alcohol and sexual victimization: a longitudinal study of Norwegian girls. *Addiction*, 1996, 91:565–581.

110. Olsson A et al. Sexual abuse during childhood and adolescence among Nicaraguan men and women: a population-based survey. *Child Abuse & Neglect*, 2000, 24:1579–1589.

111. Jewkes R, Penn-Kekana L, Levin J. Risk factors for domestic violence: findings from a South African cross-sectional study. *Social Science and Medicine* (in press).

112. Jewkes R. Intimate partner violence: causes and prevention. *Lancet*, 2002, 359:1423–1429.

113. Omorodion FI, Olusanya O. The social context of reported rape in Benin City, Nigeria. *African Journal of Reproductive Health*, 1998, 2:37–43.

114. Faune MA. Centroamerica: los costos de la guerra y la paz. [Central America: the costs of war and of peace.] *Perspectivas*, 1997, 8:14–15.

115. International Clinical Epidemiologists Network. *Domestic violence in India: a summary report of a multi-site household survey.* Washington, DC, International Center for Research on Women, 2000.

116. Heise L, Moore K, Toubia N. *Sexual coercion and women's reproductive health: a focus on research.* New York, NY, Population Council, 1995.

117. *Violence against women: a priority health issue.* Geneva, World Health Organization, 1997 (document WHO/FRH/WHD/97.8).

118. Miczek KA et al. Alcohol, drugs of abuse, aggression and violence. In: Reiss AJ, Roth JA, eds. *Understanding and preventing violence. Vol. 3. Social influences.* Washington, DC, National Academy Press, 1993:377–570.

119. Grisso JA et al. Violent injuries among women in an urban area. *New England Journal of Medicine*, 1999, 341:1899–1905.

120. Abby A, Ross LT, McDuffie D. Alcohol's role in sexual assault. In: Watson RR, ed. *Drug and alcohol reviews. Vol. 5. Addictive behaviors in women.* Totowa, NJ, Humana Press, 1995.

121. McDonald M, ed. *Gender, drink and drugs.* Oxford, Berg Publishers, 1994.

122. Drieschner K, Lange A. A review of cognitive factors in the aetiology of rape: theories, empirical studies and implications. *Clinical Psychology Review*, 1999, 19:57–77.

123. Dean KE, Malamuth NM. Characteristics of men who aggress sexually and of men who imagine aggressing: risk and moderating variables. *Journal of Personality and Social Psychology*, 1997, 72:449–455.

124. Malamuth NM, Addison T, Koss MP. Pornography and sexual aggression: are there reliable effects and how can we understand them? *Annual Review of Sex Research*, 2000, 11:26–91.

125. Malamuth NM. A multidimensional approach to sexual aggression: combining measures of past behavior and present likelihood. *Annals of the New York Academy of Science*, 1998, 528:113–146.

126. Ouimette PC, Riggs D. Testing a mediational model of sexually aggressive behavior in nonincarcerated perpetrators. *Violence and Victims*, 1998, 13:117–130.

127. Malamuth NM et al. The characteristics of aggressors against women: testing a model using a national sample of college students. *Journal of Consulting and Clinical Psychology*, 1991, 59:670–681.

128. Lisak D, Roth S. Motives and psychodynamics of self-reported, unincarcerated rapists. *Journal of Personality and Social Psychology*, 1990, 55:584–589.

129. Bourgois P. *In search of respect: selling crack in El Barrio.* Cambridge, Cambridge University Press, 1996.

130. Petty GM, Dawson B. Sexual aggression in normal men: incidence, beliefs and personality characteristics. *Personality and Individual Differences*, 1989, 10:355–362.

131. Borowsky IW, Hogan M, Ireland M. Adolescent sexual aggression: risk and protective factors. *Pediatrics*, 1997, 100:E7.

132. Gwartney-Gibbs PA, Stockard J, Bohmer S. Learning courtship aggression: the influence of parents, peers and personal experiences. *Family Relations*, 1983, 35:276–282.

133. Jenkins C. Sexual behaviour in Papua New Guinea. In: *Report of the Third Annual Meeting of the International Network on Violence Against Women, January 1998.* Washington, DC, International Network on Violence Against Women, 1998.

134. Watkins B, Bentovim A. The sexual abuse of male children and adolescents: a review of current research. *Journal of Child Psychology and Psychiatry*, 1992, 33:197–248.

135. Dobash E, Dobash R. *Women, violence and social change.* London, Routledge, 1992.

136. Wood K, Maepa J, Jewkes R. *Adolescent sex and contraceptive experiences: perspectives of teenagers and clinic nurses in the Northern Province.* Pretoria, Medical Research Council, 1997 (Technical Report).

137. Hadidi M, Kulwicki A, Jahshan H. A review of 16 cases of honour killings in Jordan in 1995. *International Journal of Legal Medicine*, 2001, 114:357–359.

138. Bourgois P. In search of masculinity: violence, respect and sexuality among Puerto Rican crack dealers in East Harlem. *British Journal of Criminology*, 1996, 36:412–427.

139. Wood K, Jewkes R. "Dangerous" love: reflections on violence among Xhosa township youth. In: Morrell R, ed. *Changing men in Southern Africa.* Pietermaritzburg, University of Natal Press, 2001.

140. Silberschmidt M. Disempowerment of men in rural and urban East Africa: implications for male identity and sexual behavior. *World Development*, 2001, 29:657–671.

141. Madge C. Public parks and the geography of fear. *Tijdschrift voor Economische en Sociale Geografie*, 1997, 88:237–250.

142. Pain RH. Social geographies of women's fear of crime. *Transactions of the Institute of British Geographers*, 1997, 22:231– 244.

143. Rozee PD. Forbidden or forgiven? Rape in cross-cultural perspective. *Psychology of Women Quarterly*, 1993, 17:499–514.

144. Ariffin RE. *Shame, secrecy and silence: study of rape in Penang.* Penang, Women's Crisis Centre, 1997.

145. Bennett L, Manderson L, Astbury J. *Mapping a global pandemic: review of current literature on rape, sexual assault and sexual harassment of women.* Melbourne, University of Melbourne, 2000.

146. Sen P. *Ending the presumption of consent: non-consensual sex in marriage.* London, Centre for Health and Gender Equity, 1999.

147. Buckley T, Gottlieb A. *Blood magic: the anthropology of menstruation.* Berkeley, CA, University of California, 1998.

148. Sanday P. The socio-cultural context of rape: a cross-cultural study. *Journal of Social Issues*, 1981, 37:5–27.

149. Gartner R. The victims of homicide: a temporal and cross-national comparison. *American Sociological Review*, 1990, 55:92–106.

150. Briggs CM, Cutright P. Structural and cultural determinants of child homicide: a cross-national analysis. *Violence and Victims*, 1994, 9:3–16.

151. Smutt M, Miranda JLE. El Salvador: socialización y violencia juvenil. [El Salvador: socialization and juvenile violence.] In: Ramos CG, ed. *America Central en los noventa: problemas de juventud. [Central America in the 90s: youth problems.]* San Salvador, Latin American Faculty of Social Sciences, 1998:151–187.

152. Watts C, Zimmerman C. Violence against women: global scope and magnitude. *Lancet*, 2002, 359:1232–1237.

153. Antrobus P. Reversing the impact of structural adjustment on women's health. In: Antrobus P et al., eds. *We speak for ourselves: population and development.* Washington, DC, Panos Institute, 1994:6–8.

154. Mulugeta E, Kassaye M, Berhane Y. Prevalence and outcomes of sexual violence among high school students. *Ethiopian Medical Journal*, 1998, 36:167–174.

155. *Evaluación de proyecto para educación, capacitación y atención a mujeres y menores de edad en materia de violencia sexual, enero a diciembre 1990. [An evaluation of a project to provide education, training and care for women and minors affected by sexual violence, January–December 1990.]* Mexico City, Asociación Mexicana contra la Violencia a las Mujeres, 1990.

156. *Carpeta de información básica para la atención solidaria y feminista a mujeres violadas. [Basic information file for mutually supportive feminist care for women rape victims.]* Mexico City, Centro do Apoyo a Mujeres Violadas, 1985.

157. Roosa MW et al. The relationship of childhood sexual abuse to teenage pregnancy. *Journal of Marriage and the Family*, 1997, 59:119–130.

158. Stock JL et al. Adolescent pregnancy and sexual risk-taking among sexually abused girls. *Family Planning Perspectives*, 1997, 29:200–227.

159. Jenny C et al. Sexually transmitted diseases in victims of rape. *New England Journal of Medicine*, 1990, 322:713–716.

160. Wingood G, DiClemente R, Raj A. Adverse consequences of intimate partner abuse among women in non-urban domestic violence shelters. *American Journal of Preventive Medicine*, 2000, 19:270–275.

161. Anteghini M et al. Health risk behaviors and associated risk and protective factors among Brazilian adolescents in Santos, Brazil. *Journal of Adolescent Health*, 2001, 28:295–302.

162. Mullen PE et al. Impact of sexual and physical abuse on women's mental health. *Lancet*, 1988, i:841–845.

163. Choquet M et al. Self-reported health and behavioral problems among adolescent victims of rape in France: results of a cross-sectional survey. *Child Abuse & Neglect*, 1997, 21:823–832.

164. Kimerling R, Calhoun KS. Somatic symptoms, social support and treatment seeking among sexual assault victims. *Journal of Consulting and Clinical Psychology*, 1994, 62:333–340.

165. Foa EB et al. A comparison of exposure therapy, stress inoculation training, and their combination for reducing post-traumatic stress disorder in female assault victims. *Journal of Consulting and Clinical Psychology*, 1999, 67:194–200.

166. Tarrier N et al. Cognitive therapy or imaginal exposure in the treatment of post-traumatic stress disorder: twelve-month follow-up. *British Journal of Psychiatry*, 1999, 175:571–575.

167. Kilpatrick DG, Edmonds CN, Seymour AK. *Rape in America: a report to the nation*. Arlington, VA, National Victim Center, 1992.

168. Davidson JR et al. The association of sexual assault and attempted suicide within the community. *Archives of General Psychiatry*, 1996, 53:550–555.

169. Luster T, Small SA. Sexual abuse history and problems in adolescence: exploring the effects of moderating variables. *Journal of Marriage and the Family*, 1997, 59:131–142.

170. McCauley J et al. Clinical characteristics of women with a history of childhood abuse: unhealed wounds. *Journal of the American Medical Association*, 1997, 277:1362–1368.

171. Nagy S, Adcock AG, Nagy MC. A comparison of risky health behaviors of sexually active, sexually abused, and abstaining adolescents. *Pediatrics*, 1994, 93:570–575.

172. Romans SE et al. Sexual abuse in childhood and deliberate self-harm. *American Journal of Psychiatry*, 1995, 152:1336–1342.

173. Wiederman MW, Sansone RA, Sansone LA. History of trauma and attempted suicide among women in a primary care setting. *Violence and Victims*, 1998, 13:3–9.

174. Statham DJ et al. Suicidal behaviour: an epidemiological and genetic study. *Psychological Medicine*, 1998, 28:839–855.

175. Heise L. Violence against women: the missing agenda. In: Koblinsky M, Timyan J, Gay J, eds. *The health of women: a global perspective*. Boulder, CO, Westview Press, 1993.

176. Ahmad K. Public protests after rape in Pakistani hospital. *Lancet*, 1999, 354:659.

177. Foa EB, Hearst-Ikeda D, Perry KJ. Evaluation of a brief cognitive-behavioural program for the prevention of chronic PTSD in recent assault victims. *Journal of Consulting and Clinical Psychology*, 1995, 63:948–955.

178. Foa EB, Street GP. Women and traumatic events. *Journal of Clinical Psychiatry*, 2001, 62 (Suppl. 17):29–34.

179. Meyer CB, Taylor SE. Adjustment to rape. *Journal of Personality and Social Psychology*, 1986, 50:1226–1234.

180. Christofides N. *Evaluation of Soul City in partnership with the National Network on Violence Against Women (NNVAW): some initial findings*. Johannesburg, Women's Health Project, University of the Witwatersrand, 2000.

181. Kelly L, Radford J. Sexual violence against women and girls: an approach to an international overview. In: Dobash E, Dobash R, eds. *Rethinking violence against women*. London, Sage, 1998.

182. Kaufman M. Building a movement of men working to end violence against women. *Development*, 2001, 44:9–14.

183. Welbourn A. *Stepping Stones*. Oxford, Strategies for Hope, 1995.

184. *Men as partners*. New York, NY, AVSC International, 1998.

185. Gordon G, Welbourn A. *Stepping Stones and men*. Washington, DC, Inter-Agency Gender Working Group, 2001.

186. Schwartz IL. Sexual violence against women: prevalence, consequences, societal factors and prevention. *American Journal of Preventive Medicine*, 1991, 7:363–373.

187. Du Mont J, Parnis D. Sexual assault and legal resolution: querying the medical collection of forensic evidence. *Medicine and Law*, 2000,19:779–792.

188. McGregor MJ et al. Examination for sexual assault: is the documentation of physical injury associated with the laying of charges? *Journal of the Canadian Medical Association*, 1999, 160:1565–1569.

189. Chaudhry S et al. Retrospective study of alleged sexual assault at the Aga Khan Hospital, Nairobi. *East African Medical Journal*, 1995, 72:200–202.

190. Harrison JM, Murphy SM. A care package for managing female sexual assault in genitourinary medicine. *International Journal of Sexually Transmitted Diseases and AIDS*, 1999, 10:283–289.

191. Parnis D, Du Mont J. An exploratory study of post-sexual assault professional practices: examining the standardised application of rape kits. *Health Care for Women International* (in press).

192. Resnick H et al. Prevention of post-rape psychopathology: preliminary findings of a controlled acute rape treatment study. *Journal of Anxiety Disorders*, 1999, 13:359–370.

193. Ramos-Jimenez P. *Philippine strategies to combat domestic violence against women*. Manila, Social Development Research Center and De La Salle University, 1996.

194. *Violence against women and HIV/AIDS: setting the research agenda*. Geneva, World Health Organization, 2001 (document WHO/FCH/GWH/01.08).

195. Case–control study of HIV seroconversion in health care workers after percutaneous exposure to HIV-infected blood: France, United Kingdom, and United States, January 1988 to August 1994. *Morbidity and Mortality Weekly Report*, 1995, 44:929–933.

196. Ippolito G et al. The risk of occupational HIV in health care workers. *Archives of Internal Medicine*, 1993, 153:1451–1458.

197. Wiebe ER et al. Offering HIV prophylaxis to people who have been sexually assaulted: 16 months' experience in a sexual assault service. *Canadian Medical Association Journal*, 2000, 162:641–645.

198. Du Mont J, MacDonald S, Badgley R. *An overview of the sexual assault care and treatment centres of Ontario*. Toronto, The Ontario Network of Sexual Assault Care and Treatment Centres, 1997.

199. Njovana E, Watts C. Gender violence in Zimbabwe: a need for collaborative action. *Reproductive Health Matters*, 1996, 7:46–54.

200. *Safe and secure: eliminating violence against women and girls in Muslim societies*. Montreal, Sisterhood Is Global Institute, 1998.

201. Mehrotra A et al. *A life free of violence: it's our right*. New York, NY, United Nations Development Fund for Women, 2000.

202. Flood M. Men's collective anti-violence activism and the struggle for gender justice. *Development*, 2001, 44:42–47.

203. Du Mont J, Myhr TL. So few convictions: the role of client-related characteristics in the legal processing of sexual assaults. *Violence Against Women*, 2000, 6:1109–1136.

204. *Further actions and initiatives to implement the Beijing Declaration and Platform for Action*. New York, NY, Women, Peace and Development, United Nations, 2000 (Outcome Document, United Nations General Assembly Special Session, Women 2000: Beijing Plus Five).

205. *Reproductive rights 2000: moving forward*. New York, NY, Center for Reproductive Law and Policy, 2000.

206. Bedont B, Martinez KH. Ending impunity for gender crimes under the International Criminal Court. *The Brown Journal of World Affairs*, 1999, 6:65–85.

207. Coomaraswamy R. *Integration of the human rights of women and the gender perspective. Violence against women*. New York, NY, United Nations Economic and Social Council, Commission on Human Rights, 2000 (Report of the Special Rapporteur on violence against women).

208. Khafagi F. Breaking cultural and social taboos: the fight against female genital mutilation in Egypt. *Development*, 2001, 44:74–78.

209. *Reproductive health effects of gender-based violence*. New York, NY, United Nations Population Fund, 1998 (available on the Internet at http://www.unfpa.org/about/report/report98/ppgenderbased.htm.) (Annual Report 1998: programme priorities).

210. *Sierra Leone: rape and other forms of sexual violence against girls and women*. London, Amnesty International, 2000.

211. *Sexual violence against refugees: guidelines on prevention and response*. Geneva, Office of the United Nations High Commissioner for Refugees, 1995.

212. *Sexual and gender-based violence programme in Guinea*. Geneva, Office of the United Nations High Commissioner for Refugees, 2001.

CHAPTER 7

Self-directed violence

Background

In the year 2000 an estimated 815 000 people died from suicide around the world. This represents an annual global mortality rate of about 14.5 per 100 000 population – or one death about every 40 seconds. Suicide is the thirteenth leading cause of death worldwide (see Statistical annex). Among those aged 15–44 years, self-inflicted injuries are the fourth leading cause of death and the sixth leading cause of ill-health and disability (1).

Deaths from suicide are only a part of this very serious problem. In addition to those who die, many more people survive attempts to take their own lives or harm themselves, often seriously enough to require medical attention (2). Furthermore, every person who kills himself or herself leaves behind many others – family and friends – whose lives are profoundly affected emotionally, socially and economically. The economic costs associated with self-inflicted death or injuries are estimated to be in the billions of US dollars a year (3).

How is suicide defined?

Suicidal behaviour ranges in degree from merely thinking about ending one's life, through developing a plan to commit suicide and obtaining the means to do so, attempting to kill oneself, to finally carrying out the act ("completed suicide").

The term "suicide" in itself evokes direct reference to violence and aggressiveness. Apparently, Sir Thomas Browne was the first to coin the word "suicide" in his *Religio medici* (1642). A physician and a philosopher, Browne based the word on the Latin *sui* (of oneself) and *caedere* (to kill). The new term reflected a desire to distinguish between the homicide of oneself and the killing of another (4).

A well-known definition of suicide is the one that appears in the 1973 edition of the Encyclopaedia Britannica, quoted by Shneidman: "the human act of self-inflicting one's own life cessation" (5). Certainly in any definition of suicide, the intention to die is a key element. However, it is often extremely difficult to reconstruct the thoughts of people who commit suicide unless they have made clear statements before their death about their intentions or left a suicide note. Not all those who survive a suicidal act intended to live, nor are all suicidal deaths planned. To make a correlation between intent and outcome can therefore be problematic. In many legal systems, a death is certified as suicide if the circumstances are consistent with suicide and if murder, accidental death and natural causes can all be ruled out.

There has been much disagreement about the most suitable terminology to describe suicidal behaviour. Recently, the outcome-based term "fatal suicidal behaviour" has been proposed for suicidal acts that result in death – and similarly "non-fatal suicidal behaviour" for suicidal actions that do not result in death (6). Such actions are also often called "attempted suicide" (a term common in the United States of America), "parasuicide" and "deliberate self-harm" (terms which are common in Europe).

The term "suicidal ideation" is often used in the technical literature, and refers to thoughts of killing oneself, in varying degrees of intensity and elaboration. In the literature, the term also refers to a feeling of being tired of life, a belief that life is not worth living, and a desire not to wake from sleep (7, 8). Although these different feelings – or ideations – express different degrees of severity, there is not necessarily a continuum between them. Furthermore, the intention to die is not a necessary criterion for non-fatal suicidal behaviour.

Another common form of self-directed violence is self-mutilation. This is the direct and deliberate destruction or alteration of parts of the body without conscious suicidal intention. Favazza (9) has proposed three main categories:

- Major self-mutilation – including self-blinding and the amputation of fingers, hands, arms, limbs, feet or genitalia.

- Stereotypical self-mutilation – such as banging one's head, biting oneself, hitting one's arm, gouging one's eyes or throat, or pulling one's hair.

- Superficial-to-moderate self-mutilation – such as cutting, scratching or burning one's skin, sticking needles into one's skin, or pulling one's hair compulsively.

Self-mutilation involves very different factors from suicidal behaviour and will not be discussed here further. For an extensive review of self-mutilation, see Favazza (*9*).

The extent of the problem

Fatal suicidal behaviour

National suicide rates vary considerably (see Table 7.1). Among countries reporting suicide to the World Health Organization, the highest suicide rates are found in Eastern European countries (for example, Belarus 41.5 per 100 000, Estonia 37.9 per 100 000, Lithuania 51.6 per 100 000 and the Russian Federation 43.1 per 100 000). High rates of suicide have also been reported in Sri Lanka (37 per 100 000 in 1996), based on data from the WHO Regional Office for South-East Asia (*10*). Low rates are found mainly in Latin America (notably Colombia 4.5 per 100 000 and Paraguay 4.2 per 100 000) and some countries in Asia (for example, the Philippines 2.1 per 100 000 and Thailand 5.6 per 100 000). Countries in other parts of Europe, in North America, and parts of Asia and the Pacific tend to fall somewhere in between these extremes (for example, Australia 17.9 per 100 000, Belgium 24.0 per 100 000, Canada 15.0 per 100 000, Finland 28.4 per 100 000, France 20.0 per 100 000, Germany 14.3 per 100 000, Japan 19.5 per 100 000, Switzerland 22.5 per 100 000 and the United States

TABLE 7.1

Age-adjusted suicide rates by country, most recent year available[a]

Country or area	Year	Total number of suicides	Suicide rate per 100 000 population			
			Total	Male	Female	Male: female ratio
Albania	1998	165	7.1	9.5	4.8	2.0
Argentina	1996	2 245	8.7	14.2	3.9	3.6
Armenia	1999	67	2.3	3.6	—[b]	—[b]
Australia	1998	2 633	17.9	28.9	7.0	4.1
Austria	1999	1 555	20.9	32.7	10.2	3.2
Azerbaijan	1999	54	1.1	1.7	—[b]	—[b]
Belarus	1999	3 408	41.5	76.5	11.3	6.7
Belgium	1995	2 155	24.0	36.3	12.7	2.9
Bosnia and Herzegovina	1991	531	14.8	25.3	4.2	6.1
Brazil	1995	6 584	6.3	10.3	2.5	4.1
Bulgaria	1999	1 307	16.4	26.2	7.7	3.4
Canada	1997	3 681	15.0	24.1	6.1	3.9
Chile	1994	801	8.1	15.0	1.9	8.1
China						
Hong Kong SAR	1996	788	14.9	19.5	10.4	1.9
Selected rural and urban areas	1999	16 836	18.3	18.0	18.8	1.0
Colombia	1995	1 172	4.5	7.4	1.8	4.1
Costa Rica	1995	211	8.8	14.4	3.0	4.7
Croatia	1999	989	24.8	40.6	11.6	3.5
Cuba	1997	2 029	23.0	32.1	14.2	2.3
Czech Republic	1999	1 610	17.5	30.1	6.3	4.8
Denmark	1996	892	18.4	27.2	10.1	2.7
Ecuador	1996	593	7.2	10.4	4.1	2.5
El Salvador	1993	429	11.2	16.3	6.8	2.4
Estonia	1999	469	37.9	68.5	12.0	5.7
Finland	1998	1 228	28.4	45.8	11.7	3.9
France	1998	10 534	20.0	31.3	9.9	3.2
Georgia	1992	204	5.3	8.7	2.5	3.4
Germany	1999	11 160	14.3	22.5	6.9	3.3
Greece	1998	403	4.2	6.7	1.8	3.7
Hungary	1999	3 328	36.1	61.5	14.4	4.3
Ireland	1997	466	16.8	27.4	6.3	4.3
Israel	1997	379	8.7	14.6	3.3	4.4
Italy	1997	4 694	8.4	13.4	3.8	3.5
Japan	1997	23 502	19.5	28.0	11.5	2.4
Kazakhstan	1999	4 004	37.4	67.3	11.6	5.8
Kuwait	1999	47	2.0	2.2	—[b]	—[b]
Kyrgyzstan	1999	559	18.7	31.9	6.3	5.1
Latvia	1999	764	36.5	63.7	13.6	4.7
Lithuania	1999	1 552	51.6	93.0	15.0	6.2
Mauritius	1999	174	19.2	26.5	12.1	2.2
Mexico	1997	3 369	5.1	9.1	1.4	6.3
Netherlands	1999	1 517	11.0	15.2	7.1	2.1
New Zealand	1998	574	19.8	31.2	8.9	3.5
Nicaragua	1996	230	7.6	11.2	4.3	2.6
Norway	1997	533	14.6	21.6	8.0	2.7
Panama (excluding Canal Zone)	1997	145	7.8	13.2	2.3	5.7
Paraguay	1994	109	4.2	6.5	1.8	3.6
Philippines	1993	851	2.1	2.5	1.6	1.6
Poland	1995	5 499	17.9	31.0	5.6	5.5
Portugal	1999	545	5.4	9.0	2.4	3.8

TABLE 7.1 *(continued)*

Country or area	Year	Total number of suicides	Suicide rate per 100 000 population			
			Total	Male	Female	Male: female ratio
Puerto Rico	1998	321	10.8	20.9	2.0	10.4
Republic of Korea	1997	6 024	17.1	25.3	10.1	2.5
Republic of Moldova	1999	579	20.7	37.7	6.3	6.0
Romania	1999	2 736	14.3	24.6	4.8	5.1
Russian Federation	1998	51 770	43.1	77.8	12.6	6.2
Singapore	1998	371	15.7	18.8	12.7	1.5
Slovakia	1999	692	15.4	27.9	4.3	6.5
Slovenia	1999	590	33.0	53.9	14.4	3.7
Spain	1998	3 261	8.7	14.2	3.8	3.8
Sweden	1996	1 253	15.9	22.9	9.2	2.5
Switzerland	1996	1 431	22.5	33.7	12.3	2.7
Tajikistan	1995	199	7.1	10.9	3.4	3.2
Thailand	1994	2 333	5.6	8.0	3.3	2.4
The former Yugoslav Republic of Macedonia	1997	155	10.0	15.2	5.2	2.9
Trinidad and Tobago	1994	148	16.9	26.1	6.8	3.8
Turkmenistan	1998	406	13.7	22.2	5.4	4.1
Ukraine	1999	14 452	33.8	61.8	10.1	6.1
United Kingdom	1999	4 448	9.2	14.6	3.9	3.8
England and Wales	1999	3 690	8.5	13.4	3.6	3.7
Northern Ireland	1999	121	9.9	17.0	—[b]	—[b]
Scotland	1999	637	15.7	25.3	6.3	4.0
United States	1998	30 575	13.9	23.2	5.3	4.4
Uruguay	1990	318	12.8	22.0	4.8	4.6
Uzbekistan	1998	1 620	10.6	17.2	4.4	3.9
Venezuela	1994	1 089	8.1	13.7	2.7	5.0

SAR: Special Administrative Region.

[a] Most recent year available between 1990 and 2000 for countries with ≥ 1 million population.

[b] Fewer than 20 deaths reported; rate and rate ratio not calculated.

13.9 per 100 000). Unfortunately, little information is available on suicide from countries in Africa (*11*).

Two countries, Finland and Sweden, have data on suicide rates dating from the 18th century and both show a trend for increasing suicide rates over time (*12*). During the 20th century, Finland, Ireland, the Netherlands, Norway, Scotland, Spain and Sweden experienced a significant increase in suicides, while England and Wales (combined data), Italy, New Zealand and Switzerland experienced a significant decrease. There was no significant change in Australia (*12*). During the period 1960–1990, at least 28 countries or territories had rising suicide rates, including Bulgaria, China (Province of Taiwan), Costa Rica, Mauritius and Singapore, while eight had declining rates, including Australia, and England and Wales (combined data) (*12*).

Rates of suicide are not distributed equally throughout the general population. One important demographic marker of suicide risk is age. Globally, suicide rates tend to increase with age, although some countries such as Canada have also recently seen a secondary peak in young people aged 15–24 years. Figure 7.1 shows the global rates recorded by age and sex in 1995. The rates ranged from 0.9 per 100 000 in the group aged 5–14 years to 66.9 per 100 000 among people aged 75 years and older. In general, suicide rates among those aged 75 years and older are approximately three times higher than those of young people aged 15–24 years. This trend is found for both sexes, but is more marked among men. For women, suicide rates present differing patterns. In some cases, female suicide rates increase steadily with age, in others the rates peak in middle age, and in yet others, particularly in developing countries and among minority groups, female rates peak among young adults (*13*).

Although suicide rates are generally higher among older people, the absolute number of cases recorded is actually higher among those under 45 years of age than among those over 45 years, given demographic distributions (see Table 7.2). This is a remarkable change from just 50 years ago, when the absolute number of cases of suicide roughly increased with age. It is not explained in terms of the overall ageing of the global population; in fact, it runs counter to this demographic trend. At present, suicide rates are already higher among people under 45 years of age than among those over 45 years in approximately one-third of all countries, a phenomenon that appears to exist in all continents and is not correlated to levels of industrialization or wealth. Examples of countries

BOX 7.1

Suicide among indigenous peoples: the cases of Australia and Canada

In the past 20 to 30 years, suicide rates have increased strikingly among indigenous peoples in both Australia and Canada. In Australia, suicide among the Aboriginal and Torres Strait Islander populations used to be considered very uncommon. Slightly over a quarter of these people live in the state of Queensland. The overall suicide rate in Queensland for the period 1990–1995 was 14.5 per 100 000, while the rate for Aboriginal and Torres Strait Islander peoples was 23.6 per 100 000.

Suicides among indigenous Australians are heavily concentrated among young men. In Queensland, 84% of all indigenous suicides were among men aged between 15 and 34 years, and the rate for indigenous men aged 15–24 years was 112.5 per 100 000 (*22*). By far the most common method of suicide among young indigenous men is by hanging.

In Canada's Arctic north, suicide rates among the Inuit of between 59.5 and 74.3 per 100 000 have been reported in various studies, compared with around 15.0 per 100 000 in the overall population. Young Inuit men are at the highest risk for suicide, and their suicide rate is rising. Rates as high as 195 per 100 000 have been recorded among those aged 15–25 years (*23*).

Various explanations have been put forward for the high rates of suicide and suicidal behaviour among indigenous peoples. Among the proposed underlying causes are the enormous social and cultural turmoil created by the policies of colonialism and the difficulties faced ever since by indigenous peoples in adjusting and integrating into the modern-day societies.

In Australia, aboriginal groups were the object of stringent racial laws and discrimination as late as the 1960s. When these laws, including the restrictions on alcohol sales, were lifted within a short period in the 1970s, the rapid social changes in the previously oppressed indigenous peoples gave rise to instability in community and family life. This instability has continued ever since, with high rates of crime, delinquency and imprisonment, violence and accidents, alcohol dependence and substance abuse, and a homicide rate that is tenfold that among the general population.

In the Canadian Arctic in the early 19th century, epidemics swept the region as the first outsiders — whalers and fur traders — arrived, taking tens of thousands of lives and leaving a population reduced in size by two-thirds by 1900. By the 1930s the fur trade had collapsed, and Canada introduced a welfare state in the Arctic. In the 1940s and 1950s missionaries came to the Arctic and there was an attempt to assimilate the Inuit. Feverish exploration for oil, starting in 1959, further added to the social disintegration.

Research on suicide among the Canadian Inuit has identified several factors as likely indirect causes of suicide, including:
— poverty;
— childhood separation and loss;
— accessibility to firearms;
— alcohol abuse and dependence;
— a history of personal or familial health problems;
— past sexual or physical abuse.

Efforts are being made in both Australia and Canada to address suicidal behaviour among indigenous populations. In Australia, the national strategy to prevent suicides among young people includes a number of programmes for indigenous youths. These programmes are designed to address the specific needs of indigenous youths and are conducted in partnership with organizations representing the interests of indigenous peoples such as the Aboriginal Coordinating Council.

Constructive measures to prevent suicide in the Canadian Arctic include improved responses to crises, widespread community redevelopment and progress toward self-government in the indigenous areas. The new and vast territory of Nunavut was created on 1 April 1999, giving the Inuit people local self-determination and returning to them some of their rights and heritage.

records provide useful data for research and prevention purposes, since those who attempt suicide are at high risk for subsequent suicidal behaviour, both fatal and non-fatal. Public health officials also rely on reviews of hospital records, population surveys and special studies, sources that often include data lacking in mortality data systems.

Available figures show – both relative to their population size and in absolute numbers – that non-fatal suicidal behaviour is more prevalent among younger people than among older people. The ratio of fatal to non-fatal suicidal behaviour in those over the age of 65 years is usually estimated to be of the order of 1:2–3, while in young people under 25 years the ratio may reach 1:100–200 (*32, 33*). Although suicidal behaviour is less frequent in the elderly, the probability of a fatal outcome is much higher (*28, 34*). On average, suicide attempts in old age are, in psychological and medical terms, more serious and the "failure" of a suicide attempt is often the result of chance. Also, as a general trend, rates of non-fatal suicidal behaviour tend to be 2–3 times higher in women than in men. Finland, though, is a remarkable exception to this pattern (*35*).

Data from an ongoing, cross-national study of non-fatal suicidal behaviour in 13 countries, show that in the period 1989–1992 the highest average age-standardized rate of suicide attempts in men was found in Helsinki, Finland (314 per 100 000), while the lowest rate (45 per 100 000) was in Guipúzcoa, Spain – a sevenfold difference (*35*). The highest average age-standardized rate for women was in Cergy-Pontoise, France (462 per 100 000) and the lowest (69 per 100 000) was again in Guipúzcoa. With only one exception, that of Helsinki, the rates of suicide attempts were higher among women than among men. In the majority of centres, the highest rates were found in the younger age groups, while the rates among people aged 55 years and over were generally the lowest. The most common method used was poisoning, followed by cutting. More than half of those attempting suicide made more than one attempt, with nearly 20% of second attempts being made within 12 months of the first.

Data from a longitudinal, representative sample of nearly 10 000 adolescents aged 12–20 years in Norway found that 8% had at one time attempted suicide and 2.7% had made such an attempt during the 2 years of the study period. Logistic regression analyses of the data showed that there was a greater likelihood of attempted suicide if the person had made an earlier suicide attempt, was female, was around the age of puberty, had suicidal ideation, consumed alcohol, did not live with both parents, or had a low level of self-esteem (*36*).

Suicidal ideation is more common than both attempted and completed suicide (*8*). However, its extent is still unclear. A review of studies published after 1985 on adolescent populations (particularly secondary-school students) suggested that between 3.5% and 52.1% of adolescents report suicidal thoughts (*31*). It is possible that these large percentage differences could be explained by the use of different definitions of suicidal ideation and by the different time periods to which the studies referred. There is evidence that women, including those in old age, are more prone to suicidal thoughts than are men (*37*). Overall, the prevalence of suicidal ideation among older adults of both sexes has been estimated at between 2.3% (for those having had suicidal thoughts in the past 2 weeks) and 17% (for those ever having had suicidal thoughts) (*38*). However, compared with other forms of suicidal behaviours, such as attempted suicide, suicidal ideation may not be a useful indicator of which adolescents or adults are most in need of preventive services.

What are the risk factors for suicidal behaviour?

Suicidal behaviour has a large number of underlying causes. The factors that place individuals at risk for suicide are complex and interact with one another. Identifying these factors and understanding their roles in both fatal and non-fatal suicidal behaviour are central to preventing suicides. Epidemiologists and experts in suicide have described a number of specific characteristics that are closely associated with a heightened risk for suicidal behaviour. Apart from demographic factors – such as age and sex, both already mentioned above – these include psychiatric, biological, social

share 50% of their genes (*54*). However, there have as yet been no studies on monozygotic twins reared apart – a prerequisite for a methodologically sound study – and none of the studies on twins have carefully controlled for psychiatric disorders. It could be that it is a psychiatric disorder that is inherited, rather than a genetic predisposition to suicidal behaviour, and that this disorder makes suicidal behaviour in related individuals more likely.

Findings from a case–control study of adopted children showed that those who committed suicide tended to have biological relatives who committed suicide (*55*). These suicides were largely independent of the presence of a psychiatric disorder, suggesting that there is a genetic predisposition for suicide independent of – or possibly in addition to – the major psychiatric disorders associated with suicide. Other social and environmental factors probably also interact with family history to increase the risk of suicide.

Further evidence suggesting a biological basis for suicide comes from studies of neurobiological processes that underlie many psychiatric conditions, including those that predispose individuals to suicide. Some studies, for example, have found altered levels of serotonin metabolites in the cerebrospinal fluid of adult psychiatric patients who committed suicide (*56, 57*). Serotonin is a very important neurohormone that controls mood and aggression. Low levels of serotonin and blunted responses to those tests that interfere with its metabolism have been shown to persist for some time after episodes of illness (*58, 59*). An impaired functioning of those neurons that contain serotonin in the prefrontal cortex of the brain may be an underlying cause of a person's reduced ability to resist impulses to act on suicidal thoughts (*60, 61*).

Suicide may also be the consequence of a severe and painful illness, especially one that is disabling. The prevalence of physical illness in those who commit suicide is estimated to be at least 25%, though it may be as high as 80% among elderly people who commit suicide (*62*). In more than 40% of cases, physical illness is considered an important contributory factor to suicidal behaviour and ideation, especially if there are also mood disorders or depressive symptoms (*63*). It is understandable that the prospect of unbearable suffering and humiliating dependency might lead people to consider ending their life. However, several investigations have shown that people suffering from a physical illness rarely commit suicide in the absence of any psychiatric symptoms (*42*).

Life events as precipitating factors

Certain life events may serve as precipitating factors for suicide. Particular events that a small number of studies have tried to link to risk of suicide include personal loss, interpersonal conflict, a broken or disturbed relationship, and legal or work-related problems (*64–67*).

The loss of a loved one, whether through divorce, separation or death, may trigger intense depressive feelings, especially if the person lost was a partner or was exceptionally close. Conflicts in interpersonal relationships in the home, or in places of study or work can also unleash feelings of hopelessness and depression. In a study of over 16 000 adolescents in Finland, for example, researchers found an increased prevalence of depression and severe suicidal ideation both among those who were bullied in school and among those who were perpetrators of bullying (*68*). A retrospective study in south-east Scotland that controlled for age, sex and mental disorders found adverse interpersonal conflict to be independently associated with suicides (*69*). In a review of all suicides over a 2-year period in Ballarat, Australia, researchers found that social and personal difficulties were associated with suicide in over one-third of the cases (*70*). Research has also indicated a greater likelihood of depression and suicide attempts among victims of violence between intimate partners (*71–74*).

A history of physical or sexual abuse in childhood can increase the risk of suicide in adolescence and adulthood (*75–77*). Humiliation and shame are commonly felt by victims of sexual abuse (*2*). Those who were abused during childhood and adolescence often feel mistrustful in interpersonal relationships and have difficulty in maintaining such relationships. They experience persistent sexual difficulties and intense feelings of inadequacy and inferiority. Researchers in the Netherlands examined the relationship between sexual abuse and suicidal behaviour in 1490 adolescent students, and found that those who had experienced abuse displayed significantly more suicidal behaviour, as well as other emotional and behavioural problems, than their non-abused peers (*78*). An ongoing 17-year longitudinal study of 375 subjects in the United States found that 11% had reported physical or sexual abuse before the age of 18 years. Subjects aged between 15 and 21 years who had been abused reported more suicidal behaviour, depression, anxiety, psychiatric disorders, and other emotional and behavioural problems than those who had not been abused (*79*).

Sexual orientation may also be related to an increased risk for suicide in adolescents and young adults (*80, 81*). Estimates of the prevalence of suicide among gay and lesbian youths, for example, range from 2.5% to 30% (*82, 83*). The factors that may contribute to suicides and attempted suicide here include discrimination, stress in interpersonal relations, drugs and alcohol, anxiety about HIV/AIDS and limited sources of support (*84, 85*).

Being in a stable marital relationship, on the other hand, would seem generally to be a "protective" factor against suicide. Responsibilities for bringing up children confer an additional protective element (*86*). Studies on the relationship between marital status and suicide reveal high rates of suicide among single or never-married people in Western cultures, even higher rates among widowed people, and some of the highest rates among people who are separated or divorced (*87, 88*). This last phenomenon is particularly evident in males, especially in the first few months after their loss or separation (*89*).

In an exception to the generally protective effect of marriage, those who marry early (before 20 years of age) have higher rates of suicidal behaviour than their unmarried peers, according to some studies (*90, 91*). Furthermore, marriage is not protective in all cultures. Higher rates of both fatal and non-fatal suicidal behaviour have been reported among married women in Pakistan, compared with both married men and single women (*92, 93*). This may be because social, economic and legal discrimination creates psychological stress that predisposes these women to suicidal behaviour (*92*). Higher rates of suicide have also been reported among married women over the age of 60 years in Hong Kong SAR, China, compared with widowed and divorced women in this age group (*90*).

While problems in interpersonal relationships may increase the risk of suicidal behaviour, social isolation can also be a precipitating factor for suicidal behaviour. Social isolation lay behind Durkheim's concepts of "egoistic" and "anomic" suicide (*94*), both of which were related to the idea of inadequate social connectedness. A large body of literature suggests that individuals who experience isolation in their lives are more vulnerable to suicide than those who have strong social ties with others (*95–98*). Following the death of a loved one, for example, a person may attempt suicide if there is insufficient support provided during the grieving period by those close to the bereaved person.

In a comparative study of social behaviour between groups of people who have attempted suicide, people who have completed suicide and people dying of natural causes, Maris (*99*) found that those who completed suicide had participated less in social organization, were often without friends and had shown a progressive decline in interpersonal relationships leading to a state of total social isolation. Psychological autopsy studies show that social withdrawal frequently precedes the suicidal act (*99*). This was also brought out in a study by Negron et al. (*100*), who found that people who attempted suicide were more likely to isolate themselves during an acute suicidal phase than those with suicidal ideation. Wenz (*101*) identified anomie – the feeling of alienation from society caused by the perceived absence of a supporting social framework – as one factor in the suicidal behaviour of widows, along with actual and expected social isolation. Social isolation has frequently been identified as a contributing factor in suicidal ideation among the elderly (*102, 103*). A study of suicide attempts among

163. Oliver RG, Hetzel BS. Rise and fall of suicide rates in Australia: relation to sedative availability. *Medical Journal of Australia*, 1972, 2:919–923.

164. Kreitman N. The coal gas history: United Kingdom suicide rates, 1960–1971. *British Journal of Preventive and Social Medicine*, 1972, 30:86–93.

165. Lester D. Preventing suicide by restricting access to methods for suicide. *Archives of Suicide Research*, 1998, 4:7–24.

166. Clarke RV, Lester D. Toxicity of car exhausts and opportunity for suicide. *Journal of Epidemiology and Community Health*, 1987, 41:114–120.

167. Lester D, Murrell ME. The influence of gun control laws on suicidal behaviour. *American Journal of Psychiatry*, 1980, 80:151–154.

168. Kellerman AL et al. Suicide in the home in relation to gun ownership. *New England Journal of Medicine*, 1992, 327:467–472.

169. Carrington PJ, Moyer MA. Gun control and suicide in Ontario. *American Journal of Psychiatry*, 1994, 151:606–608.

170. Reed TJ. *Goethe*. Oxford, Oxford University Press, 1984 (Past Masters Series).

171. *Preventing suicide: a resource for media professionals*. Geneva, World Health Organization, 2000 (document WHO/MNH/MBD/00.2).

172. *Preventing suicide: how to start a survivors group*. Geneva, World Health Organization, 2000 (document WHO/MNH/MBD/00.6).

173. *Prevention of suicide: guidelines for the formulation and implementation of national strategies*. New York, NY, United Nations, 1996 (document ST/SEA/245).

174. *Preventing suicide: a resource for general physicians*. Geneva, World Health Organization, 2000 (document WHO/MNH/MBD/00.1).

175. *Preventing suicide: a resource for teachers and other school staff*. Geneva, World Health Organization, 2000 (document WHO/MNH/MBD/00.3).

176. *Preventing suicide: a resource for primary health care workers*. Geneva, World Health Organization, 2000 (document WHO/MNH/MBD/00.4).

177. *Preventing suicide: a resource for prison officers*. Geneva, World Health Organization, 2000 (document WHO/MNH/MBD/00.5).

178. *The world health report 2001. Mental health: new understanding, new hope*. Geneva, World Health Organization, 2001.

179. United States Public Health Service. *The Surgeon General's call to action to prevent suicide*. Washington, DC, United States Department of Health and Human Services, 1999.

180. Isacsson G. Suicide prevention: a medical breakthrough? *Acta Psychiatrica Scandinavica*, 2000, 102:113–117.

181. Rutz W. The role of family physicians in preventing suicide. In: Lester D, ed. *Suicide prevention: resources for the millennium*. Philadelphia, PA, Brunner-Routledge, 2001:173–187.

182. De Leo D. Cultural issues in suicide and old age. *Crisis*, 1999, 20:53–55.

183. Schmidtke A et al. Suicide rates in the world: an update. *Archives of Suicide Research*, 1999, 5:81–89.

CHAPTER 8

Collective violence

middle-income countries in the WHO Eastern Mediterranean Region (8.2 per 100 000) and WHO European Region (7.6 per 100 000), respectively.

Casualties of conflicts

Between the 16th and 20th centuries, the estimated totals of conflict-related deaths per century were, respectively, 1.6 million, 6.1 million, 7.0 million, 19.4 million and 109.7 million (*12, 13*). Such figures naturally conceal the circumstances in which people died. Six million people, for instance, are estimated to have lost their lives in the capture and transport of slaves over four centuries, and 10 million indigenous people in the Americas died at the hands of European colonists.

According to one estimate (*14*), some 191 million people lost their lives directly or indirectly in the 25 largest instances of collective violence in the 20th century, 60% of those deaths occurring among people not engaged in fighting. Besides the First World War and the Second World War, two of the most catastrophic events in terms of lives lost were the period of Stalinist terror and the millions of people who perished in China during the Great Leap Forward (1958–1960). Both events are still surrounded by uncertainty over the scale of human losses. Conflict-related deaths in the 25 largest events included some 39 million soldiers and 33 million civilians. Famine related to conflict or genocide in the 20th century killed a further 40 million people.

A relatively new development in armed conflicts is the increasing number of violent deaths of civilian United Nations employees and workers from nongovernmental organizations in conflict zones. In the period 1985–1998, over 380 deaths occurred among humanitarian workers (*15*), with more United Nations civilian personnel than United Nations peacekeeping troops being killed.

Torture and rape

Torture is a common practice in many conflicts (see Box 8.1). Because victims are inclined to hide the trauma they have suffered and because there are also political pressures to conceal the use of torture, it is difficult to estimate how widespread it is.

Rape as a weapon of war has also been documented in numerous conflicts. Though women form the overwhelming majority of those targeted, male rape also occurs in conflicts. Estimates of the number of women raped in Bosnia and Herzegovina during the conflict between 1992 and 1995 range from 10 000 to 60 000 (*22*). Reports of rape during violent conflicts in recent decades have also been documented from Bangladesh, Liberia, Rwanda and Uganda, amongst others (see Chapter 6). Rape is often used to terrorize and undermine communities, to force people to flee, and to break up community structures. The physical and psychological effects on the victims are far-reaching (*23, 24*).

The nature of conflicts

Since the Second World War, there have been a total of 190 armed conflicts, only a quarter of which were between states. In fact, modern-day conflicts are increasingly within rather than between states. Most of the armed conflicts since the Second World War have been shorter than 6 months in duration. Those that lasted longer often went on for many years. For example, in Viet Nam, violent conflict spanned more than two decades. Other examples include the conflicts in Afghanistan and Angola. The total number of armed conflicts in progress was less than 20 in the 1950s, over 30 in both the 1960s and 1970s, and rose to over 50 during the late 1980s. While there were fewer armed conflicts in progress after 1992, those that took place were, on average, of longer duration.

While conflicts within states are most common, conflicts between states still occur. The war between Iraq and the Islamic Republic of Iran in 1980–1988 is estimated to have left 450 000 soldiers and 50 000 civilians dead (*13*). The conflict between Eritrea and Ethiopia at the end of the 20th century was largely fought between two conventional armies, using heavy weaponry and trench warfare, and claimed tens of thousands of lives. There have also been coalitions of multinational forces engaged in conflict by means of massive air attacks – as in the Gulf War against Iraq in 1991 and in the North Atlantic Treaty Organization (NATO) campaign against the Federal Republic of Yugoslavia in 1999.

BOX 8.1

Torture

A number of international treaties have defined torture. The United Nations Convention against Torture and Other Cruel, Inhuman or Degrading Treatment or Punishment of 1984 refers to an "act by which severe pain or suffering, whether physical or mental, is intentionally inflicted on a person", for a purpose such as obtaining information or a confession, punishment, intimidation or coercion, "or for any reason based on discrimination of any kind". The Convention is concerned with torture by public officials or others acting in an official capacity.

In preparing its 2000 report on torture (*16*), the human rights organization Amnesty International found reports of torture or ill-treatment by officials in more than 150 countries. In more than 70 countries, the practice was apparently widespread and in over 80 countries, people reportedly died as a result of torture. Most of the victims appeared to have been people suspected or convicted of criminal offences, and most of the torturers were police officers.

The prevalence of torture against criminal suspects is most likely to be underreported, as the victims are generally less able to file complaints. In some countries, a long-standing practice of torturing common criminals attracts attention only when more overt political repression has declined. In the absence of proper training and investigative mechanisms, police may resort to torture or ill-treatment to extract confessions quickly and obtain convictions.

In some instances of torture, the purpose is to extract information, to obtain a confession (whether true or false), to force collaboration or to "break" the victim as an example to others. In other cases, punishment and humiliation are the primary aim. Torture is also sometimes employed as a means of extortion. Once established, a regime of torture can perpetuate itself.

Torture has serious implications for public health, as it damages the mental and physical health of populations. The victims may stay in their own country, adapting as best they can, with or without medical and psychosocial support. If their needs are not properly attended to they risk becoming increasingly alienated or dysfunctional members of society. The same is true if they go into exile. Existing data on asylum-seekers, some of whom have undergone torture in their home country, suggest that they have significant health needs (*17, 18*).

Failure to control the use of torture encourages poor practice by the police and security forces and an increased tolerance of human rights abuses and violence. Various organizations of health professionals have taken a vigorous stand against torture, seeing its prevention as closely linked to their medical calling and to the good of public health (*19*). Nongovernmental organizations have also promoted prevention (*20*).

One particular control mechanism — the inspection system of the Council of Europe — has been recommended for use at the global level. A draft "Optional Protocol" to the United Nations Convention on Torture would provide for a similar such inspection system in places of detention. To date, progress in elaborating an Optional Protocol has been slow.

Initiatives to investigate and document torture have grown in recent years. The United Nations guidelines on assessing and recording medical evidence of torture, known as the "Istanbul Protocol", were drawn up in 1999 by forensic scientists, doctors, human rights monitors and lawyers from 15 countries and published 2 years later (*21*).

Many of the conflicts since the end of the Second World War have been in developing countries. After the collapse of communist regimes in Eastern Europe and the former Soviet Union in the late 1980s and early 1990s, there was a sharp increase, for a while, in armed conflicts taking place in Europe.

The size of the area of conflict has changed radically in the past two centuries. Until the early

19th century, warfare between states took place on a "field of battle". The mobilization of citizen-soldiers during the Napoleonic wars created larger, but essentially similar battlefields. With the development in the 19th century of railways and the mechanization of mass transport, mobile warfare with rapidly moving positions in large geographical areas became possible. Subsequently, the development of tanks, submarines, fighter/bombers and laser-guided missiles laid the foundations for battle-fields without geographical limits. Recent conflicts, such as the one waged in 1999 by NATO against the Federal Republic of Yugoslavia, have been referred to as "virtual wars" (*25*), given the extent to which these conflicts are fought with missiles controlled from a distance, without the involvement of troops on the ground.

What are the risk factors for collective violence?

Good public health practice requires identifying risk factors and determinants of collective violence, and developing approaches to resolve conflicts without resorting to violence. A range of risk factors for major political conflicts has been identified. In particular, the Carnegie Commission on Preventing Deadly Conflict (*26*) has listed indicators of states at risk of collapse and internal conflict (see Table 8.1). In combination, these factors interact with one another to create conditions for violent conflict. On their own, none of them may be sufficient to lead to violence or disintegration of a state.

The risk factors for violent conflicts include:
- Political factors:
  — a lack of democratic processes;
  — unequal access to power.
- Economic factors:

— grossly unequal distribution of resources;
— unequal access to resources;
— control over key natural resources;
— control over drug production or trading.
- Societal and community factors:
  — inequality between groups;
  — the fuelling of group fanaticism along ethnic, national or religious lines;
  — the ready availability of small arms and other weapons.
- Demographic factors:
  — rapid demographic change.

Many of these risk factors can be identified before overt collective violence takes place.

Political and economic factors

The grossly unequal distribution of resources, particularly health and education services, and of access to these resources and to political power –

TABLE 8.1

Indicators of states at risk of collapse and internal conflict

Indicator	Signs
Inequality	• Widening social and economic inequalities – especially those between, rather than within, distinct population groups
Rapidly changing demographic characteristics	• High rates of infant mortality • Rapid changes in population structure, including large-scale movements of refugees • Excessively high population densities • High levels of unemployment, particularly among large numbers of young people • An insufficient supply of food or access to safe water • Disputes over territory or environmental resources that are claimed by distinct ethnic groups
Lack of democratic processes	• Violations of human rights • Criminal behaviour by the state • Corrupt governments
Political instability	• Rapid changes in regimes
Ethnic composition of the ruling group sharply different from that of the population at large	• Political and economic power exercised – and differentially applied – according to ethnic or religious identity • Desecration of ethnic or religious symbols
Deterioration in public services	• A significant decline in the scope and effectiveness of social safety nets designed to ensure minimum universal standards of service
Severe economic decline	• Uneven economic development • Grossly unequal gains or losses between different population groups or geographical areas resulting from large economic changes • Massive economic transfers or losses over short periods of time
Cycles of violent revenge	• A continued cycle of violence between rival groups

whether by geographical area, social class, religion, race or ethnicity – are important factors that can contribute to conflict between groups. Undemocratic leadership, especially if it is repressive and if power stems from ethnic or religious identity, is a powerful contributor to conflict. A decline in public services, usually affecting the poorest segments of society most severely, may be an early sign of a deteriorating situation.

Conflict is less likely in situations of economic growth than in contracting economies, where competition over resources is intensified.

Globalization

Trends in the global economy have accelerated the pace of global integration and economic growth for some countries, and for some groups within countries, and at the same time have contributed to the fragmentation and economic marginalization of others. Other possible risk factors for conflict that may be linked to globalization are financial (the frequently large and rapid movements of currencies around the world) and cultural (individual and collective aspirations raised by the global media that cannot realistically be met). It is still unknown whether current trends in globalization are likely to lead to more conflict and greater violence within or between states. Figure 8.1 shows potential links between trends in globalization and the occurrence of conflict (27).

Natural resources

Struggles over access to key natural resources frequently play a role in fuelling and prolonging conflicts. Examples from conflicts in the past two decades are those related to diamonds in Angola, the Democratic Republic of the Congo and Sierra Leone; to oil in Angola and southern Sudan; and to timber and gems in Cambodia. In other places, including Afghanistan, Colombia and Myanmar, the desire to control the production and distribution of drugs has contributed to violent conflicts.

Societal and community factors

A particularly important risk factor associated with the occurrence of conflict is the existence of inter-group inequalities, especially if these are widening (28) and are seen to reflect the unequal allocation of resources within a society. Such a factor is often seen in countries where the government is dominated by one community, that wields political, military and economic power over quite distinct communities.

The ready availability of small arms or other weapons in the general population can also heighten the risk of conflict. This is particularly

---

FIGURE 8.1

Possible linkages between globalization, inequalities and conflict

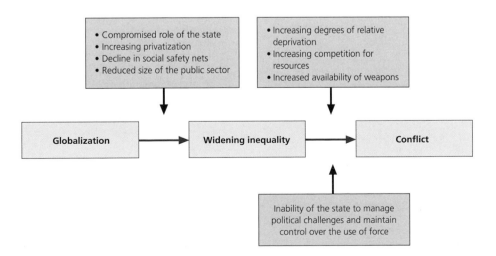

problematic in places where there have previously been conflicts, and where programmes of demobilization, decommissioning of weapons and job creation for former soldiers are inadequate or where such measures have not been established.

Demographic factors

Rapid demographic change – including an increased population density and a greater proportion of young people – combined with the inability of a country to match the population increase with correspondingly more jobs and schools, may contribute to violent conflict, particularly where other risk factors are also present. In these conditions, large population movements may occur as desperate people seek a more sustainable life elsewhere, and this in turn may increase the risk of violence in the areas into which people move.

Technological factors

The level of weapons technology does not necessarily affect the risk of a conflict, but it does determine the scale of any conflict and the amount of destruction that will take place. Many centuries ago, the progression from the arrow to the crossbow increased the range and destructive force of projectile weapons. Much later, simple firearms were developed, followed by rifles, machine guns and submachine guns. The ability to fire more bullets, more quickly, and with greater range and accuracy, has greatly increased the potential destructive power of such weapons.

Nonetheless, even basic weapons, such as the machete, can contribute to the occurrence of massive human destruction, as was seen in the genocide in Rwanda in 1994 (*29*). In the acts of terrorism in the United States on 11 September 2001, where hijacked passenger aircraft were deliberately crashed into the World Trade Center Towers and the Pentagon, killing several thousand people, conventional weapons were not a major feature of the incidents.

The consequences of collective violence

Impact on health

The impact of conflict on health can be very great in terms of mortality, morbidity and disability (see Table 8.2).

Infant mortality

In times of conflict, infant mortality generally increases. Preventable diseases such as measles, tetanus and diphtheria may become epidemic. In

TABLE 8.2
Examples of the direct impact of conflict on health

Health impact	Causes
Increased mortality	• Deaths due to external causes, mainly related to weapons • Deaths due to infectious diseases (such as measles, poliomyelitis, tetanus and malaria) • Deaths due to noncommunicable diseases, as well as deaths otherwise avoidable through medical care (including asthma, diabetes and emergency surgery)

Increased morbidity	• Injuries from external causes, such as those from weapons, mutilation, anti-personnel landmines, burns and poisoning
	• Morbidity associated with other external causes, including sexual violence
	• Infectious diseases:
	  — water-related (such as cholera, typhoid and dysentery due to *Shigella* spp.)
	  — vector-borne (such as malaria and onchocerciasis)
	  — other communicable diseases (such as tuberculosis, acute respiratory infections, HIV infection and other sexually transmitted diseases)
	• Reproductive health:
	  — a greater number of stillbirths and premature births, more cases of low birth weight and more delivery complications
	  — longer-term genetic impact of exposure to chemicals and radiation
	• Nutrition:
	  — acute and chronic malnutrition and a variety of deficiency disorders
	• Mental health:
	  — anxiety
	  — depression
	  — post-traumatic stress disorder
	  — suicidal behaviour

Increased disability	• Physical • Psychological • Social

the mid-1980s, infant mortality in Uganda rose above 600 per 1000 in some conflict-affected areas (*30*). According to the United Nations Children's Fund, reductions in infant mortality were reported for all countries in southern Africa over the period 1960–1986, with the exception of Angola and Mozambique, both of which were subject to ongoing conflicts (*31*). Efforts to eradicate infectious diseases such as poliomyelitis are hampered by residues of the disease in conflict-affected areas.

In Zepa, Bosnia and Herzegovina – a United Nations-controlled "safe area" subsequently overrun by Bosnian Serb forces – perinatal and childhood mortality rates doubled after only one year of conflict. In Sarajevo, deliveries of premature babies had doubled and average birth weights fallen by 20% by 1993.

Communicable diseases

The increased risk during conflicts of communicable diseases stems generally from:

— the decline in immunization coverage;
— population movements and overcrowding in refugee camps;
— greater exposure to vectors and environmental hazards, such as polluted water;
— the reduction in public health campaigns and outreach activities;
— the lack of access to health care services.

During the fighting in Bosnia and Herzegovina in 1994, fewer than 35% of children were immunized, compared with 95% before hostilities broke out (*32, 33*). In Iraq, there were sharp declines in immunization coverage after the Gulf War of 1991 and the subsequent imposition of economic and political sanctions. However, recent evidence from El Salvador indicates that it is possible, with selective health care interventions and the provision of adequate resources, to improve certain health problems during ongoing conflicts (*34*).

In Nicaragua in 1985–1986, a measles epidemic was attributed in large part to the declining ability of the health service to immunize those at risk in conflict-affected areas (*35*). A deterioration in malaria-control activities was linked to epidemics of malaria in Ethiopia (*36*) and Mozambique (*37*),

highlighting the vulnerability of disease control programmes during periods of conflict. The outbreak of Ebola haemorrhagic fever in Gulu, Uganda, in 2000, was widely believed to be connected with the return of troops from fighting in the Democratic Republic of the Congo.

In Ethiopia in the late 1980s, epidemics of typhus fever and relapsing fever – infectious diseases transmitted by infected ticks, lice or fleas – were believed to come from crowded army camps, prisons and relief camps, as well as from the sale of infected blankets and clothes to local communities by retreating soldiers (*36*). In the exodus from Rwanda in 1994, epidemics of water-related diseases, such as cholera and dysentery due to *Shigella* spp., led to the death within a month of 6–10% of the refugee population arriving in Zaire (now the Democratic Republic of the Congo) (*38*). The crude death rate of 20–35 per 10 000 population per day was 2–3 times higher than that previously reported in refugee populations.

During and in the wake of violent conflicts, there is often a greatly increased risk of transmission of HIV infection and other sexually transmitted diseases (*39*). In many armed forces, the prevalence of HIV infection has already reached high levels (*40*). In times of conflict, military forces (including sometimes also peacekeeping forces) assume the power to command sexual services from local people, either by force or payment (*41*). The transmission of HIV and other sexually transmitted diseases is further fuelled by the fact that troops have a high degree of mobility, and ultimately return to different regions after demobilization (*36, 42, 43*). Overall, refugees from conflicts and internally displaced people have an increased risk of HIV infection (*44*) because:

• They are generally more vulnerable to sexual abuse and violence.

• They are more likely to turn to prostitution – having been deprived of their normal sources of income for surviving.

• Displaced children, with little else to occupy them and possibly no one to supervise them, may become sexually active earlier than they would otherwise.

- Blood used in emergencies for transfusions may not have been screened for HIV.

Disability

Data on conflict-related disability are scant. A nationwide survey conducted in 1982 in Zimbabwe found that 13% of all physical disabilities were a direct result of the previous armed conflict. Over 30 years of armed conflict in Ethiopia led to some 1 million deaths, around half of which were among civilians (*36*). About one-third of the 300 000 soldiers returning from the front line after the end of the conflict had been injured or disabled and at least 40 000 people had lost one or more limbs in the conflict.

Landmines are a major contributor to disability. In Cambodia, 36 000 people have lost at least one limb after accidentally detonating a landmine – one in every 236 of the population (*45*). A total of 6000 people were disabled in this way in 1990 alone. Over 30 million mines were laid in Afghanistan in the 1980s.

In some conflicts, mutilation in the form of cutting off ears or lips, as practised in Mozambique during the civil war (*46*), or limbs, as more recently in Sierra Leone (*47*), has been systematically practised in order to demoralize the opposing forces.

Mental health

The impact of conflicts on mental health is influenced by a range of factors. These include (*48*):

— the psychological health of those affected, prior to the event;
— the nature of the conflict;
— the form of trauma (whether it results from living through and witnessing acts of violence or whether it is directly inflicted, as with torture and other types of repressive violence);
— the response to the trauma, by individuals and communities;
— the cultural context in which the violence occurs.

Psychological stresses related to conflicts are associated with or result from (*49*):

— displacement, whether forced or voluntary;
— loss and grief;
— social isolation;
— loss of status;
— loss of community;
— in some settings, acculturation to new environments.

Manifestations of such stress can include:

— depression and anxiety;
— psychosomatic ailments;
— suicidal behaviour;
— intra-familial conflict;
— alcohol abuse;
— antisocial behaviour.

Single and isolated refugees, as well as women who are heads of households, may be at particular risk of suffering psychological stress.

Some experts (*48, 50*) have cautioned against assuming that people do not have the ability and resilience to respond to the adverse conditions stemming from violent conflict. Others have warned of the danger (*51*) that humanitarian assistance programmes may become a substitute for political dialogue with parties to the conflict – possibly those who are its main driving force. Studies in South Africa (*52*) have found that not all those who were subject to trauma under apartheid became "victims". Instead, at least in some cases, individuals were able to respond strongly because they saw themselves as fighting for worthwhile and legitimate causes. The medical model which ascribes to individuals the condition of "post-traumatic stress syndrome" may fail to take account of the variety and complexity of human responses to stressful events (*48*). It is now becoming clearer that recovery from psychological trauma resulting from violent conflict is associated with the reconstruction of social and economic networks and cultural institutions (*50*).

Increased rates of depression, substance abuse and suicide frequently result from violent conflicts (*34*). Before its two decades of violent conflict, Sri Lanka had a much lower suicide rate overall than it does now (*53*). Similar findings have been reported from El Salvador (*34*). In both these cases, the sharp increase in suicides was at least in part a consequence of political violence.

From a mental health point of view, populations affected by violent conflict can be divided into three groups (54):

— those with disabling psychiatric illnesses;
— those with severe psychological reactions to trauma;
— those, forming the majority, who are able to adapt once peace and order are restored.

The first two groups are likely to benefit considerably from the provision of mental health care that takes into account cultural and socio-economic factors.

Impact on specific populations

The direct effect of conflict on the health of armed forces is usually recorded with some degree of precision; however, the effect of conflict on particular groups is often especially difficult to determine. Population size and density can vary greatly over short periods of time as people move to safe areas and to places where more resources are available. This fact complicates measurements of the impact of conflict on health.

Civilians

According to the 1949 Geneva Conventions, armed forces must apply the principles of proportionality and distinction in their choice of targets. *Proportionality* involves trying to minimize civilian casualties when pursuing military and related targets. *Distinction* means avoiding civilian targets wherever possible (52). Despite such attempts to regulate their impact, armed conflicts cause many deaths among civilians.

While civilian deaths may be the direct result of military operations, increased mortality rates among civilians in times of conflict are usually a reflection of the combined effects of:

— decreased access to food, leading to poor nutrition;
— increased risk of communicable diseases;
— reduced access to health services;
— reduced public health programmes;
— poor environmental conditions;
— psychosocial distress.

Refugees and internally displaced people

Refugees and internally displaced people typically experience high mortality, especially in the period immediately after their migration (55, 56). Reviews of the health of refugees and displaced populations have revealed massively raised mortality rates – at their worst, up to 60 times the expected rates during the acute phase of displacement (55, 57, 58). In Monrovia, Liberia, the death rate among civilians displaced during the conflict in 1990 was seven times greater than the pre-conflict rate (57).

Deaths from malnutrition, diarrhoea and infectious diseases occur especially in children, while other infectious diseases such as malaria, tuberculosis and HIV, as well as a range of noncommunicable diseases, injuries and violence typically affect adults. The prior health status of the population, their access to key determinants of health (such as food, shelter, water, sanitation and health services), the extent to which they are exposed to new diseases, and the availability of resources all have an important influence on the health of refugees during and after conflicts.

Demographic impact

One consequence of the shift in the methods of modern warfare, where entire communities are increasingly being targeted, has been the large numbers of displaced people. The total numbers of refugees fleeing across national borders rose from around 2.5 million in 1970 and 11 million in 1983 to 23 million in 1997 (59, 60). In the early 1990s, in addition, an estimated 30 million people were internally displaced at any one time (60), most of them having fled zones of conflict. Those displaced within countries probably have less access to resources and international support than refugees escaping across borders, and are also more likely to be at continuing risk of violence (61).

Table 8.3 shows the movements of refugees and internally displaced populations during the 1990s (62). In Africa, the Americas and Europe during this period there were far more internally displaced people than refugees, while in Asia and the Middle East the reverse was true.

had to serve much larger catchment areas. Widespread damage to water supplies, electricity and sewage disposal further reduced the ability of what remained of the health services to operate (68). In the violent conflict in East Timor in 1999 following the referendum for independence, militia forces destroyed virtually all the health care services. Only the main hospital in the principal town, Dili, was left standing.

During and in the wake of conflicts the supply of medicines is usually disrupted, causing increases in medically preventable conditions, including potentially fatal ones, such as asthma, diabetes and a range of infectious diseases. Apart from medicines, medical personnel, diagnostic equipment, electricity and water may all be lacking, seriously affecting the quality of health care available.

Human resources in the health care services are also usually seriously affected by violent conflicts. In some instances, such as in Mozambique and Nicaragua, medical personnel have been specifically targeted. Qualified personnel often retreat to safer urban areas or may leave their profession altogether. In Uganda between 1972 and 1985, half of the doctors and 80% of the pharmacists left the country for their security. In Mozambique, only 15% of the 550 doctors present during the last years of Portuguese colonial rule were still there at the end of the war of independence in 1975 (69).

What can be done to prevent collective violence?

Reducing the potential for violent conflicts

Among the policies needed to reduce the potential for violent conflicts in the world, of whatever type, are (70):

- Reducing poverty, both in absolute and relative terms, and ensuring that development assistance is targeted so as to make the greatest possible impact on poverty.
- Making decision-making more accountable.
- Reducing inequality between groups in society.
- Reducing access to biological, chemical, nuclear and other weapons.

Promoting compliance with international agreements

An important element in preventing violent conflict and other forms of collective violence is ensuring the promotion and application of internationally agreed treaties, including those relating to human rights.

National governments can help prevent conflicts by upholding the spirit of the United Nations Charter, which calls for the prevention of aggression and the promotion of international peace and security. At a more detailed level, this involves adhering to international legal instruments, including the 1949 Geneva Conventions and their 1977 Protocols.

Laws pertaining to human rights, especially those that stem from the International Covenant on Civil and Political Rights, place limits on the way governments exercise their authority over persons under their jurisdiction, and unconditionally prohibit, among other acts, torture and genocide. The establishment of the International Criminal Court will ensure a permanent mechanism for dealing with war crimes and crimes against humanity. It may also provide disincentives against violence directed at civilian populations.

Efforts to produce treaties and agreements covering collective violence, with disincentives against and sanctions for abuse, tend to be more effective concerning violence between states and generally have far less power within national borders, which is the area where conflicts are increasingly occurring.

The potential benefits of globalization

Globalization is producing new ways for raising public awareness and knowledge about violent conflicts, their causes and their consequences. The new technologies that are appearing provide new means not only to exchange ideas but also pressure decision-makers to increase the accountability and transparency of governance and reduce social inequalities and injustices.

An increasing number of international organizations – including Amnesty International, Human Rights Watch, the International Campaign to Ban

Landmines and Physicians for Human Rights – are monitoring conflicts and urging preventive or corrective actions. Individuals and groups affected by conflict can now – through these organizations and in other ways – make use of the new technologies to relate their experiences and concerns to a wide public.

The role of the health sector

Investing in health development also contributes to the prevention of violent conflict. A strong emphasis on social services can help maintain social cohesion and stability.

Early manifestations of situations that can lead to conflicts can often be detected in the health sector. Health care workers have an important role to play in drawing attention to these signs and in calling for appropriate social and health interventions to reduce the risks of conflict (see Box 8.2).

In terms of reducing inequalities between social groups and unequal access to resources – both important risk factors for violence – the health sector is well placed to detect inequalities in health status and access to health care. Identifying these inequalities early on and promoting corrective measures are important preventive actions against potential conflicts, especially so where the gaps between social groups are growing. Monitoring the distribution and trends in diseases associated with poverty, in medically preventable or treatable conditions, and in inequalities in survival, are all essential for detecting largely unrecognized, but important and possibly widening, disparities in society.

The health sector can also perform a major service by publicizing the social and economic impacts of violent conflicts and their effects on health.

Responses to violent conflicts
Service provision during conflicts

Common problems confronting humanitarian operations during periods of conflict include (*71*):
— how best to upgrade health care services for the host population in parallel with providing services for refugees;
— how to provide good-quality services, humanely and efficiently;

— how to involve communities in determining priorities and the way in which services are provided;
— how to create sustainable mechanisms through which experience from the field is used in formulating policy.

Refugees fleeing their country across borders lose their usual sources of health care. They are then dependent on whatever is available in the host country or can be provided in additional services by international agencies and nongovernmental organizations. The services of the host government may be overwhelmed if large numbers of refugees suddenly move into an area and seek to use local health services. This can be a source of antagonism between the refugees and population of the host country, that may spill over into new violence. Such antagonism may be aggravated if refugees are offered services, including health services, more easily or cheaply than are available to the local population, or if the host country does not receive resources from outside to cope with its greatly increased burden. When ethnic Albanians from Kosovo fled into Albania and The former Yugoslav Republic of Macedonia during the conflict in 1999, the World Health Organization and other agencies tried to help the existing health and welfare systems of these host countries to deal with the added load, rather than simply allowing a parallel system to be imported through the aid agencies.

When planning responses during crises, governments and agencies need to:
— assess at a very early stage who is particularly vulnerable and what their needs are;
— strictly coordinate activities between the various players;
— work towards increasing global, national and local capabilities so as to deliver effective health services during the various stages of the emergency.

The World Health Organization has developed surveillance mechanisms to help identify and respond, earlier rather than later, to conflicts. Its Health Intelligence Network for Advanced Contingency Planning provides rapid access to up-to-date information on particular countries and their

BOX 8.2

Health as a bridge for peace

The concept that health can further regional conciliation and collaboration was enshrined in 1902 in the founding principles of the Pan American Health Organization, the oldest international health organization in the world. For the past two decades, the Pan American Health Organization/WHO Regional Office for the Americas has been instrumental in applying this concept.

In 1984, PAHO/WHO, in partnership with national health ministries and other institutions, launched a strategic initiative in war-torn areas of Central America. The aim was to improve the health of the peoples of Central America, while building cooperation between and within countries of the region. Under the overall theme of "Health as a bridge for peace, solidarity and understanding", the plan consisted of a range of programmes.

In the first phase, up to 1990, there were seven priorities for collaboration:
— strengthening health services;
— developing human resources;
— essential drugs;
— food and nutrition;
— major tropical diseases;
— child survival;
— water supply and sanitation.

Within a few years, over 250 projects in these priority areas had been developed, stimulating collaboration among nations and groupings in Central America otherwise in dispute with one another. In El Salvador, for example, despite the difficulty of working in the midst of political violence, "days of tranquillity" were negotiated and fighting was suspended so that children could be immunized. This arrangement lasted from 1985 until the end of the conflict in 1992, allowing some 300 000 children to be immunized annually. The incidence of measles, tetanus and poliomyelitis dropped dramatically, that of poliomyelitis falling to zero.

Collaboration also took place in malaria control, cross-border distribution of medicines and vaccines, and training. Regional and subregional health information networks were established and a rapid-response system for natural disasters was set up. These efforts created a precedent for wider dialogue within the region, until the eventual peace accords.

During the second phase of the initiative, from 1990 to 1995, health sectors across Central America supported efforts for development and democracy. Following the peace settlements, PAHO/WHO helped in demobilization, rehabilitation and social reintegration of those most affected by the conflict — including indigenous and border populations. Health continued to be a driving factor for democratic consolidation in the third phase between 1995 and 2000.

Between 1991 and 1997, similar programmes were set up in Angola, Bosnia and Herzegovina, Croatia, Haiti and Mozambique. In each programme, representatives from the WHO regional offices worked in partnership with the government, local nongovernmental organizations and other United Nations agencies. All these programmes were instrumental in reconstructing the health sector following the end of the conflicts. In Angola and Mozambique, the World Health Organization participated in the demobilization process, promoted the reintegration into the national system of health services formerly outside the control of the central government, and retrained health workers from these regions. In Bosnia and Herzegovina and in Croatia, the World Health Organization facilitated exchanges between different ethnic groups and enabled regular contacts and collaboration between health professionals from all communities.

> **BOX 8.2 (continued)**
>
> All the experiences of this period were consolidated by the World Health Organization in 1997 under a global programme, "Health as a Bridge for Peace". Since then, new programmes have been set up in the Caucasus Region, Bosnia and Herzegovina, Indonesia, Sri Lanka and The former Yugoslav Republic of Macedonia. In Indonesia, for instance, the World Health Organization has organized teams of health professionals to operate in areas of actual or potential conflict. One such group, comprising both Muslim and Christian professionals, is working in the islands of Maluku province, an area of acute religious conflict in recent years.
>
> Through the "Health as a Bridge for Peace" programme, health workers around the world are being organized to contribute to peace, to bring about stability and reconstruction as conflicts end, and to help conciliation in divided and strife-torn communities.

health indices, as well as guidance on best practices and data on disease surveillance.

In emergencies, humanitarian organizations try in the first instance to prevent loss of life and subsequently to re-establish an environment where health promotion is possible. Many relief organizations see their primary role as saving lives that have been placed at risk as a result of atypical events, without necessarily being concerned whether their activities can be replicated or sustained over the longer term. Those agencies that adopt a specifically development-related perspective, on the other hand, attempt early on to take into account issues such as efficiency, sustainability, equality and local ownership – all of which will produce greater benefits in the longer term. This approach stresses creating local capacity and maintaining low costs. Extending the short-term responses to try to set up longer-term systems is, however, difficult.

Organizations need to work closely together if they are to maximize the use of their resources, keep to a minimum any duplication of activities, and enhance the efficiency of operations. The Code of Conduct for Humanitarian Organizations, as put forward by the International Federation of Red Cross and Red Crescent Societies (62), states a number of key principles that many humanitarian organizations see as forming a basis for their work. Such a code is voluntary, though, and there are no effective measures for enforcing its principles or evaluating whether they are being effectively implemented.

Ethical considerations of aid provision

There are ethical problems relating to interventions in emergency situations and particularly how to distribute aid. In some cases, such as the crisis in Somalia in the early 1990s, aid agencies have hired armed guards in order to be able to carry out their operations, an action which is regarded as ethically questionable. As regards the distribution of aid, there is frequently an expectation that a proportion will be diverted to the warring parties. Aid agencies have generally taken the view that some degree of "leakage" of resources is acceptable, provided that most still reach their intended destination. In some places, though, the proportion of food and other aid being siphoned off has been so great that the agencies have chosen to withdraw their services.

Other ethical concerns centre around the fact that working with warring factions indirectly confers a degree of legitimacy on them and on their activities. Questions arise concerning whether aid agencies should be silent about observed abuses or speak out, and whether they should carry on providing services in the light of continued abuses. Anderson (72), among others, discusses the broader issues of how emergency aid can help promote peace – or alternatively, prolong conflicts.

Community involvement

During periods of conflict, local community structures and activities may be seriously disrupted. People may fear actively debating such issues as social policy or campaigning on behalf of marginalized or vulnerable groups. This is likely to be even more the case under undemocratic political regimes and where state violence is being threatened against perceived opponents of the regime.

In some cases, though, there may be a positive outcome in terms of the community response, where the development of social structures, including health services, is actually made easier. This type of response would appear to be more common in conflicts based on ideology – such as those in the latter part of the 20th century in Mozambique, Nicaragua and Viet Nam. In the conflict in Ethiopia between 1974 and 1991, community-based political movements in Eritrea and Tigray were heavily involved in creating participatory local structures for decision-making and in developing health promotion strategies (73).

Re-establishing services after conflicts

There has been considerable discussion on how best to re-establish services as countries emerge from major periods of conflict (74–76). When inaccessible areas open up in the aftermath of complex emergencies, they release a backlog of public health needs that have long previously been unattended to, typically flagged by epidemics of measles. In addition, ceasefire arrangements, even if precarious, need to include special health support for demobilizing soldiers, plans for demining, and arrangements for refugees and internally displaced people to return. All these demands are likely to occur at a time when the infrastructure of the local health system is seriously weakened and when other economic resources are depleted.

More precise information is needed on interventions in various places, the conditions under which they take place, and their effects and limitations. One problem in collecting data on conflicts is defining a notional end-point. Usually, the boundary between the end of a conflict and the beginning of the post-conflict period is far from clear cut, as significant levels of insecurity and instability often persist for a considerable time.

Table 8.5 outlines some of the typical approaches to rebuilding health care systems in the aftermath of conflicts. In the past, there has been considerable emphasis on physical reconstruction and on disease control programmes, but relatively little consideration of coordinating donor responses or setting up effective policy frameworks.

Documentation, research and dissemination of information

Surveillance and documentation are core areas for public health activities relating to conflicts. While it is the case, as mentioned above, that data on collective violence are often unsatisfactory and imprecise, too rigid a concern with precision of data is not usually warranted in this field. It is essential, however, that data are valid.

Providing valid data to policy-makers is an equally important component of public health action. The United Nations, international agencies, nongovernmental organizations and health professionals all have key roles to perform in this area. The International Committee of the Red Cross (ICRC), for instance, through its extensive research and campaigning work, played a significant part in promoting the Ottawa process which led to the adoption of the anti-personnel Mine Ban Treaty that entered into force on 1 March 1999. As one ICRC staff member involved in this effort put it: "Observing and documenting the effects of weapons does not bring about changes in belief, behaviour or law unless communicated compellingly to both policy-makers and the public" (77).

Some nongovernmental organizations, such as Amnesty International, have explicit mandates to speak out about abuses of human rights. So do some United Nations bodies, such as the Office of the United Nations High Commissioner for Human Rights. Some agencies, however, are reluctant to speak out against those involved in conflicts for fear that their ability to deliver essential services could be compromised. In such cases, agencies may choose to convey information indirectly, through third parties or the media.

If dissemination is to be effective, good data are needed and the experiences from interventions must be properly analysed. Research is crucial for assessing the impact of conflicts on health and on health care systems, and for establishing which interventions are effective.

TABLE 8.5

Post-conflict health challenges

Component of post-conflict health sector activity	Typical situation at present	Actions for a more appropriate response
Setting policy	• Activities are seen as independent projects • Limited attention is given to setting up policy frameworks	• At an early stage, develop policy frameworks within which projects can be based • Encourage donor support to the Ministry of Health for policy development and for gathering and disseminating information • Facilitate communication between key participants
Donor coordination	• Donors agree in principle that coordination is desirable, but none wishes to be coordinated	• Identify areas of common interest and build on these • Strengthen the capacity of the Ministry of Health to take a leading role and to coordinate donors and nongovernmental organizations
Working with the government	• The government is often bypassed, with support being channelled through nongovernmental organizations and United Nations agencies	• Reform the international aid system so as to allow development activities to take place earlier in the period of post-conflict recovery • Consider sector-wide approaches, where donors agree to work within an agreed policy framework
Developing infrastructure	• The aim is to reconstruct exactly what existed before	• Review the needs for services and their distribution • Rationalize and make more equitable the distribution of available services • In placing new services, recognize changed population patterns
Specific disease problems	• Disease control and service delivery is narrowly focused • Donors have considerable control over programmes and provide most of the funds	• Facilitate linkages between different programmes • Ensure programmes operate through the major health system structures • Ensure that disease-focused interventions and those that are health system-oriented complement each other • Fully involve all relevant participants, including the national and local public sector, nongovernmental organizations and the private sector
Reconciliation work	• Activities are focused around temporary cessation of hostilities, so as to carry out disease control	• Recognize the symbolic value of health care in restoring relationships between communities • Recognize the promotion of justice and reconciliation as long-term goals involving the often slow rebuilding of trust between communities • Promote every reasonable opportunity for collaboration between communities • Consider innovative responses, such as truth and reconciliation commissions
Role of the private sector	• Efforts are made to diversify the range of service providers and to deregulate the private sector	• Promote the role of the state in framing policies, setting standards and monitoring the quality of services • Recognize at the same time the important role of the private sector in providing health care • Develop incentives to promote equitable access to and delivery of important public health services
Promoting an equitable society	• Usually considered important but often postponed to a later period	• Recognize that achieving equitable social structures is a prime objective but that in the short term, in the interests of stability, some reforms may need to be delayed • Build links between competing population groups and different localities as key elements of post-conflict reform
Training	• Training is often overlooked, fragmented and uncoordinated	• Recognize the importance of developing human resources • Work out ways to integrate people who have been trained under different systems • Invest in training for planners and managers
Information systems	• Information is not considered a priority • Even when information exists it is not shared	• Make documentation a priority • Set up a central repository for information • Make use of new technologies to disseminate information • Make funding conditional on sharing information

Recommendations

Various measures need to be taken to prevent the occurrence of conflict and – where it does occur – to lessen its impact. These measures fall into the following broad categories:

— obtaining more extensive information and a better understanding of conflicts;

— taking political action to predict, prevent and respond to conflicts;

— peacekeeping activities;

BOX 8.3 *(continued)*
— obsessive thoughts of revenge;
— feelings of estrangement from others.

In addition, the "militarized behaviour" of the children may lead to a low level of acceptance of the norms of civilian society. As the World Health Organization pointed out in its contribution to the United Nations study on child soldiers (*78*):

"Children going through the development stages of socialization and acquisition of moral judgement in [a military] environment are ill-prepared to be reintegrated into a non-violent society. They acquire a premature self-sufficiency, devoid of the knowledge and skills for moral judgement and for discriminating inappropriate risk behaviours — whether reflected in violence, substance abuse or sexual aggression. Their rehabilitation constitutes one of the major social and public health challenges in the aftermath of armed conflict."

Health professionals may also play a valuable educational role in helping prevent children being recruited into armies (including as volunteers), by raising awareness among children and adolescents who are at risk, as well as among their families and communities, and by stressing the associated dangers, including the severe damage to psychological and mental health.

---

familiar: discrimination, fanaticism, intolerance, persecution. The consequences are also familiar: social disaffection, separatism, micronationalism and conflict" (*80*).

Peacekeeping

Despite massive increases in peacekeeping activities by the United Nations, the effectiveness of such operations has often been questionable. The reasons include uncertainty about the mandates for such interventions, poor lines of control between the various forces contributing to a peacekeeping effort and inadequate resources for the task. In response to these problems, the Secretary-General of the United Nations created a Panel on United Nations Peace Operations to assess the shortcomings of the existing system and to make specific recommendations for change. The Panel, composed of individuals experienced in various aspects of conflict prevention, peacekeeping and peace-building, made recommendations covering operational and organizational areas for improvement, as well as politics and strategy. These recommendations were summarized in a report that is more commonly known as the "Brahimi report" (*81*).

Health sector responses

The potential – and limitations – of the health care sector in helping prevent and respond to conflicts should be more thoroughly researched and documented. More documentation of good practice is required, particularly with regard to providing effective services after conflicts – an area where new lessons are beginning to emerge.

Governments should support organizations, such as the World Health Organization and other United Nations agencies, in a global effort to devise more effective policies for the prevention of and responses to conflicts.

Humanitarian responses

Both the standards and the level of accountability of organizations responding to violent crises need to be raised. The Sphere Project, which is based in Geneva, Switzerland, is seeking to have minimum standards for humanitarian assistance agreed and acted upon. Similarly, the Humanitarian Accountability Project, a network also based in Geneva and supported by donor agencies and nongovernmental organizations, is working to raise levels of accountability, especially among potential beneficiaries of humanitarian activities. Governments and humanitarian agencies are urged to support both these efforts.

Conclusion

This chapter has focused on the impact of violent conflicts on public health and health care systems, and has attempted to describe the range of possible responses to such crises. Clearly, there is a need for a greater emphasis on primary prevention, which seeks to prevent conflicts from occurring in the first place.

There is much that needs to be learnt – and acted upon – concerning the prevention of collective violence and dealing with its underlying causes. In the first instance, this applies to the forms of collective violence that have become common in the past hundred years or more – conflicts between states or involving organized groups within a specific geographical area (such as regions in rebellion against the central state), civil wars and the various forms of state-sponsored violence against individuals or groups.

The shape of collective violence is changing, though. At the start of the 21st century, new forms of collective violence are emerging, involving organized but highly dispersed organizations and networks of organizations – groups without a "fixed address", whose very aims, strategies and psychology differ radically from earlier ones. These groups make full use of the high technologies and modern financial systems that the globalized world order has created. Their weaponry is also new, as they seek to exploit such forms as biological, chemical and possibly nuclear weapons in addition to more conventional explosives and missiles. Their goals are physical as well as psychological, involving both mass destruction and the creation of widespread fear.

The world will need to learn quickly how to combat the new threat of global terrorism in all of its forms, while at the same time showing a high degree of determination to prevent and lessen the impact of conventional forms of collective violence, which continue to cause the overwhelming proportion of deaths, illness, injuries and destruction. A strong will is needed, together with a generous commitment of resources, not only to reach a much deeper understanding of the problems of violent conflict, but also to find solutions.

References

1. WHA34.38. In: *Handbook of resolutions and decisions of the World Health Assembly and the Executive Board, Volume II, 1973–1984.* Geneva, World Health Organization, 1985:397–398.

2. *Handbook for emergencies.* Geneva, Office of the United Nations High Commissioner for Refugees, 2001.

3. Leaning J. Introduction. In: Leaning J et al., eds. *Humanitarian crises: the medical and public health response.* Cambridge, MA, Harvard University Press, 1999:1–11.

4. Goodhand J, Hulme D. From wars to complex political emergencies: understanding conflict and peace-building in the new world disorder. *Third World Quarterly*, 1999, 20:13–26.

5. Kaldor M. *New and old wars: organized violence in a global era.* Cambridge, Polity Press, 1999.

6. Cornish P. Terrorism, insecurity and underdevelopment. *Conflict – Security – Development*, 2001, 1:147–151.

7. Zwi A, Ugalde A, Richards P. The effects of war and political violence on health services. In: Kurtz L, ed. *Encyclopedia of violence, peace and conflict.* San Diego, CA, Academic Press, 1999:679–690.

8. Ball P, Kobrak P, Spirer H. *State violence in Guatemala, 1960–1996: a quantitative reflection.* Washington, DC, American Academy for the Advancement of Science, 1999.

9. Roberts L et al. *Mortality in eastern Democratic Republic of Congo: results from eleven mortality surveys.* New York, NY, International Rescue Committee, 2001.

10. *International classification of diseases*, ninth revision. Geneva, World Health Organization, 1978.

11. *International statistical classification of diseases and related health problems*, tenth revision. *Volume 1: Tabular list; Volume 2: Instruction manual; Volume 3: Index.* Geneva, World Health Organization, 1992–1994.

12. Sivard RL. *World military and social expenditures*, 14th ed. Washington, DC, World Priorities, 1991.

13. Sivard RL. *World military and social expenditures*, 16th ed. Washington, DC, World Priorities, 1996.

14. Rummel RJ. *Death by government: genocide and mass murder since 1900.* New Brunswick, NJ, and London, Transaction Publications, 1994.

15. Sheil M et al. Deaths among humanitarian workers. *British Medical Journal*, 2000, 321:166–168.

16. *Take a step to stamp out torture.* London, Amnesty International, 2000.

17. Burnett A, Peel M. Asylum-seekers and refugees in Britain: health needs of asylum-seekers and refugees. *British Medical Journal*, 2001, 322:544–547.

18. Harris MF, Telfer BL. The health needs of asylum-seekers living in the community. *Medical Journal of Australia*, 2001, 175:589–592.

19. British Medical Association. *The medical profession and human rights: handbook for a changing agenda.* London, Zed Books, 2001.

20. *12-point program for the prevention of torture by agents of the state.* London, Amnesty International, 2000.

21. *Istanbul Protocol: manual on the effective investigation and documentation of torture and other cruel, inhuman or degrading treatment or punishment.* New York, NY, Office of the United Nations High Commissioner for Human Rights, 2001 (available on the Internet at http://www.unhchr.ch/pdf/8istprot.pdf).

22. Ashford MW, Huet-Vaughn Y. The impact of war on women. In: Levy BS, Sidel VW, eds. *War and public health.* Oxford, Oxford University Press, 1997:186–196.

23. Turshen M, Twagiramariya C, eds. *What women do in wartime: gender and conflict in Africa.* London, Zed Books, 1998.

24. Stiglmayer A, ed. *Mass rape: the war against women in Bosnia–Herzegovina.* Lincoln, NE, University of Nebraska Press, 1994.

25. Ignatieff M. *Virtual war: Kosovo and beyond.* London, Chatto & Windus, 2000.

26. Carnegie Commission on Preventing Deadly Conflict. *Preventing deadly conflict: final report.* New York, NY, Carnegie Corporation, 1997.

27. Zwi AB, Fustukian S, Sethi D. Globalisation, conflict and the humanitarian response. In: Lee K, Buse K, Fustukian S, eds. *Health policy in a globalising world.* Cambridge, Cambridge University Press, 2002.

28. Stewart F. The root causes of humanitarian emergencies. In: Nafziger EW, Stewart F, Väyrynen R, eds. *War, hunger and displacement: the origin of humanitarian emergencies.* Oxford, Oxford University Press, 2000.

29. Prunier G. *The Rwanda crisis 1959–1994: history of a genocide.* London, Hurst, 1995.

30. Dodge CP. Health implications of war in Uganda and Sudan. *Social Science and Medicine,* 1990, 31:691–698.

31. *Children on the front line: the impact of apartheid, destabilization and warfare on children in southern and South Africa,* 3rd ed. New York, NY, United Nations Children's Fund, 1989.

32. Mann J et al. Bosnia: the war against public health. *Medicine and Global Survival,* 1994, 1:130–146.

33. Horton R. On the brink of humanitarian disaster. *Lancet,* 1994, 343:1053.

34. Ugalde A et al. The health costs of war: can they be measured? Lessons from El Salvador. *British Medical Journal,* 2000, 321:169–172.

35. Garfield RM, Frieden T, Vermund SH. Health-related outcomes of war in Nicaragua. *American Journal of Public Health,* 1987, 77:615–618.

36. Kloos H. Health impacts of war in Ethiopia. *Disasters,* 1992, 16:347–354.

37. Cliff J, Noormahomed AR. Health as a target: South Africa's destabilization of Mozambique. *Social Science and Medicine,* 1988, 27:717–722.

38. Goma Epidemiology Group. Public health impact of Rwandan refugee crisis: what happened in Goma, Zaire, in July 1994? *Lancet,* 1995, 345:339–344.

39. Zwi AB, Cabral AJ. High-risk situations for AIDS prevention. *British Medical Journal,* 1991, 303:1527–1529.

40. *AIDS and the military: UNAIDS point of view.* Geneva, Joint United Nations Programme on HIV/AIDS, 1998 (UNAIDS Best Practice Collection).

41. Mann JM, Tarantola DJM, Netter TW, eds. *AIDS in the world.* Cambridge, MA, Harvard University Press, 1992.

42. Khaw AJ et al. HIV risk and prevention in emergency-affected populations: a review. *Disasters,* 2000, 24:181–197.

43. Smallman-Raynor M, Cliff A. Civil war and the spread of AIDS in central Africa. *Epidemiology of Infectious Diseases,* 1991, 107:69–80.

44. *Refugees and AIDS: UNAIDS point of view.* Geneva, Joint United Nations Programme on HIV/AIDS, 1997 (UNAIDS Best Practice Collection).

45. Stover E et al. The medical and social consequences of land mines in Cambodia. *Journal of the American Medical Association,* 1994, 272:331–336.

46. *The causes of conflict in Africa.* London, Department for International Development, 2001.

47. *Getting away with murder, mutilation, rape: new testimony from Sierra Leone.* New York, NY, Human Rights Watch, 1999 (Vol. 11, No. 3(A)).

48. Summerfield D. The psychosocial effects of conflict in the Third World. *Development in Practice,* 1991, 1:159–173.

49. Quirk GJ, Casco L. Stress disorders of families of the disappeared: a controlled study in Honduras. *Social Science and Medicine,* 1994, 39:1675–1679.

50. Bracken PJ, Giller JE, Summerfield D. Psychological responses to war and atrocity: the limitations of current concepts. *Social Science and Medicine,* 1995, 40:1073–1082.

51. Pupavac V. Therapeutic governance: psychosocial intervention and trauma risk. *Disasters,* 2001, 25:1449–1462.

52. Robertson G. *Crimes against humanity: the struggle for global justice.* Harmondsworth, Penguin, 1999.

53. Gururaj G et al. *Suicide prevention: emerging from darkness*. New Delhi, WHO Regional Office for South-East Asia, 2001.

54. Silove D, Ekblad S, Mollica R. The rights of the severely mentally ill in post-conflict societies. *Lancet*, 2000, 355:1548–1549.

55. Toole MJ, Waldman RJ. Prevention of excess mortality in refugee and displaced populations in developing countries. *Journal of the American Medical Association*, 1990, 263:3296–3302.

56. Toole MJ, Waldman RJ, Zwi AB. Complex humanitarian emergencies. In: Black R, Merson M, Mills A. *Textbook of international health*. Gaithersburg, MD, Aspen, 2000.

57. Centers for Disease Control and Prevention. Famine-affected, refugee, and displaced populations: recommendations for public health issues. *Morbidity and Mortality Weekly Report*, 1992, 41(No. RR-13).

58. Toole MJ, Waldman RJ. Refugees and displaced persons: war, hunger and public health. *Journal of the American Medical Association*, 1993, 270:600–605.

59. Deacon B. *Global social policy, international organizations and the future of welfare*. London, Sage, 1997.

60. Reed H, Haaga J, Keely C, eds. *The demography of forced migration: summary of a workshop*. Washington, DC, National Academy Press, 1998.

61. Hampton J, ed. *Internally displaced people: a global survey*. London, Earthscan, Norwegian Refugee Council and Global IDP Survey, 1998.

62. International Federation of Red Cross and Red Crescent Societies. *World disasters report 1999*. Dordrecht, Martinus Nijhoff, 1999.

63. Hodes RM, Kloos H. Health and medical care in Ethiopia. *New England Journal of Medicine*, 1988, 319:918–924.

64. Brauer J, Gissy WG, eds. *Economics of conflict and peace*. Aldershot, Avebury, 1997.

65. Cranna M, ed. *The true cost of conflict*. London, Earthscan and Saferworld, 1994.

66. Kumaranayake L, Zwi A, Ugalde A. Costing the direct health burden of political violence in developing countries. In: Brauer J, Gissy W, eds. *Economics of conflict and peace*. Aldershot, Avebury, 1997:292–301.

67. Macrae J, Zwi A. Famine, complex emergencies and international policy in Africa: an overview. In: Macrae J, Zwi A, eds. *War and hunger: rethinking international responses to complex emergencies*. London, Zed Books, 1994:6–36.

68. Lee I, Haines A. Health costs of the Gulf War. *British Medical Journal*, 1991, 303:303–306.

69. Walt G, Cliff J. The dynamics of health policies in Mozambique 1975–85. *Health Policy and Planning*, 1986, 1:148–157.

70. Addison T. Aid and conflict. In: Tarp F, ed. *Foreign aid and development: lessons learnt and directions for the future*. London, Routledge, 200:392–408.

71. Banatvala N, Zwi A. Public health and humanitarian interventions: improving the evidence base. *British Medical Journal*, 2000, 321:101–105.

72. Anderson MB. *Do no harm. How aid can support peace – or war*. Boulder, CO, and London, Lynne Rienner, 1999.

73. Barnabas GA, Zwi AB. Health policy development in wartime: establishing the Baito health system in Tigray, Ethiopia. *Health Policy and Planning*, 1997, 12:38–49.

74. Kumar K, ed. *Rebuilding societies after civil war*. Boulder, CO, and London, Lynne Rienner, 1997.

75. Kumar K et al. *The international response to conflict and genocide: lessons from the Rwanda experience. Study 4: rebuilding post-war Rwanda*. Copenhagen, Steering Committee of the Joint Evaluation of Emergency Assistance to Rwanda, 1996.

76. *Post-conflict reconstruction: the role of the World Bank*. Washington, DC, World Bank, 1998.

77. Coupland RM. The effects of weapons and the Solferino cycle. *British Medical Journal*, 1999, 319:864–865.

78. Machel G. *Impact of armed conflict on children: report of the Expert Group of the Secretary-General*. New York, NY, United Nations, 1996 (document A/51/306).

79. Laurence EJ. *Arms watching: integrating small arms and light weapons into the early warning of violent conflict*. London, Saferworld, 2000.

80. Boutros-Ghali B. *An agenda for development*. New York, NY, United Nations, 1995.

81. *Report of the Panel on United Nations Peace Operations*. New York, NY, United Nations General Assembly Security Council, 2000 (document A/55/305, S/2000/809).

The way forward: recommendations for action

- The Convention Against Torture and Other Cruel, Inhuman or Degrading Treatment or Punishment (1984).
- The Convention on the Rights of the Child (1989) and its two Optional Protocols on the Involvement of Children in Armed Conflict (2000) and on the Sale of Children, Child Prostitution and Child Pornography (2000).
- The Rome Statute of the International Criminal Court (1998).

There are also other important agreements that are highly pertinent to various aspects of violence, such as the African Charter on Human and Peoples' Rights (1981) and the Inter-American Convention on the Prevention, Punishment and Eradication of Violence Against Women (1994).

While many national governments have made progress in harmonizing legislation with their obligations and commitments, others have not. Some do not have the resources or expertise to put the provisions of such international instruments into practice. Where the obstacle is the scarcity of resources or information, the international community should do more to assist. In other cases, strong campaigning will be necessary to bring about changes in legislation and practice.

Recommendation 9.
Seek practical, internationally agreed responses to the global drugs trade and the global arms trade

The global drugs trade and the global arms trade are integral to violence in both developing and industrialized countries, and come within the purview of both the national and the international levels. From the evidence provided in various parts of this report, even modest progress on either front will contribute to reducing the amount and degree of violence suffered by millions of people. To date, however – and despite their high profile in the world arena – no solutions seem to be in sight for these problems. Public health strategies could help reduce the health impacts of both in a variety of settings at the local and national levels, and should therefore be allotted a much higher profile in global-level responses.

Conclusion

Violence is not inevitable. We can do much to address and prevent it. The individuals, families and communities whose lives each year are shattered by it can be safeguarded, and the root causes of violence tackled to produce a healthier society for all.

The world has not yet fully measured the size of this task and does not yet have all the tools to carry it out. But the global knowledge base is growing and much useful experience has already been gained.

This report attempts to contribute to the knowledge base. It is hoped that the report will inspire and facilitate increased cooperation, innovation and commitment to preventing violence around the world.

References

1. WHO Collaborating Centre on Injury Surveillance. *International classification for external causes of injuries.* Amsterdam, Consumer Safety Institute, 2001.
2. Holder Y et al., eds. *Injury surveillance guidelines.* Geneva, World Health Organization (published in collaboration with the United States Centers for Disease Control and Prevention), 2001 (document WHO/NMH/VIP/01.02).

The way forward: recommendations for action

Background

Violence leaves no continent, no country and few communities untouched. Although it appears everywhere, violence is not an inevitable part of the human condition, nor is it an intractable problem of "modern life" that cannot be overcome by human determination and ingenuity.

Earlier chapters of this report have supplied considerable detail about specific types of violence and the public health interventions that may be applied in an attempt to reduce both their occurrence and their consequences. This final chapter highlights a number of global patterns and themes that cut across the various types of violence. It reiterates the case for a public health approach and provides a set of recommendations for decision-makers and practitioners at all levels.

Responding to violence: what is known so far?

Major lessons to date

Although important gaps exist in the information base, and much research needs to be done, useful lessons have been learned about preventing and reducing the consequences of violence.

Predictable and preventable

Violence is often predictable and preventable. As this report has shown, certain factors appear to be strongly predictive of violence within given populations, even if direct causality is sometimes difficult to establish. These range from individual and family factors – such as impulsivity, depression, poor monitoring and supervision of children, rigid gender roles and marital conflict – to macro-level factors, such as rapid changes in social structures and sharp economic downturns, bringing high unemployment and deteriorating public services. There are also local factors, specific to a given place and time, such as an increased presence of weapons or changing patterns of drug dealing in a particular neighbourhood. Identifying and measuring these factors can provide timely warning to decision-makers that action is required.

At the same time, the array of tools with which to take action is growing as public health-oriented research advances. In each category of violence examined in this report, examples have been cited of interventions that show promise for reducing violence and its consequences. These range from small-scale individual and community efforts to country-level policy changes that have achieved reductions in violence. While the majority of such interventions that have been documented and formally evaluated are to be found in wealthier parts of the world, many innovative interventions also exist in developing countries.

Upstream investment, downstream results

There is a tendency worldwide for authorities to act only after cases of highly visible violence occur, and then to invest resources for a short time on programmes for small, easily identified groups of people. Periodic police "crackdowns" on areas with high levels of violence are classic examples of this, usually following a much-publicized incident. In contrast, public health emphasizes prevention, especially primary prevention efforts operating "upstream" of problems – efforts that try to stop violent incidents from occurring in the first place or that prevent violent conditions from resulting in serious injury. Primary prevention approaches operate on the basis that even small investments may have large and long-lasting benefits.

Understanding the context of violence

All societies experience violence, but its context – the circumstances in which it occurs, its nature and its social acceptability – varies greatly from one setting to another. Wherever prevention programmes are planned, the context of violence must be understood in order to tailor the intervention to the targeted population.

Chapters 4 (intimate partner violence) and 6 (sexual violence) provide a wealth of examples in which the cultural context exacerbates the consequences of violence, creating formidable problems for prevention. One example is the belief in many societies that men have the right to discipline their wives – including through the use of physical force – for a variety of reasons, including the refusal to have sex. Behaviour resulting from such a belief puts these

244 • WORLD REPORT ON VIOLENCE AND HEALTH

women at risk not only of immediate physical and psychological violence, but also of unwanted pregnancy and sexually transmitted diseases. Another example is the approval of harsh, physical punishment in child-rearing, which is deeply ingrained in some societies. Interventions are unlikely to be successful unless they take into account the strength of these beliefs and attitudes, and the way they relate to other aspects of local culture.

At the same time, cultural traditions can also be protective; researchers and programme designers must be prepared to identify and make use of them in interventions. For example, Chapter 7 (self-directed violence) describes the contribution that religious affiliation appears to make in reducing the risk of suicide, and discusses the reasons – such as identification with a religion and specific prohibitions against suicide – why this may be so.

Exploiting linkages

Different types of violence are linked to each other in many important ways, often sharing similar risk factors. An example can be seen in Chapter 3 (child abuse and neglect by parents and other caregivers), where the list of common risk factors overlaps to a large degree with those for other types of violence. Some of these factors include:

- Poverty – linked with all forms of violence.
- Family or personal histories marked by divorce or separation – a factor also associated with youth violence, intimate partner violence, sexual violence and suicide.
- Alcohol and substance abuse – associated with all interpersonal forms of violence, as well as suicide.
- A history of family violence – linked to youth violence, intimate partner violence, sexual violence and suicide.

The overlap between the set of risk factors for different types of violence suggests a strong potential for partnerships between groups with a major interest in both primary and secondary prevention: local government and community officials, social housing planners, the police, social workers, women's and human rights groups, the medical profession and researchers working in each specific field. Partnerships may be advantageous in a variety of ways, including:

- improving the effectiveness of interventions;
- avoiding a duplication of efforts;
- increasing the resources available through a pooling of funds and personnel in joint actions;
- allowing research and prevention activities to be conducted in a more collective and coordinated way.

Unfortunately, research and prevention efforts for the various types of violence have often been developed in isolation from one another. If this fragmentation can be overcome, there is considerable scope in the future for more comprehensive and effective interventions.

Focusing on the most vulnerable groups

Violence, like many health problems, is not neutral. While all social classes experience violence, research consistently suggests that people with the lowest socioeconomic status are at greatest risk. More often it is the factors related to poverty, rather than poverty itself, that increase the risk for violence. Chapter 2, for instance, discusses the roles of poor housing, lack of education, unemployment, and other poverty-related conditions in youth violence – and how these factors place some young people at heightened risk of being influenced by delinquent peers and participation in criminal activities. The rate at which people enter into poverty – losing resources that were previously available – and the differential way in which they experience poverty (that is, their relative deprivation within a particular setting rather than their absolute level of poverty) are also important.

Chapter 6 (sexual violence) describes how poverty exacerbates the vulnerability of women and girls. In carrying out everyday tasks such as working in the fields, collecting water alone or walking home from work late at night, poor women and girls in rural or economically depressed areas are often at risk of rape. The conditions of poverty make them vulnerable to sexual exploitation in situations as diverse as seeking employment, engaging in trade or obtaining an education. Poverty is also a leading factor that pushes women into prostitution and forces families to sell children to sexual traffickers. Chapter 8 (collective violence) broadens the discussion further, pointing out that poverty and inequality are among the driving forces in violent conflict and that long periods of conflict may increase poverty – in turn creating the conditions that give rise to other forms of violence.

The neglect of poor people is not new: the poorest people in most societies are generally those least served by the state's various protection and care services. However, the fact that violence is linked with poverty may be an additional reason why policy-makers and government authorities have neglected public health approaches to violence – approaches that would mean a greater proportion of services and resources going to poor families and communities – in favour of policing and prisons. This neglect must be corrected if violence is to be prevented.

Combating complacency

Something that greatly encourages violence – and is a formidable obstacle in responding to it – is complacency. This is particularly true of the attitude that regards violence – like the closely related problem of gender inequality – as something that has always been present in human society and will therefore always continue to be so. Often, this complacency is strongly reinforced by self-interest. The social acceptance, for instance, of the right of men to "correct" their wives clearly benefits men more than it does women. The drug trade thrives on its illegal status, in which violence is an acceptable way for those involved to settle disputes or increase their market share.

In describing some of the elements that create a culture of violence, several chapters in this report emphasize that such a culture is often supported by both laws and attitudes. Both may be at work in factors such as the glorification of violence by the media, the tolerance of sexual assault or violence against intimate partners, harsh physical disciplining of children by parents in the home, bullying in schools and playgrounds, the use of unacceptable

levels of force by police, and the prolonged exposure of children and adolescents to armed conflict. Achieving significant reductions in both interpersonal and collective violence will be difficult unless the complacency surrounding such issues is abolished.

Gaining commitment from decision-makers

While much can be achieved by grassroots organizations, individuals and institutions, much of the success of public health efforts ultimately depends on political commitment. Support from political leaders is not only necessary to ensure proper funding and effective legislation, but also to give prevention efforts increased legitimacy and a higher profile within the public consciousness. Commitment is as important at national level – where policy and legislative decisions are made – as at provincial, district and municipal levels, where the day-to-day functioning of many interventions is controlled.

Gaining the strong commitment necessary for addressing violence is often the result of sustained efforts by many sectors of society. Public health practitioners and researchers have an important contribution to make to this process by providing decision-makers with solid information on the prevalence, consequences and impact of violence, and by carefully documenting the proven and promising practices that can lead to its prevention or management.

Why should the health sector be involved?

Until recently, the responsibility for remedying or containing violence in most modern societies fell on the judicial system, police and correctional services, and in some cases the military. The health sector, both public and private, was relegated to the role of providing care after the event, when the victims of violence came forward for treatment.

Assets and comparative advantages

Today, the health sector is an active and valuable ally in the global response to violence and brings a variety of advantages and assets to this work. One such asset is its closeness to, and therefore familiarity with the problem. The personnel of hospitals and clinics, and other health care providers dedicate a great amount of time to the victims of violence.

Another important asset is the information that the health sector has at its disposal to facilitate research and prevention work. Possession of data means that the sector is uniquely placed to draw attention to the health burden imposed by violence. When combined sensitively with the human stories the health sector witnesses every day, such information can provide a powerful tool both for advocacy and for action.

A special responsibility

The health sector's role in preventing violence stems from its responsibility to the public – the people who ultimately pay for services and for the governmental structures that organize them. With this responsibility and its various assets and advantages, the health sector has the potential to take a much more proactive role in violence prevention – ideally, in collaboration with other sectors – than it has done in the past. On a day-to-day basis, doctors, nurses and other health care personnel are well placed to identify cases of abuse, and to refer victims to other services for follow-up treatment or protection. At the programme level, hospitals and other health care facilities can serve as useful settings for interventions, using their resources and infrastructure for prevention activities. Equally important, the design and implementation of interventions can be enhanced by the close cooperation of health care professionals and institutions with other institutions or sectors concerned with violence, including nongovernmental organizations and research bodies.

These functions of the health sector are already being carried out in many parts of the world, though sometimes in a tentative or piecemeal fashion. The time has now come for more decisive and coordinated action, and for extending efforts to places where they do not yet exist, despite being sorely needed. Anything less will be a failure of the health sector.

Assigning responsibilities and priorities

Given the multifaceted nature of violence and its complex roots, governments and relevant organizations at all levels of decision-making – local, national and international – must be engaged in its prevention. Complementary and coordinated action across sectors will enhance the effectiveness of violence prevention activities.

In addition to working at their own level of government or authority, decision-makers and practitioners can and must work together across levels for significant progress to be made. The various components of civil society – such as the media, community organizations, professional associations, labour organizations, religious institutions and traditional structures – may contain a great volume of relevant knowledge and experience.

Each country has its own particular governing structure, from a highly centralized unitary state to a federal system that divides powers between local, regional and national governments. Whatever the structure, however, strategic planning processes – usually led by national governments but including other levels and sectors – may be useful for creating consensus, setting objectives and timetables, and assigning responsibilities to all those with something to contribute. Certain United Nations organizations and bilateral development agencies have considerable expertise in strategic planning for public health issues in developing countries, which could profitably contribute to violence prevention.

Recommendations

The following recommendations aim to mobilize action in response to violence. All recommendations need to be addressed by a range of sectors and stakeholders if they are to achieve their objectives.

These recommendations must obviously be applied with flexibility and with proper understanding of local conditions and capacities. Countries currently experiencing collective violence, or with scarce financial and human resources, will find it difficult or impossible to apply some of the national and local recommendations on their own. Under such circumstances, they may be able to work with international organizations or nongovernmental organizations operating within their borders that are able to support or implement some of the recommendations.

Recommendation 1.
Create, implement and monitor a national action plan for violence prevention

The development of a multisectoral national action plan is a key element for sustained violence prevention efforts. It may not always be easy to achieve, given understandable public demands for immediate action to deal with the more visible effects of violence. National leaders, though, must understand that the benefits of a sustained public health approach will be more substantial and longer-lasting than short-term, reactive policies. Such an action plan will require visible political commitment and the investment of moral authority.

A national action plan to prevent violence should include objectives, priorities, strategies and assigned responsibilities, as well as a timetable and evaluation mechanism. It should be based on a consensus developed by a wide range of governmental and nongovernmental actors, including appropriate stakeholder organizations. The plan should take into account the human and financial resources that are and will be made available for its implementation. It should include elements such as the review and reform of existing legislation and policy, building data collection and research capacity, strengthening services for victims, and developing and evaluating prevention responses. To ensure that the plan moves beyond words to action, it is essential that a specific organization be mandated to monitor and report periodically on progress made in these and other elements of the plan.

Coordinating mechanisms at the local, national and international level will be required to enable fruitful collaboration between such sectors as criminal justice, education, labour, health, social welfare, and others potentially involved in the development and implementation of the plan. Mechanisms such as national task forces, inter-ministerial committees and United Nations working groups may be able to facilitate such coordination. At the local level, councils, community-based task forces and networks can be created or utilized to help build and implement the plan.

Recommendation 2.
Enhance capacity for collecting data on violence

The national action plan for violence prevention must include establishing or enhancing national capacity to collect and analyse data covering the scope, causes and consequences of violence. These data are necessary in order to set priorities, guide programme design, and monitor the progress of the action plan. As described throughout the report, in all countries at least some data collection efforts are under way, but the quality and the sharing of the data could be strengthened.

In some countries, it may be most efficient for the national government to designate an institution, agency or government unit to be responsible for collating and comparing information from health, law enforcement and other authorities that maintain regular contact with the victims and perpetrators of violence. Such an institution could be a "centre of excellence", with responsibility for documenting the extent of violence within the country, promoting or carrying out research, and training people for these functions. It should liaise with other comparable institutions and agencies in order to exchange data, research tools and methods. In countries with limited resources, it may also assume the monitoring function described under Recommendation 1.

Data collection is important at all levels, but it is at the local level that the quality and completeness of data will be determined. Systems must be designed that are simple and cost-effective to implement, appropriate to the level of skills of the staff using them, and conforming to both national and international standards. In addition, there should be procedures to share data between the relevant authorities (such as those responsible for health, criminal justice and social policy) and interested parties, and the capability to carry out comparative analysis.

At the international level, the world currently lacks internationally accepted standards for data collection on violence to enhance the comparison of data across nations and cultures. This is serious, not least because current gaps in information make it difficult to quantify the magnitude of violence worldwide, and therefore to undertake global-level research or develop interventions. While many of these gaps are simply the result of missing data, others result from differences in the way data are classified by different countries (and sometimes by different agencies within individual countries). This can and should be remedied by the development and propagation of internationally accepted standards for data collection. The *International classification for external causes of injuries* (*1*) and the *Injury surveillance guidelines* developed by the World Health Organization and the United States Centers for Disease Control and Prevention (*2*) are steps in that direction.

Recommendation 3.
Define priorities for, and support research on, the causes, consequences, costs and prevention of violence

Although the report has shown that progress has been made in understanding violence among different population groups and in various settings, additional research is urgently needed. There are many reasons to undertake such research, but a main priority is to gain a better understanding of the problem in different cultural contexts so that appropriate responses can be developed and evaluated.

At the national level, and as part of the plan of action, a research agenda can be advanced by government policy, by direct involvement of government institutions (many social service or interior ministries, as well as criminal justice agencies, have in-house research programmes), and by funding to academic institutions and independent researchers.

Research can and should also be undertaken at the local level. Local research is first and foremost valuable for its use in local violence prevention activities, but it is also an important component in the larger research effort required to tackle violence on a global scale. For maximum benefit, local authorities should involve all partners possessing relevant expertise, including university faculties (such as medicine, social sciences, criminology and

epidemiology), research facilities and nongovernmental organizations.

While the bulk of research required to prevent violence must be carried out at the local level, in response to local conditions and needs, some high-priority issues of global importance call for cross-national research at the international level. These issues include: the relationship between violence and various aspects of globalization, including economic, environmental and cultural impacts; risk and protective factors common to different cultures and societies; and promising prevention approaches applicable in a variety of contexts.

Some aspects of globalization have an important impact on different types of violence in different settings, but little is known about precisely what factors cause the violence or how these might be mitigated. Not enough research has been done about risk factors that are shared across different settings, and even less has been done on the potentially highly rewarding area of protective factors. In addition, although there is considerable information about individual interventions from a variety of countries (some of the most promising are described in this report), few have been evaluated.

Recommendation 4.
Promote primary prevention responses

The importance of primary prevention is a theme echoed throughout this report. Research suggests that primary prevention is most effective when carried out early, and among people and groups known to be at higher risk than the general population – though even efforts directed at the general population can have beneficial effects. Yet as the various chapters in this report indicate, not enough emphasis is being given at any level to primary prevention. This situation must be redressed.

Some of the important primary prevention interventions for reducing violence include:

— prenatal and perinatal health care for mothers as well as preschool enrichment and social development programmes for children and adolescents;

— training for good parenting practices and improved family functioning;

— improvements to urban infrastructure (both physical and socioeconomic);

— measures to reduce firearm injuries and improve firearm-related safety;

— media campaigns to change attitudes, behaviour and social norms.

The first two interventions are important for reducing child abuse and neglect as well as violence perpetrated during adolescence and adulthood.

Important contributions can also be made through improvements to infrastructure (both physical and socioeconomic). Specifically, this means addressing environmental factors within communities: identifying locations where violence frequently occurs, analysing the factors that make a given place dangerous (for example, bad lighting, isolation, or being near an establishment where alcohol is consumed), and modifying or removing these factors. It also calls for an improvement to the socioeconomic infrastructure of local communities through greater investment and improved educational and economic opportunities.

Another issue for both national and local interventions is prevention of firearm injuries and improvement of firearm-related safety measures. Firearms are an important risk factor in many types of violence, including youth and collective violence and suicide. Interventions to reduce injuries from guns – whether accidental or intentional – include, for example, legislation on gun sales and ownership, programmes to collect and decommission illegal weapons in areas of frequent gun-related violence, programmes to demobilize militia and soldiers after conflicts, and measures to improve safe storage of weapons. Further research is needed to determine the effectiveness of these and other types of interventions. This is a prime area in which multisectoral collaboration between legislative, policing and public health authorities will be important in achieving overall success.

The media have considerable potential as both negative and positive forces in violence prevention. While no conclusive research results are yet available on how exposure to violence through the media affects many types of violence, there is evidence for a relationship between reporting of suicides and subsequent suicides. The media can be used to change violence-related attitudes and behaviour as well as social norms by printing or broadcasting anti-violence information, or by incorporating anti-violence messages into entertainment formats such as soap operas (see Box 9.1).

Depending on conditions in specific locations, most of these primary interventions can also have important mutual reinforcing effects.

Recommendation 5.
Strengthen responses for victims of violence

The health, social and legal services provided to victims of violence should be strengthened in all countries. This requires a review of services currently provided, better training of staff, and improved integration of health, social and legal support.

The health system as a whole should have as a national goal to strengthen the capacity and funding to provide high-quality care to victims of all types of violence, as well as the rehabilitation and support services needed to prevent further complications. Priorities include:

— improvements to emergency response systems and the ability of the health care sector to treat and rehabilitate victims;

— recognition of signs of violent incidents or ongoing violent situations, and referral of victims to appropriate agencies for follow-up and support;

— ensuring that health, judicial, policing and social services avoid a renewed victimization of earlier victims, and that these services effectively deter perpetrators from re-offending;

— social support, prevention programmes, and other services to protect families at risk of violence and reduce stress on caregivers;

— incorporation of modules on violence prevention into curricula for medical and nursing students.

Each of these responses can help minimize the impact of violence on individuals and the cost to health and social systems. Emergency response systems and pre-hospital care can significantly

BOX 9.1

Health promotion, violence prevention and the media: the *Soul City* campaign

In South Africa, the Institute for Health and Development Communication (IHDC) has won acclaim for the innovative way in which it uses the power of the mass media to promote health and development. The nongovernmental organization's project intertwines social and health issues into prime-time television and radio dramas, reaching audiences of millions throughout the country. By closely involving its viewers and listeners on an emotional level, the format of the programmes aims to change basic attitudes and social norms, and ultimately to change behaviour. One broadcast series, called *Soul City*, targets the general public, while a second, *Soul Buddyz*, is for children aged 8–12 years. *Soul City* is one of the most popular programmes on South African television, reaching almost 80% of its target audience of some 16 million people, and *Soul Buddyz* is viewed by two-thirds of all children in South Africa.

To accompany the broadcast programmes, IHDC has produced booklets providing further information on the topics covered, with illustrations of popular characters from the television dramas. The project has also produced audio and video tapes for use in a variety of formal and informal educational settings.

Violence is a major public health priority in South Africa, and the broadcast series have dealt with this issue in most of their programmes. Particular topics covered have included general interpersonal violence, bullying, gang violence, domestic violence, rape and sexual harassment. The project aims to prevent violence by:

— making audiences fully aware of the extent of violence in their society and its consequences;
— persuading people that they are in a position to do something about violence, both as individuals and as members of the community;
— encouraging better parenting, through the use of role models, and better communications and relationships between parents and children.

The IHDC project also runs a toll-free telephone helpline for audiences of the programmes, providing crisis counselling and referring people where necessary to community-based support services. It has also developed training materials on violence against women for counsellors and health workers, the police and legal officials.

An evaluation of the first series of *Soul Buddyz* is currently being conducted. Evaluations of the adult *Soul City* series have found increased knowledge and awareness, and shifts in attitudes and social norms concerning domestic violence and gender relations. Furthermore, there has been a significant increase in the willingness to change behaviour and take action against violence, both in urban and rural areas and among both men and women.

reduce the risk of death or disability resulting from physical trauma. Less tangible but equally important are measures such as changing the attitudes of the police and other public officials, educating them about intimate partner and sexual violence, and training them to recognize and respond to cases of violence.

Where health ministries provide guidelines for curricula within medical and nursing schools, national policy should see that all health personnel – while they are students – receive training on violence, its consequences and its prevention. Having graduated, health personnel should be able to recognize signs of violence and should be intent on doing so. Such measures can be particularly helpful to people who are unable to communicate what has happened to them, such as small children or incapacitated elderly people, or else are afraid to do so – for instance, victims of domestic violence, sex workers or undocumented migrants.

The practical application of these policies must be carefully implemented and evaluated in order to avoid creating renewed victimization of victims of violence. For example, if staff ascertain that a patient has suffered violence, procedures to pursue that evidence should not place the patient at risk of further violence from the perpetrator, censure from his or her family or community, or other negative consequences.

Recommendation 6.
Integrate violence prevention into social and educational policies, and thereby promote gender and social equality

Much violence has links with gender and social inequalities that place large sections of the population at increased risk. The experience of countries that have improved the status of women and reduced social discrimination suggests that an array of interventions will be required. At the national level, these will include legislative and legal reforms, communications campaigns aimed at public awareness of the problem, training and monitoring of the police and public officials, and educational or economic incentives for disadvantaged groups. Cultural and social research will be necessary in developing these interventions, so that they will be feasible and effective.

At the same time, social protection policies and programmes, both for the general population and for disadvantaged groups, need to be strengthened. These measures are under considerable strain in many parts of the world as a result of a range of factors, including the impacts of globalization, debt and structural adjustment policies, the transformation from planned to market economies, and armed conflicts. Many countries have seen real wages fall, basic infrastructure deteriorate – particularly in urban areas – and steady reductions in the quality and quantity of health, education and social services. Because of the established links between such conditions and violence, governments should do their utmost to keep social protection services operational, if necessary reordering the priorities in their national budgets.

Recommendation 7.
Increase collaboration and exchange of information on violence prevention

Working relations and communications between international agencies, governmental agencies, researchers, networks and nongovernmental organizations engaged in the prevention of violence should be assessed in order to achieve better sharing of knowledge, agreement on prevention goals, and coordination of action. All have important roles to play in violence prevention (see Box 9.2).

A number of international agencies, regional institutions and United Nations bodies are either currently working in violence prevention or have mandates or activities highly relevant to reducing violence, including those dealing with economic matters, human rights, international law and sustainable development. To date, coordination across all these agencies is still insufficient. This should be remedied in order to avoid much needless duplication and to benefit from the economies of pooling expertise, networks, funding and in-country facilities. Mechanisms to improve cooperation should be explored, possibly starting on a small scale and involving a small number of organizations with both a mandate and practical experience in violence prevention (see Box 9.3).

The vastly improved communications technology of recent years is a positive aspect of globalization, which has permitted thousands of networks in a whole variety of fields. In violence prevention and related fields, networks of researchers and practitioners have greatly enhanced the world's knowledge base by proposing a range of prevention models, discussing methodologies and critically examining research results. Their exchange of information and ideas is crucial to future progress, alongside the work of government authorities, service providers and advocacy groups.

Advocacy groups are also important partners in public health. Advocacy groups concerned with violence against women and abuses of human rights (notably torture and war crimes) are prime examples. These groups have proved their ability to mobilize resources, gather and convey information

---

BOX 9.2

Responding to the threat of violence: the Inter-American Coalition for the Prevention of Violence

In countries on the American continent, as throughout the world, public safety is an issue of urgent concern for governments. From a national economic standpoint, violence affects foreign and domestic investment, impeding long-term growth and development. Violence also causes citizens to feel insecure and to lose faith in their criminal justice and political systems.

As a response to this concern, five international and regional bodies and one national organization joined forces in June 2000 to set up an initiative called the Inter-American Coalition for the Prevention of Violence. The participating organizations were:

— the Inter-American Development Bank;
— the Organization of American States;
— the Pan American Health Organization;
— the United Nations Educational, Scientific and Cultural Organization;
— the United States Centers for Disease Control and Prevention;
— the World Bank.

The Coalition believes that it can give effective support to national initiatives — whether by governments, civil society or the private sector — in preventing violence, particularly by mobilizing new partners and resources. While its activities are based on the principle of cooperation, it respects the freedom of individual countries to make their own decisions regarding the prevention of violence.

The main actions planned by the Coalition include:

— sponsoring campaigns to raise public awareness of the importance of violence prevention;
— supporting efforts to gather and publish reliable data on violence and crime, at local and national levels;
— setting up a web site on violence prevention, with a database of best practices;
— providing information on violence prevention to policy-makers and decision-makers throughout the region;
— organizing regional seminars and workshops on violence prevention, as well as study tours and initiatives between twinned cities;
— working with the media;
— working with government ministers and city mayors, and other national and local officials;
— working with the private sector, nongovernmental organizations, and ethnic and religious communities;
— providing technical support in the design, implementation and evaluation of national programmes to prevent violence.

This is the first violence prevention effort of its kind on the American continent, and it may provide a model for similar regional initiatives in other parts of the world.

---

about important problems, and mount campaigns that have had an impact on decision-makers. Groups focusing on other issues, notably abuse of the elderly and suicide, have also become prominent in recent years. The value of advocacy groups should be recognized. This can be achieved by practical measures such as offering them official status at key international conferences and including them in official working groups.

Another important area where progress could be made is in the sharing of information between experts working on the different types of violence. Experts working on issues such as child abuse, youth violence, violence against intimate partners,

---

BOX 9.3

United Nations efforts to prevent interpersonal violence

Much work is currently being done by United Nations agencies to prevent interpersonal violence, particularly through initiatives addressing specific types of violence in particular settings. However, until recently, a large proportion of this work was being carried out in isolation.

In November 2001, representatives from ten United Nations agencies met in Geneva, Switzerland, to discuss their work on interpersonal violence and to find ways to coordinate future efforts in this field. Although United Nations agencies had previously collaborated successfully on conflict-related violence, little interagency work had been done to prevent everyday acts of violence and crime — incidents that affect individuals, families, communities and institutions such as schools and workplaces. Considerable benefits were envisaged if greater collaboration could take place on this complex problem, within and particularly between United Nations agencies. The meeting was the first step in that direction.

In a message to the representatives, United Nations Secretary-General Kofi Annan stated: "Men and women everywhere have the right to live their lives and raise their children free from the fear of violence. We must help them enjoy that right by making it clearly understood that violence is preventable, and by working together to identify and address its underlying causes."

Participants outlined a range of collaborative activities they would undertake. For the short term, these include the preparation of a guide to United Nations resources and activities for the prevention of interpersonal violence, highlighting the core competencies of each agency in preventing interpersonal violence and identifying areas not currently addressed by United Nations organizations. Based on this guide, a web site will be developed to help participating agencies exchange information and to serve as a resource for other United Nations agencies, governments, nongovernmental organizations, researchers and donors. For the medium and longer term, collaborative efforts will include advocacy work, data collection and analysis, research and prevention initiatives.

---

abuse of the elderly or suicide prevention often collaborate closely with experts working on the same type of violence, but much less successfully with those working on other types of violence. As this report has shown, the different types of violence share common risk factors and prevention strategies. Therefore, much could be gained by developing platforms that will facilitate the exchange of information, as well as joint research and advocacy work.

Recommendation 8.
Promote and monitor adherence to international treaties, laws and other mechanisms to protect human rights

Over the past half-century, national governments have signed a variety of international legal agreements that have direct relevance to violence and its prevention. Such agreements set standards for national legislation and establish norms and limits of behaviour. Some of the most important in the context of this report are:

- The Convention on the Prevention and Punishment of the Crime of Genocide (1948).

- The Convention for the Suppression of the Traffic in Persons and of the Exploitation of the Prostitution of Others (1949).

- The Convention on the Elimination of All Forms of Racial Discrimination (1965).

- The International Covenant on Economic, Social and Cultural Rights (1966).

- The International Covenant on Civil and Political Rights (1966).

- The Convention on the Elimination of All Forms of Discrimination against Women (1979).

- The Convention Against Torture and Other Cruel, Inhuman or Degrading Treatment or Punishment (1984).
- The Convention on the Rights of the Child (1989) and its two Optional Protocols on the Involvement of Children in Armed Conflict (2000) and on the Sale of Children, Child Prostitution and Child Pornography (2000).
- The Rome Statute of the International Criminal Court (1998).

There are also other important agreements that are highly pertinent to various aspects of violence, such as the African Charter on Human and Peoples' Rights (1981) and the Inter-American Convention on the Prevention, Punishment and Eradication of Violence Against Women (1994).

While many national governments have made progress in harmonizing legislation with their obligations and commitments, others have not. Some do not have the resources or expertise to put the provisions of such international instruments into practice. Where the obstacle is the scarcity of resources or information, the international community should do more to assist. In other cases, strong campaigning will be necessary to bring about changes in legislation and practice.

Recommendation 9.
Seek practical, internationally agreed responses to the global drugs trade and the global arms trade

The global drugs trade and the global arms trade are integral to violence in both developing and industrialized countries, and come within the purview of both the national and the international levels. From the evidence provided in various parts of this report, even modest progress on either front will contribute to reducing the amount and degree of violence suffered by millions of people. To date, however – and despite their high profile in the world arena – no solutions seem to be in sight for these problems. Public health strategies could help reduce the health impacts of both in a variety of settings at the local and national levels, and should therefore be allotted a much higher profile in global-level responses.

Conclusion

Violence is not inevitable. We can do much to address and prevent it. The individuals, families and communities whose lives each year are shattered by it can be safeguarded, and the root causes of violence tackled to produce a healthier society for all.

The world has not yet fully measured the size of this task and does not yet have all the tools to carry it out. But the global knowledge base is growing and much useful experience has already been gained.

This report attempts to contribute to the knowledge base. It is hoped that the report will inspire and facilitate increased cooperation, innovation and commitment to preventing violence around the world.

References

1. WHO Collaborating Centre on Injury Surveillance. *International classification for external causes of injuries.* Amsterdam, Consumer Safety Institute, 2001.
2. Holder Y et al., eds. *Injury surveillance guidelines.* Geneva, World Health Organization (published in collaboration with the United States Centers for Disease Control and Prevention), 2001(document WHO/NMH/VIP/01.02).

Statistical annex

Background

Each year, over 100 countries send detailed information on the number of deaths from various diseases, illnesses or injuries to the World Health Organization (WHO). Data from these WHO Member States are compiled from vital registration systems using the International Classification of Diseases (ICD) codes (*1, 2*). National vital registration systems capture about 17 million deaths that occur annually throughout the world. Data from these registration systems, as well as from surveys, censuses and epidemiological studies, are analysed by the World Health Organization to determine patterns of causes of death for countries, regions and the world.

WHO has also used these data, along with other information, to assess the global burden of disease. First published in 1996, these estimates represent the most comprehensive examination of global mortality and morbidity ever produced (*3*). A new assessment of the global burden of disease for the year 2000 is in progress (*4*). Estimates of the global burden of injury for the year 2000 are presented here. A description of the tables included in the annex and the data used to produce the 2000 estimates of violence-related deaths is provided below.

Types of tables

The statistical annex includes three types of tables:
— global and regional estimates of mortality;
— the ten leading causes of death and disability-adjusted life years (DALYs) for all WHO Member States combined and for each of the WHO regions;
— country-level rates of mortality.

Global and regional estimates of mortality

Table A.1 provides an overview of the population counts used to estimate global and regional rates of mortality. Tables A.2–A.5 contain estimates of violence-related mortality for the year 2000. Table A.2 presents mortality estimates for all intentional injuries, by sex, age group, WHO region and income level. Estimates for homicide, suicide and war, by sex, age group, WHO region and income level, are given separately in Tables A.3–A.5.

Cause of death and DALY rankings

Table A.6 presents the ten leading causes of death and DALYs for the year 2000, as well as the rankings for violence-related deaths and DALYs. These rankings are given for all WHO Member States combined and for each of the WHO regions.

Country-level rates of mortality

Tables A.7–A.9, respectively, present the numbers and rates of deaths due to intentional injury, homicide and suicide, while Table A.10 provides the corresponding figures for firearm-related mortality, categorized by manner of death. In these tables, the absolute numbers and rates per 100 000 population are presented by sex and age group for countries reporting data to WHO.

Methods
Categories

Deaths and non-fatal injuries are categorically attributed to one underlying cause using the rules and conventions of the International Classification of Diseases (*1, 2*). The cause list for the Global Burden of Disease project for 2000 (GBD 2000 project) has four levels of disaggregation and includes 135 specific diseases and injuries (*5*). Unintentional and intentional injury categories are defined in terms of external cause codes. For instance, the codes for intentional injuries are as follows:[1]

- Homicide – ICD-9 E960–E969 or ICD-10 X85–Y09.
- Suicide – ICD-9 E950–E959 or ICD-10 X60–X84.
- War-related injuries – ICD-9 E990–E999 or ICD-10 Y36.
- Legal intervention – ICD-9 E970–E978 or ICD-10 Y35.
- All intentional injury – ICD-9 E950–E978, E990–E999 or ICD-10 X60–Y09, Y35, Y36.

Absolute numbers and rates per 100 000 in the population are presented by sex and WHO region for

---

[1] Based on the *International classification of diseases*, ninth revision (ICD-9) (*1*) and the *International statistical classification of diseases and related health problems*, tenth revision (ICD-10) (*2*).

six age groups: 0–4 years, 5–14 years, 15–29 years, 30–44 years, 45–59 years and 60 years or older.

WHO regions

WHO Member States are grouped in six regions: the African Region, the Region of the Americas, the South-East Asia Region, the European Region, the Eastern Mediterranean Region and the Western Pacific Region. The countries included in each region are indicated in Table A.1.

Countries within the six WHO regions in Tables A.1–A.5 are further divided by income level based on 1996 estimates of gross national product (GNP) per capita (now referred to as gross national income) compiled by the World Bank and used in the *World health report 1999* (*6*). On the basis of the GNP per capita, economies are classified as low income (US$ 785 or less), middle income (US$ 786–9635) or high income (US$ 9636 or more).

Global estimates of mortality

The GBD 2000 project uses the latest population estimates for WHO Member States prepared by the United Nations Population Division (*7*). New life tables for the year 2000 have been constructed for all 191 WHO Member States (*8, 9*). The results for injuries reported here from Version 1 of the GBD 2000 project are based on an extensive analysis of mortality data for all regions of the world, together with systematic reviews of epidemiological studies and health service data (*4*). Complete or incomplete vital registration data together with sample registration systems cover 72% of global mortality. Survey data and indirect demographic techniques provide information on levels of child and adult mortality for the remaining 28% of estimated global mortality.

Data on causes of death have been analysed to take into account incomplete coverage of vital registration in countries and the likely differences in cause-of-death patterns that would be expected in the uncovered and often poorer subpopulations (*4*). For example, the patterns of causes of death in China and India were based on existing mortality registration systems. In China, the disease surveillance points system and the vital registration system

of the Ministry of Health were used. In India, mortality data from the medical certificate of cause of death were used for urban areas and the annual survey of cause of death was employed for rural areas.

For all other countries lacking vital registration data, cause-of-death models were used for an initial estimate of the maximum likelihood distribution of deaths across the broad categories of communicable and noncommunicable diseases and injuries, based on estimated total mortality rates and income. A regional model pattern of specific causes of death was then constructed based on local vital registration and verbal autopsy data and this proportionate distribution was then applied within each broad group of causes. Finally, the resulting estimates were adjusted based on other epidemiological evidence from studies on specific diseases and injuries.

Special attention has been paid to problems of misattribution or miscoding of causes of death. The category "Injury undetermined whether accidentally or purposely inflicted" (E980–E989 in the 3-digit ICD-9 codes or Y10–Y34 in ICD-10) can often include a significant share of deaths due to injury. Except where more detailed local information is available, these deaths have been proportionately allocated to the other injury causes of death.

Global and regional rankings of DALYs

The DALY measure is used to quantify the burden of disease (*3, 10*). The DALY is a health-gap measure that combines information on the number of years of life lost from premature death with the loss of health from disability.

Years lived with disability (YLDs) are the disability component of DALYs. YLDs measure the equivalent healthy years of life lost as a result of disabling sequelae of diseases and injuries. They require estimation of incidence, average duration of disability and disability weights (in the range 0–1).

Many sources of information were used to estimate YLDs for diseases and injuries in the GBD 2000 project. These included national and international surveillance data and disease registries, health survey data, data on use of hospital and medical services, and international and country-specific epidemiological studies (*4*).

The analysis of the burden of injury in the GBD 2000 project is based on methods developed for the 1990 project. These methods define a case of injury as one severe enough to warrant medical attention or one that leads to death. Estimation of YLDs resulting from injuries was based on analysis of databases of health facility data that recorded both type and nature of injury codes. National databases in Australia, Chile, Mauritius, Sweden and the United States of America were used to develop ratios of death to incidence. These ratios were then applied to extrapolate YLDs from injury deaths for all regions of the world. The death:incidence ratios were quite consistent for developed and developing countries. The proportion of incident cases resulting in long-term disabling sequelae was estimated for each nature of injury category from a review of long-term epidemiological studies of injury outcomes.

To produce the rankings in Table A.6, deaths and disabilities were first divided into three broad groups:

— communicable diseases, maternal causes and conditions arising in the perinatal period, and nutritional deficiencies;

— noncommunicable diseases;

— injuries.

Next, deaths and disabilities were grouped into categories. For example, injuries were divided between unintentional and intentional injuries. Following this level of disaggregation, deaths and disabilities were further divided into subcategories. Unintentional injuries, for example, were subdivided into road traffic injuries, poisonings, falls, fires, drowning and other unintentional injuries, while intentional injuries were subdivided into self-inflicted injuries, interpersonal violence and war-related injuries. The rankings were produced by ordering the subcategories.

The ten leading causes of death and DALYs are reported in Table A.6 for all WHO Member States combined and for each of the six WHO regions. In regions where violence-related deaths and DALYs rank below the ten leading causes, the actual rank

order is reported. The DALYs reported in Table A.6 use the standard rates of time discounting (3%) and standard age weights (*3*).

Country-level rates of mortality

The numbers and rates of violence-related mortality reported in Tables A.7–A.10 are for the most recent year between 1990 and 2000 reported to WHO by countries with a population greater than 1 million. For countries with populations under 1 million, an average rate based on the last 3 years of data reported to WHO between 1990 and 2000 is given.

Rates were not calculated where the number of deaths in a particular category was less than 20, though the number of deaths is reported. Age-specific and age-standardized rates are reported. Age-standardized rates are calculated by applying the age-specific rates to the World Standard Population (*11*) and they allow comparison of rates in populations with different age structures.

The population counts used to estimate the rates of mortality for each country in Tables A.7–A.10 are available from the World Health Organization at http://www3.who.int/whosis/whsa/ftp/download.htm.

References

1. *International classification of diseases*, ninth revision. Geneva, World Health Organization, 1978.

2. *International statistical classification of diseases and related health problems*, tenth revision. *Volume 1: Tabular list; Volume 2: Instruction manual; Volume 3: Index*. Geneva, World Health Organization, 1992–1994.

3. Murray CJL, Lopez AD. *The Global Burden of Disease: a comprehensive assessment of mortality and disability from diseases, injuries and risk factors in 1990 and projected to 2020*. Cambridge, MA, Harvard School of Public Health, 1996 (Global Burden of Disease and Injury Series, Vol. I).

4. Murray CJL et al. *The Global Burden of Disease 2000 project: aims, methods and data sources*. Geneva, World Health Organization, 2001 (GPE Discussion Paper, No. 36).

5. Murray CJL, Lopez AD. Progress and directions in refining the global burden of disease approach: response to Williams. *Health Economics*, 2000, 9:69–82.

6. *World health report 1999 – making a difference.* Geneva, World Health Organization, 1999.

7. *World population prospects: the 2000 revision.* New York, NY, United Nations, 2001.

8. Lopez AD et al. *Life tables for 191 countries for 2000: data, methods, results.* Geneva, World Health Organization, 2001 (GPE Discussion Paper, No. 40).

9. *World health report 2000 – health systems: improving performance.* Geneva, World Health Organization, 2000.

10. Murray CJ, Lopez AD. *Global health statistics.* Cambridge, MA, Harvard School of Public Health, 1996 (Global Burden of Disease and Injury Series, Vol. II).

11. Ahmad OA et al. *Age standardization of rates: a new WHO standard.* Geneva, World Health Organization, 2000 (GPE Discussion Paper, No. 31).

TABLE A.1

Population (in thousands) by sex and age group, for all WHO Member States, 2000[a]

Member States by WHO region and income level	Total[b]	Males						
		All ages	0–4 years	5–14 years	15–29 years	30–44 years	45–59 years	≥60 years
All	6 045 172	3 045 375	314 256	615 986	797 048	643 148	404 000	270 937
High-income	915 866	451 069	27 970	59 366	94 800	106 787	86 747	75 398
Low-income and middle-income	5 129 306	2 594 306	286 286	556 619	702 249	536 361	317 253	195 539
African Region (low-income and middle-income)[c]	639 631	318 751	54 547	87 461	88 948	48 416	25 515	13 865
Algeria	30 291	15 346	1 798	3 601	4 724	2 959	1 425	839
Angola	13 134	6 499	1 300	1 867	1 683	888	493	269
Benin	6 272	3 092	557	900	839	441	227	127
Botswana	1 541	755	113	214	234	118	50	26
Burkina Faso	11 535	5 576	1 114	1 713	1 531	658	332	227
Burundi	6 356	3 088	559	955	837	423	211	104
Cameroon	14 876	7 405	1 182	2 046	2 099	1 089	609	381
Cape Verde	427	199	31	54	62	38	5	9
Central African Republic	3 717	1 811	304	494	489	268	158	98
Chad	7 885	3 900	749	1 087	1 031	557	302	174
Comoros	706	354	59	95	104	55	27	13
Congo	3 018	1 478	282	413	391	212	113	68
Côte d'Ivoire	16 013	8 206	1 219	2 166	2 317	1 301	785	417
Democratic Republic of the Congo	50 948	25 245	5 043	7 427	6 522	3 414	1 834	1 005
Equatorial Guinea	457	225	40	60	58	35	20	12
Eritrea	3 659	1 817	311	496	488	287	156	78
Ethiopia	62 908	31 259	5 628	8 629	8 284	4 730	2 617	1 372
Gabon	1 230	609	98	150	147	95	69	49
Gambia	1 303	644	103	159	165	118	66	32
Ghana	19 306	9 613	1 421	2 555	2 836	1 526	823	452
Guinea	8 154	4 102	733	1 087	1 129	646	338	169
Guinea-Bissau	1 199	591	105	156	154	93	53	31
Kenya	30 669	15 273	2 367	4 333	4 697	2 251	1 023	602
Lesotho	2 035	1 009	148	256	281	167	99	59
Liberia	2 913	1 465	277	347	499	183	99	61
Madagascar	15 970	7 943	1 436	2 140	2 122	1 248	646	350
Malawi	11 308	5 617	1 038	1 609	1 534	783	420	233
Mali	11 351	5 624	1 081	1 552	1 531	778	394	287
Mauritania	2 665	1 321	236	354	361	203	110	56
Mauritius	1 161	579	48	103	154	145	84	45
Mozambique	18 292	9 042	1 589	2 426	2 475	1 377	753	421
Namibia	1 757	868	142	245	242	132	64	44
Niger	10 832	5 459	1 157	1 584	1 457	746	352	162
Nigeria	113 862	57 383	9 996	16 068	15 825	8 410	4 546	2 538
Rwanda	7 609	3 765	642	1 040	1 137	540	267	140
Sao Tome and Principe	138	64	10	17	20	12	2	3
Senegal	9 421	4 697	805	1 303	1 296	731	385	178
Seychelles	80	40	3	7	11	10	6	3
Sierra Leone	4 405	2 165	403	568	580	336	185	94
South Africa	43 309	21 323	2 608	4 784	6 334	4 340	2 270	986
Swaziland	925	456	70	123	130	72	39	22
Togo	4 527	2 248	386	620	628	335	178	100
Uganda	23 300	11 625	2 358	3 393	3 181	1 515	774	403
United Republic of Tanzania	35 119	17 422	3 015	4 937	4 960	2 552	1 319	639
Zambia	10 421	5 236	954	1 497	1 501	701	369	214
Zimbabwe	12 627	6 315	1 030	1 831	1 864	898	418	273
Region of the Americas (high-income)	314 291	155 035	11 201	23 350	32 303	37 526	28 679	21 977
Bahamas	304	150	15	30	42	35	17	11
Canada	30 757	15 229	920	2 095	3 166	3 817	2 953	2 277
United States of America	283 230	139 655	10 265	21 225	29 095	33 674	25 709	19 689

Member States by WHO region and income level	Females						
	All ages	0–4 years	5–14 years	15–29 years	30–44 years	45–59 years	⩾60 years
All	2 999 797	297 863	582 630	761 707	621 685	402 225	333 687
High-income	464 797	26 478	56 255	90 803	103 963	87 204	100 094
Low-income and middle-income	2 535 000	271 385	526 375	670 904	517 722	315 021	233 593
African Region (low-income and middle-income)[c]	320 880	53 609	86 331	88 370	48 701	27 079	16 790
Algeria	14 945	1 721	3 435	4 515	2 891	1 392	992
Angola	6 635	1 292	1 867	1 700	919	534	324
Benin	3 180	551	899	849	503	242	137
Botswana	787	111	211	232	121	68	44
Burkina Faso	5 959	1 096	1 694	1 642	779	417	331
Burundi	3 268	555	955	857	459	272	170
Cameroon	7 471	1 163	2 021	2 088	1 097	652	451
Cape Verde	228	30	53	65	48	14	18
Central African Republic	1 907	304	497	511	286	181	128
Chad	3 985	743	1 085	1 043	574	328	212
Comoros	352	57	92	103	55	29	16
Congo	1 540	281	420	405	223	126	86
Côte d'Ivoire	7 807	1 202	2 157	2 279	1 141	648	380
Democratic Republic of the Congo	25 703	4 984	7 392	6 532	3 479	2 012	1 304
Equatorial Guinea	231	40	60	58	36	22	15
Eritrea	1 842	306	494	490	293	165	94
Ethiopia	31 649	5 568	8 589	8 287	4 815	2 787	1 602
Gabon	621	97	149	148	96	73	58
Gambia	658	103	159	169	123	69	36
Ghana	9 692	1 397	2 527	2 827	1 545	871	525
Guinea	4 052	715	1 057	1 101	637	348	194
Guinea-Bissau	608	105	156	156	96	57	37
Kenya	15 396	2 330	4 301	4 697	2 284	1 103	681
Lesotho	1 026	145	250	276	170	109	75
Liberia	1 448	274	346	491	168	97	72
Madagascar	8 028	1 430	2 137	2 122	1 258	675	406
Malawi	5 692	1 016	1 576	1 513	811	485	291
Mali	5 727	1 061	1 540	1 527	788	445	365
Mauritania	1 344	234	352	360	210	117	70
Mauritius	583	47	100	149	140	88	59
Mozambique	9 251	1 589	2 434	2 482	1 407	825	515
Namibia	889	140	242	238	136	77	56
Niger	5 373	1 128	1 532	1 410	737	372	193
Nigeria	56 479	9 688	15 549	15 357	8 304	4 700	2 881
Rwanda	3 844	642	1 047	1 150	537	289	179
Sao Tome and Principe	73	10	17	21	15	4	6
Senegal	4 723	787	1 281	1 292	741	405	218
Seychelles	40	3	7	10	10	6	4
Sierra Leone	2 239	403	575	591	350	203	116
South Africa	21 986	2 569	4 773	6 369	4 356	2 443	1 476
Swaziland	469	69	123	132	75	42	27
Togo	2 279	381	617	629	340	192	120
Uganda	11 676	2 333	3 382	3 171	1 480	827	482
United Republic of Tanzania	17 697	2 960	4 889	5 020	2 637	1 425	767
Zambia	5 185	933	1 465	1 466	669	393	259
Zimbabwe	6 313	1 021	1 826	1 841	858	446	320
Region of the Americas (high-income)	159 256	10 666	22 263	31 189	36 916	29 301	28 922
Bahamas	154	15	29	41	36	20	14
Canada	15 527	874	1 993	3 040	3 773	2 987	2 860
United States of America	143 575	9 777	20 240	28 108	33 108	26 294	26 048

TABLE A.1 *(continued)*

Member States by WHO region and income level	Total[b]	Males						
		All ages	0–4 years	5–14 years	15–29 years	30–44 years	45–59 years	⩾60 years
Region of the Americas (low-income and middle-income)	**513 081**	**254 252**	**27 942**	**54 610**	**72 444**	**51 530**	**29 507**	**18 219**
Antigua and Barbuda	65	32	3	7	9	7	4	3
Argentina	37 032	18 163	1 779	3 436	4 785	3 454	2 612	2 098
Barbados	267	130	9	19	33	35	19	14
Belize	226	115	15	29	34	20	10	7
Bolivia	8 329	4 144	617	1 063	1 155	683	393	233
Brazil	170 406	84 169	8 145	16 804	24 344	18 495	10 440	5 941
Chile	15 211	7 531	734	1 469	1 865	1 737	1 057	669
Colombia	42 105	20 786	2 429	4 608	5 758	4 375	2 318	1 297
Costa Rica	4 024	2 040	226	441	557	438	236	142
Cuba	11 199	5 611	368	850	1 310	1 432	918	733
Dominica	71	35	3	7	9	7	4	3
Dominican Republic	8 373	4 254	479	950	1 215	876	466	268
Ecuador	12 646	6 350	747	1 429	1 857	1 239	668	410
El Salvador	6 278	3 082	407	731	954	495	293	201
Grenada	94	46	5	9	13	10	6	4
Guatemala	11 385	5 741	942	1 593	1 637	828	448	292
Guyana	761	369	41	76	118	74	36	23
Haiti	8 142	3 989	578	1 099	1 179	601	326	206
Honduras	6 417	3 230	491	874	935	524	252	153
Jamaica	2 576	1 270	134	278	370	242	132	113
Mexico	98 872	48 926	5 705	11 012	14 605	9 374	5 094	3 136
Nicaragua	5 071	2 523	408	691	741	389	189	105
Panama	2 856	1 441	154	303	393	302	176	113
Paraguay	5 496	2 772	394	711	761	509	267	129
Peru	25 662	12 726	1 475	2 877	3 743	2 399	1 368	865
Saint Kitts and Nevis	38	19	2	4	5	4	2	2
Saint Lucia	148	72	9	16	22	14	7	5
Saint Vincent and the Grenadines	113	56	6	11	15	12	7	5
Suriname	417	207	20	44	65	45	17	15
Trinidad and Tobago	1 294	644	45	119	188	143	91	57
Uruguay	3 337	1 619	145	278	396	318	244	239
Venezuela	24 170	12 161	1 429	2 771	3 371	2 449	1 404	737
South-East Asia Region (low-income and middle-income)[c]	**1 535 634**	**786 265**	**90 144**	**172 450**	**218 856**	**160 218**	**90 548**	**54 049**
Bangladesh	137 439	70 858	9 562	17 773	20 431	13 252	6 434	3 405
Bhutan	2 085	1 054	167	287	281	157	98	64
Democratic People's Republic of Korea	22 268	11 179	987	2 030	2 789	2 728	1 644	1 001
India	1 008 937	520 312	60 014	114 668	142 803	105 142	60 892	36 792
Indonesia	212 092	106 379	11 094	22 082	31 038	22 647	12 123	7 394
Maldives	291	149	24	41	41	23	12	8
Myanmar	47 749	23 729	2 740	5 246	6 885	4 655	2 696	1 507
Nepal	23 043	11 811	1 833	3 052	3 184	1 923	1 150	669
Sri Lanka	18 924	9 718	794	1 734	2 629	2 214	1 449	898
Thailand	62 806	31 078	2 928	5 536	8 776	7 476	4 049	2 312
European Region (high-income)	**394 607**	**193 120**	**10 797**	**23 462**	**39 208**	**46 232**	**37 098**	**36 323**
Andorra	86	45	2	5	10	13	8	7
Austria	8 080	3 942	209	481	768	1 046	759	680
Belgium	10 249	5 020	282	624	978	1 198	971	966
Denmark	5 320	2 633	169	330	499	607	564	464
Finland	5 172	2 523	148	329	492	569	566	420
France	59 238	28 856	1 862	3 817	6 081	6 431	5 526	5 138
Germany	82 017	40 148	1 965	4 583	7 254	10 564	7 897	7 885
Greece	10 610	5 230	259	565	1 161	1 158	965	1 122

Member States by WHO region and income level	Females						
	All ages	0–4 years	5–14 years	15–29 years	30–44 years	45–59 years	⩾60 years
Region of the Americas (low-income and middle-income)	**258 829**	**26 872**	**52 717**	**71 810**	**53 591**	**31 566**	**22 273**
Antigua and Barbuda	33	3	6	8	7	4	3
Argentina	18 868	1 720	3 330	4 691	3 509	2 780	2 839
Barbados	138	8	19	33	35	21	22
Belize	112	14	28	34	20	9	7
Bolivia	4 185	593	1 026	1 149	711	426	280
Brazil	86 238	7 860	16 268	24 223	19 206	11 301	7 380
Chile	7 680	707	1 418	1 821	1 742	1 110	882
Colombia	21 319	2 331	4 438	5 727	4 669	2 555	1 599
Costa Rica	1 983	216	420	528	426	235	158
Cuba	5 588	350	809	1 258	1 423	953	796
Dominica	36	3	7	9	8	5	4
Dominican Republic	4 119	461	915	1 150	841	468	284
Ecuador	6 296	719	1 383	1 812	1 231	684	466
El Salvador	3 196	390	707	949	573	327	250
Grenada	47	4	9	12	10	6	5
Guatemala	5 645	903	1 527	1 593	852	460	310
Guyana	392	40	75	119	86	43	30
Haiti	4 153	557	1 072	1 187	683	402	253
Honduras	3 187	472	844	910	526	261	173
Jamaica	1 307	129	270	367	268	139	134
Mexico	49 946	5 463	10 590	14 694	10 008	5 483	3 707
Nicaragua	2 548	393	669	742	414	203	127
Panama	1 415	147	290	384	302	174	118
Paraguay	2 725	379	688	740	495	259	164
Peru	12 935	1 421	2 794	3 727	2 560	1 442	992
Saint Kitts and Nevis	19	2	4	5	4	3	2
Saint Lucia	75	8	15	22	15	8	7
Saint Vincent and the Grenadines	57	5	11	15	12	8	6
Suriname	210	20	43	63	46	20	19
Trinidad and Tobago	651	43	116	185	147	93	67
Uruguay	1 718	139	266	383	331	265	334
Venezuela	12 009	1 368	2 659	3 271	2 433	1 421	857
South-East Asia Region (low-income and middle-income)[c]	**749 369**	**85 306**	**162 342**	**204 600**	**149 046**	**88 487**	**59 589**
Bangladesh	66 582	9 090	16 765	19 111	12 132	6 093	3 391
Bhutan	1 032	160	276	271	153	99	71
Democratic People's Republic of Korea	11 090	945	1 940	2 675	2 629	1 665	1 236
India	488 626	56 384	106 854	131 070	95 662	58 596	40 060
Indonesia	105 713	10 688	21 367	30 239	22 054	12 615	8 750
Maldives	142	23	39	39	22	11	7
Myanmar	24 020	2 667	5 154	6 866	4 752	2 848	1 734
Nepal	11 232	1 730	2 839	2 968	1 878	1 125	692
Sri Lanka	9 206	767	1 681	2 546	2 113	1 238	861
Thailand	31 728	2 851	5 426	8 815	7 650	4 197	2 788
European Region (high-income)	**201 490**	**10 224**	**22 287**	**37 512**	**45 016**	**37 338**	**49 109**
Andorra	41	2	4	9	12	7	7
Austria	4 138	198	456	739	992	758	996
Belgium	5 229	269	596	944	1 159	959	1 302
Denmark	2 687	159	314	481	581	553	600
Finland	2 649	141	315	472	549	560	612
France	30 382	1 771	3 648	5 875	6 483	5 584	7 021
Germany	41 869	1 861	4 330	6 838	9 876	7 778	11 184
Greece	5 380	242	532	1 104	1 158	982	1 361

TABLE A.1 *(continued)*

Member States by WHO region and income level	Total[b]	Males						
		All ages	0–4 years	5–14 years	15–29 years	30–44 years	45–59 years	≥60 years
European Region (high-income) *(continued)*								
Iceland	279	140	11	23	32	31	24	19
Ireland	3803	1890	136	286	502	384	324	258
Israel	6040	2980	316	560	773	561	429	341
Italy	57530	27902	1350	2870	5665	6676	5434	5908
Luxembourg	437	215	14	28	42	53	42	36
Monaco	33	16	1	2	3	4	3	3
Netherlands	15864	7862	480	1005	1520	1992	1616	1249
Norway	4469	2213	149	305	437	509	437	376
Portugal	10016	4819	288	569	1159	1065	860	879
San Marino	27	13	1	1	3	3	3	3
Spain	39910	19511	939	2088	4657	4634	3454	3738
Sweden	8842	4375	226	599	817	941	921	870
Switzerland	7170	3546	187	424	619	896	764	655
United Kingdom	59415	29242	1804	3972	5733	6896	5529	5307
European Region (low-income and middle-income)	**478968**	**230651**	**15396**	**38477**	**59421**	**51974**	**36583**	**28800**
Albania	3134	1603	159	326	418	365	203	131
Armenia	3787	1834	106	356	496	433	231	212
Azerbaijan	8041	3959	314	886	1083	935	392	350
Belarus	10187	4746	241	732	1153	1150	793	677
Bosnia and Herzegovina	3977	1968	106	283	462	521	342	254
Bulgaria	7949	3864	162	479	890	813	773	747
Croatia	4654	2253	138	292	486	527	434	377
Czech Republic	10272	4995	231	633	1229	1045	1096	761
Estonia	1393	649	31	95	155	150	118	99
Georgia	5262	2512	153	399	611	575	379	395
Hungary	9968	4756	251	613	1149	1001	983	758
Kazakhstan	16172	7844	648	1570	2131	1807	1011	676
Kyrgyzstan	4921	2413	265	579	676	486	230	177
Latvia	2421	1116	48	168	261	265	203	171
Lithuania	3696	1743	95	272	412	423	289	252
Malta	390	193	12	28	44	40	40	28
Poland	38605	18761	1024	2767	4772	4143	3498	2557
Republic of Moldova	4295	2054	133	375	539	453	325	229
Romania	22438	10977	584	1511	2760	2376	1930	1816
Russian Federation	145491	68130	3254	10103	16713	16737	11983	9339
Slovakia	5399	2625	148	391	686	590	479	331
Slovenia	1988	966	46	116	222	230	201	151
Tajikistan	6087	3032	393	822	852	551	232	182
The former Yugoslav Republic of Macedonia	2034	1017	75	162	249	226	172	133
Turkey	66668	33676	3614	6581	10002	6843	4024	2612
Turkmenistan	4737	2345	305	598	653	463	197	128
Ukraine	49568	23019	1122	3397	5549	5281	4011	3659
Uzbekistan	24881	12357	1407	3182	3538	2436	1045	749
Yugoslavia	10552	5248	332	762	1226	1109	970	848
Eastern Mediterranean Region (high-income)	**5870**	**3594**	**230**	**597**	**783**	**1000**	**763**	**221**
Cyprus	784	391	28	66	89	85	69	55
Kuwait	1914	1115	73	231	287	261	205	57
Qatar	565	366	27	50	62	141	74	13
United Arab Emirates	2606	1722	102	250	345	513	414	97
Eastern Mediterranean Region (low-income and middle-income)	**475785**	**242847**	**34697**	**62275**	**67412**	**41988**	**23809**	**12666**
Afghanistan	21765	11227	1954	2923	3018	1814	1008	510

Member States by WHO region and income level	Females						
	All ages	0–4 years	5–14 years	15–29 years	30–44 years	45–59 years	⩾60 years
European Region (high-income) *(continued)*							
Iceland	139	10	21	31	31	23	23
Ireland	1 913	128	270	481	393	321	321
Israel	3 060	298	533	737	581	458	453
Italy	29 628	1 271	2 726	5 460	6 631	5 603	7 937
Luxembourg	222	13	26	41	52	40	49
Monaco	17	1	2	3	4	3	4
Netherlands	8 002	457	960	1 464	1 904	1 567	1 649
Norway	2 256	141	289	420	487	422	498
Portugal	5 197	272	542	1 132	1 098	943	1 210
San Marino	14	1	1	3	3	3	4
Spain	20 400	877	1 970	4 462	4 584	3 555	4 952
Sweden	4 467	214	569	781	898	896	1 109
Switzerland	3 624	178	405	589	837	743	871
United Kingdom	30 173	1 719	3 778	5 447	6 704	5 578	6 947
European Region (low-income and middle-income)	**248 317**	**14 736**	**36 869**	**57 486**	**52 418**	**40 312**	**46 495**
Albania	1 531	150	305	391	346	189	150
Armenia	1 953	101	336	479	477	274	286
Azerbaijan	4 082	296	836	1 024	996	437	493
Belarus	5 441	227	704	1 147	1 205	911	1 248
Bosnia and Herzegovina	2 009	99	266	437	511	357	339
Bulgaria	4 086	155	457	852	815	831	976
Croatia	2 401	131	279	469	518	442	562
Czech Republic	5 276	220	602	1 178	1 015	1 136	1 125
Estonia	745	30	91	151	151	140	182
Georgia	2 750	146	379	587	611	437	591
Hungary	5 212	239	586	1 099	995	1 084	1 209
Kazakhstan	8 329	625	1 520	2 094	1 818	1 141	1 131
Kyrgyzstan	2 508	259	567	670	497	249	266
Latvia	1 305	46	160	254	269	242	334
Lithuania	1 953	91	261	400	427	341	434
Malta	197	12	26	41	39	40	38
Poland	19 844	970	2 634	4 594	4 080	3 724	3 843
Republic of Moldova	2 242	126	360	533	485	379	358
Romania	11 461	553	1 447	2 659	2 351	2 044	2 406
Russian Federation	77 361	3 108	9 657	16 269	16 974	13 768	17 584
Slovakia	2 773	141	374	662	580	515	501
Slovenia	1 022	44	110	212	228	198	230
Tajikistan	3 055	381	801	836	573	232	233
The former Yugoslav Republic of Macedonia	1 017	70	153	238	220	176	160
Turkey	32 992	3 494	6 332	9 528	6 659	3 960	3 019
Turkmenistan	2 393	296	583	646	477	212	179
Ukraine	26 549	1 068	3 254	5 399	5 527	4 775	6 526
Uzbekistan	12 524	1 354	3 079	3 487	2 506	1 089	1 009
Yugoslavia	5 305	308	710	1 148	1 068	988	1 083
Eastern Mediterranean Region (high-income)	**2 276**	**219**	**563**	**627**	**440**	**289**	**137**
Cyprus	393	26	62	85	83	70	68
Kuwait	800	71	224	262	126	88	28
Qatar	199	26	48	46	51	23	5
United Arab Emirates	884	96	229	234	180	108	37
Eastern Mediterranean Region (low-income and middle-income)	**232 939**	**33 023**	**59 158**	**64 526**	**39 940**	**22 641**	**13 650**
Afghanistan	10 538	1 852	2 736	2 796	1 679	955	519

TABLE A.1 *(continued)*

Member States by WHO region and income level	Total[b]	Males						
		All ages	0–4 years	5–14 years	15–29 years	30–44 years	45–59 years	≥60 years
Eastern Mediterranean Region (low-income and middle-income) *(continued)*								
Bahrain	640	368	29	63	75	120	64	16
Djibouti	632	297	52	86	80	38	28	14
Egypt	67 884	34 364	4 096	8 182	9 788	6 652	3 721	1 925
Iraq	22 946	11 666	1 817	3 063	3 329	1 939	1 018	501
Islamic Republic of Iran	70 330	35 998	3 882	9 640	10 578	6 420	3 702	1 776
Jordan	4 913	2 554	390	618	780	459	194	113
Lebanon	3 496	1 711	171	384	498	357	163	137
Libyan Arab Jamahiriya	5 290	2 741	329	589	877	473	316	157
Morocco	29 878	14 964	1 832	3 441	4 457	2 948	1 429	856
Oman	2 538	1 347	206	363	334	223	166	55
Pakistan	141 256	72 622	11 427	18 985	19 041	11 856	7 234	4 080
Saudi Arabia	20 346	10 872	1 630	2 835	2 682	1 731	1 471	523
Somalia	8 778	4 358	897	1 216	1 154	619	314	158
Sudan	31 095	15 639	2 412	3 943	4 390	2 645	1 456	792
Syrian Arab Republic	16 189	8 200	1 146	2 228	2 488	1 400	575	363
Tunisia	9 459	4 776	430	1 013	1 441	986	511	396
Yemen	18 349	9 142	1 996	2 703	2 402	1 308	439	294
Western Pacific Region (high-income)	**201 099**	**99 320**	**5 743**	**11 957**	**22 505**	**22 029**	**20 208**	**16 878**
Australia	19 138	9 529	648	1 368	2 127	2 176	1 788	1 421
Brunei Darussalam	328	173	18	36	41	44	25	9
Japan	127 096	62 212	3 159	6 424	13 293	12 493	14 004	12 839
New Zealand	3 778	1 861	142	302	393	424	335	265
Republic of Korea	46 740	23 522	1 631	3 517	6 239	6 309	3 679	2 147
Singapore	4 018	2 023	145	310	412	583	376	197
Western Pacific Region (low-income and middle-income)	**1 486 206**	**761 540**	**63 560**	**141 345**	**195 168**	**182 236**	**111 291**	**67 940**
Cambodia	13 104	6 389	1 070	1 846	1 700	1 050	518	205
China	1 282 437	659 410	51 092	116 265	165 941	162 699	101 353	62 059
Cook Islands	20	10	1	2	3	2	1	1
Federated States of Micronesia	123	64	9	15	16	12	7	4
Fiji	814	414	50	90	118	85	49	22
Kiribati	83	43	6	10	11	8	5	3
Lao People's Democratic Republic	5 279	2 636	426	722	719	420	210	139
Malaysia	22 218	11 255	1 350	2 541	3 029	2 286	1 357	692
Marshall Islands	51	26	4	6	7	5	3	2
Mongolia	2 533	1 268	139	315	387	259	105	63
Nauru	12	6	1	2	2	1	1	<1
Niue	2	1	<1	<1	<1	<1	<1	<1
Palau	19	10	1	2	2	2	1	1
Papua New Guinea	4 809	2 507	366	635	746	436	223	101
Philippines	75 653	38 092	5 031	9 474	10 973	6 925	3 785	1 903
Samoa	159	83	11	23	27	12	6	5
Solomon Islands	447	230	41	63	66	33	18	10
Tonga	99	52	6	12	15	10	6	3
Tuvalu	10	5	1	1	2	1	1	<1
Vanuatu	197	101	16	27	27	17	9	5
Viet Nam	78 137	38 938	3 939	9 293	11 379	7 973	3 633	2 722

Source: United Nations, 2001.

[a] Numbers are rounded to the nearest 1000. Any apparent discrepancies in total sums are a result of rounding.

[b] Combined total for males and females.

[c] No high-income countries in the region.

Member States by WHO region and income level	Females						
	All ages	0–4 years	5–14 years	15–29 years	30–44 years	45–59 years	⩾60 years
Eastern Mediterranean Region (low-income and middle-income) *(continued)*							
Bahrain	272	28	60	68	72	30	14
Djibouti	335	51	85	83	53	43	21
Egypt	33 521	3 915	7 811	9 197	6 367	3 871	2 359
Iraq	11 280	1 739	2 935	3 178	1 875	1 001	553
Islamic Republic of Iran	34 332	3 672	9 107	10 154	6 007	3 496	1 895
Jordan	2 359	372	588	713	392	184	110
Lebanon	1 786	164	370	489	404	197	162
Libyan Arab Jamahiriya	2 549	314	563	848	444	248	133
Morocco	14 914	1 764	3 318	4 307	2 966	1 511	1 049
Oman	1 191	198	352	325	170	94	52
Pakistan	68 634	10 783	17 826	18 240	11 178	6 547	4 065
Saudi Arabia	9 474	1 556	2 713	2 590	1 330	831	453
Somalia	4 420	890	1 206	1 164	639	336	184
Sudan	15 457	2 316	3 803	4 284	2 641	1 507	905
Syrian Arab Republic	7 988	1 093	2 144	2 417	1 340	593	401
Tunisia	4 682	403	964	1 387	1 005	522	402
Yemen	9 207	1 914	2 575	2 285	1 378	680	375
Western Pacific Region (high-income)	**101 778**	**5 368**	**11 142**	**21 475**	**21 591**	**20 276**	**21 926**
Australia	9 608	615	1 296	2 052	2 179	1 762	1 705
Brunei Darussalam	156	17	34	38	39	19	8
Japan	64 884	2 993	6 118	12 730	12 229	14 135	16 679
New Zealand	1 917	135	288	383	452	337	323
Republic of Korea	23 218	1 474	3 118	5 883	6 107	3 653	2 984
Singapore	1 995	135	289	388	585	370	227
Western Pacific Region (low-income and middle-income)	**724 667**	**57 838**	**128 958**	**184 113**	**174 027**	**104 936**	**74 795**
Cambodia	6 715	1 037	1 797	1 681	1 170	665	366
China	623 027	45 892	104 807	155 577	154 205	94 679	67 867
Cook Islands	9	1	2	3	2	1	1
Federated States of Micronesia	59	8	15	15	11	6	4
Fiji	400	47	85	112	82	50	25
Kiribati	40	6	10	10	7	4	3
Lao People's Democratic Republic	2 643	410	698	705	441	231	157
Malaysia	10 964	1 280	2 405	2 925	2 269	1 314	771
Marshall Islands	25	4	6	6	4	3	2
Mongolia	1 265	133	305	380	262	108	78
Nauru	6	1	1	1	1	1	<1
Niue	1	<1	<1	<1	<1	<1	<1
Palau	9	1	2	2	2	1	1
Papua New Guinea	2 303	344	583	637	422	217	98
Philippines	37 561	4 800	9 090	10 641	6 901	3 837	2 293
Samoa	75	11	21	22	9	6	6
Solomon Islands	217	38	59	61	34	17	9
Tonga	47	6	11	13	9	5	4
Tuvalu	5	1	1	1	1	1	<1
Vanuatu	96	14	25	26	17	8	5
Viet Nam	39 199	3 804	9 034	11 295	8 179	3 782	3 106

TABLE A.2

Estimated mortality caused by intentional injury,[a] by sex, age group, WHO region and income level, 2000

Absolute numbers (in thousands)[b]

WHO region	Income level	Total[c]	Males						
			All ages	0–4 years	5–14 years	15–29 years	30–44 years	45–59 years	≥60 years
All	all	1 659	1 153	41	54	351	320	205	182
	high	149	111	1	1	24	31	27	27
	low and middle	1 510	1 042	40	54	326	288	178	156
African Region[d]	low and middle	311	225	17	23	72	57	31	25
Region of the Americas	all	228	196	2	3	87	60	28	17
	high	56	44	<1	1	13	14	9	7
	low and middle	171	152	1	2	74	46	19	10
South-East Asia Region[d]	low and middle	317	216	5	15	69	59	38	29
European Region	all	303	239	2	5	53	78	58	44
	high	55	41	<1	<1	7	11	10	12
	low and middle	248	198	2	5	46	67	48	31
Eastern Mediterranean Region	all	95	62	14	5	20	11	7	5
	high	1	<1	<1	<1	<1	<1	<1	<1
	low and middle	95	61	14	5	20	11	7	5
Western Pacific Region	all	405	216	1	4	50	55	44	62
	high	37	26	<1	<1	4	6	8	7
	low and middle	368	190	1	4	45	48	36	55

Rate per 100 000 population

WHO region	Income level	Total[c, e]	Males						
			All ages[e]	0–4 years	5–14 years	15–29 years	30–44 years	45–59 years	≥60 years
All	all	28.8	40.5	13.0	8.8	44.0	49.7	50.7	67.4
	high	14.4	22.1	2.2	1.5	25.7	29.4	31.3	35.8
	low and middle	32.1	44.8	14.1	9.6	46.5	53.8	56.0	79.6
African Region[d]	low and middle	60.9	94.6	31.2	25.9	80.9	118.0	119.7	182.5
Region of the Americas	all	27.7	48.6	3.8	3.4	83.2	67.2	48.0	43.1
	high	17.2	27.6	4.0	2.4	41.8	36.3	30.7	33.7
	low and middle	34.3	62.1	3.8	3.8	101.7	89.7	64.9	54.5
South-East Asia Region[d]	low and middle	22.8	31.3	6.0	8.9	31.7	36.6	41.8	54.1
European Region	all	32.0	52.5	6.5	7.9	53.7	79.6	78.1	67.0
	high	11.5	17.8	0.9	0.7	16.6	24.7	26.7	34.3
	low and middle	49.6	83.7	10.4	12.4	78.1	128.4	130.2	108.3
Eastern Mediterranean Region	all	21.6	27.4	39.9	7.3	29.1	26.6	27.2	40.8
	high	10.3	13.9	3.9	3.3	19.0	17.6	12.3	20.2
	low and middle	21.8	27.7	40.2	7.3	29.2	26.9	27.7	41.2
Western Pacific Region	all	24.3	26.5	1.9	2.8	22.7	26.7	33.6	72.9
	high	15.4	22.3	1.1	1.2	18.7	27.9	41.3	41.8
	low and middle	26.2	27.7	2.0	3.0	23.2	26.6	32.2	80.6

Proportion of all deaths due to injury (%)

WHO region	Income level	Total[c]	Males						
			All ages	0–4 years	5–14 years	15–29 years	30–44 years	45–59 years	≥60 years
All	all	32.8	33.8	15.0	20.0	39.8	38.7	34.7	31.9
	high	31.6	35.7	12.8	14.9	37.2	42.7	41.9	26.1
	low and middle	32.9	33.6	15.1	20.1	40.0	38.3	33.8	33.2
African Region[d]	low and middle	41.3	43.9	23.7	29.7	56.3	53.4	43.8	43.0
Region of the Americas	all	40.6	44.9	8.7	17.6	57.7	50.2	41.2	26.0
	high	33.1	37.9	19.6	19.6	46.2	42.8	39.9	25.7
	low and middle	43.9	47.5	7.1	17.1	60.4	52.9	41.8	26.3
South-East Asia Region[d]	low and middle	23.1	24.3	7.9	18.7	28.1	28.4	26.1	21.1
European Region	all	37.1	39.3	16.0	29.7	41.7	43.2	39.2	34.6
	high	29.4	33.7	8.1	10.0	28.9	44.0	42.8	27.1
	low and middle	39.4	40.7	17.0	31.9	44.5	43.1	38.5	38.9

Absolute numbers (in thousands)[b]

WHO region	Income level	Females						
		All ages	0–4 years	5–14 years	15–29 years	30–44 years	45–59 years	≥60 years
All	all	506	23	37	153	119	77	97
	high	38	<1	1	6	10	9	12
	low and middle	468	23	37	147	109	68	85
African Region[d]	low and middle	86	12	13	32	15	9	6
Region of the Americas	all	31	1	1	11	9	5	4
	high	12	<1	<1	3	4	3	2
	low and middle	19	1	1	8	5	2	2
South-East Asia Region[d]	low and middle	101	4	13	37	23	13	12
European Region	all	64	1	1	11	17	14	21
	high	15	<1	<1	2	3	4	6
	low and middle	50	1	1	9	13	11	15
Eastern Mediterranean Region	all	34	4	5	12	5	3	4
	high	<1	<1	<1	<1	<1	<1	<1
	low and middle	34	4	5	12	5	3	4
Western Pacific Region	all	189	1	3	50	50	33	52
	high	11	<1	<1	2	2	3	5
	low and middle	178	1	3	48	47	31	47

Rate per 100 000 population

WHO region	Income level	Females						
		All ages[e]	0–4 years	5–14 years	15–29 years	30–44 years	45–59 years	≥60 years
All	all	17.3	7.7	6.4	20.1	19.1	19.1	29.2
	high	6.9	1.8	0.9	6.7	9.2	10.3	12.2
	low and middle	19.7	8.3	7.0	21.9	21.1	21.5	36.5
African Region[d]	low and middle	29.6	21.9	14.6	36.1	31.5	32.2	36.4
Region of the Americas	all	7.5	2.7	1.8	10.5	10.1	8.4	7.2
	high	7.1	3.2	1.4	8.2	10.8	9.3	6.6
	low and middle	7.6	2.6	2.0	11.5	9.6	7.5	7.9
South-East Asia Region[d]	low and middle	14.3	4.3	8.3	18.2	15.2	14.2	19.7
European Region	all	12.5	3.3	2.1	11.3	17.2	18.4	21.6
	high	5.7	0.7	0.5	4.4	7.5	9.7	11.7
	low and middle	18.3	5.2	3.1	15.7	25.5	26.5	31.9
Eastern Mediterranean Region	all	15.5	13.1	8.7	19.1	12.9	11.6	27.2
	high	4.4	2.1	0.7	5.7	6.0	4.0	6.1
	low and middle	15.7	13.2	8.8	19.2	13.0	11.7	27.4
Western Pacific Region	all	22.5	2.2	2.4	24.5	25.3	26.6	53.3
	high	8.8	1.3	0.9	8.4	9.9	12.8	21.0
	low and middle	25.0	2.3	2.5	26.3	27.2	29.2	62.8

Proportion of all deaths due to injury (%)

WHO region	Income level	Females						
		All ages	0–4 years	5–14 years	15–29 years	30–44 years	45–59 years	≥60 years
All	all	30.7	10.3	18.1	42.9	42.3	37.3	26.0
	high	24.4	14.8	17.1	35.2	45.3	43.1	13.7
	low and middle	31.4	10.2	18.1	43.3	42.0	36.6	29.9
African Region[d]	low and middle	35.8	19.0	27.2	60.8	44.3	36.8	27.4
Region of the Americas	all	25.3	9.2	18.1	42.1	41.0	32.3	9.0
	high	22.6	22.4	19.6	32.6	39.1	35.0	8.1
	low and middle	27.3	7.1	17.7	46.3	42.6	29.6	10.3
South-East Asia Region[d]	low and middle	20.9	7.9	14.6	29.1	26.5	23.8	14.5
European Region	all	30.8	11.7	18.7	39.1	47.6	38.2	21.6
	high	21.8	8.9	12.9	31.0	50.8	48.1	12.5
	low and middle	35.1	12.1	19.5	41.0	46.8	35.7	30.1

TABLE A.2 *(continued)*

Proportion of all deaths due to injury (%) *(continued)*

WHO region	Income level	Total[c]	Males						
			All ages	0–4 years	5–14 years	15–29 years	30–44 years	45–59 years	⩾60 years
Eastern Mediterranean Region	all	28.2	28.9	41.0	17.9	33.1	28.4	23.2	21.0
	high	19.9	19.5	15.8	17.2	21.4	23.0	15.1	16.6
	low and middle	28.3	29.0	41.1	17.9	33.3	28.5	23.4	21.1
Western Pacific Region	all	33.1	28.5	1.9	7.6	29.3	31.6	33.5	39.3
	high	33.0	33.5	5.0	10.5	32.4	41.5	43.8	25.1
	low and middle	33.2	27.9	1.8	7.5	29.1	30.7	31.8	42.3

Proportion of all deaths (%)

WHO region	Income level	Total[c]	Males						
			All ages	0–4 years	5–14 years	15–29 years	30–44 years	45–59 years	⩾60 years
All	all	3.0	3.9	0.7	7.4	18.6	10.6	4.7	1.3
	high	1.9	2.7	1.4	7.3	26.4	15.7	5.2	0.8
	low and middle	3.2	4.1	0.7	7.4	18.2	10.2	4.6	1.4
African Region[d]	low and middle	2.9	4.1	0.8	10.5	13.8	6.4	5.0	2.7
Region of the Americas	all	3.9	6.2	0.6	7.4	40.3	20.3	6.0	0.9
	high	2.1	3.3	2.2	11.0	35.3	16.7	4.7	0.7
	low and middle	5.4	8.4	0.4	6.8	41.3	21.7	6.8	1.1
South-East Asia Region[d]	low and middle	2.2	2.8	0.3	5.9	12.7	7.4	3.1	0.9
European Region	all	3.1	4.8	1.2	16.2	29.5	19.7	7.0	1.3
	high	1.4	2.1	0.7	4.0	18.8	14.6	4.6	0.8
	low and middle	4.3	6.6	1.3	18.1	32.0	20.9	7.9	1.7
Eastern Mediterranean Region	all	2.4	2.9	1.8	5.9	15.3	6.9	2.6	0.7
	high	2.4	3.0	1.3	9.7	16.2	9.7	2.1	0.5
	low and middle	2.4	2.9	1.8	5.9	15.3	6.9	2.6	0.7
Western Pacific Region	all	3.6	3.4	0.2	3.8	17.3	11.4	4.5	1.6
	high	2.6	3.3	0.8	5.2	22.8	16.4	7.2	1.2
	low and middle	3.7	3.4	0.2	3.7	16.9	11.0	4.2	1.6

Source: WHO Global Burden of Disease project for 2000, Version 1.

[a] Intentional injury = ICD-10 X60–Y09, Y35, Y36 (ICD-9 E950–E978, E990–E999).

[b] Absolute numbers are rounded to the nearest 1000. Any apparent discrepancies in total sums are a result of rounding.

[c] Combined total for males and females.

[d] No high-income countries in the region.

[e] Age-standardized.

Proportion of all deaths due to injury (%) *(continued)*

WHO region	Income level	Females						
		All ages	0–4 years	5–14 years	15–29 years	30–44 years	45–59 years	≥60 years
Eastern Mediterranean Region	all	27.1	12.2	25.3	44.7	34.5	27.5	24.7
	high	22.3	13.4	9.3	34.2	26.1	18.0	13.8
	low and middle	27.1	12.2	25.3	44.7	34.6	27.5	24.8
Western Pacific Region	all	40.8	2.3	10.1	52.3	56.3	50.4	43.0
	high	32.2	7.4	17.0	46.2	52.1	48.1	22.7
	low and middle	41.5	2.2	10.0	52.6	56.5	50.6	47.1

Proportion of all deaths (%)

WHO region	Income level	Females						
		All ages	0–4 years	5–14 years	15–29 years	30–44 years	45–59 years	≥60 years
All	all	1.9	0.4	5.2	8.8	5.8	2.9	0.7
	high	1.0	1.5	4.8	18.1	10.0	3.3	0.3
	low and middle	2.1	0.4	5.2	8.6	5.6	2.8	0.8
African Region[d]	low and middle	1.7	0.6	5.7	4.1	1.9	2.0	0.6
Region of the Americas	all	1.1	0.5	5.1	13.7	6.3	1.8	0.2
	high	0.9	2.2	9.1	17.9	9.3	2.4	0.2
	low and middle	1.4	0.4	4.5	12.7	5.0	1.3	0.2
South-East Asia Region[d]	low and middle	1.6	0.2	4.8	7.5	4.2	1.5	0.4
European Region	all	1.4	0.7	6.9	17.4	11.6	4.0	0.5
	high	0.7	0.6	4.1	14.2	9.3	3.4	0.3
	low and middle	1.8	0.8	7.4	18.2	12.4	4.2	0.7
Eastern Mediterranean Region	all	1.8	0.6	6.7	9.7	4.0	1.4	0.6
	high	1.1	0.8	2.8	14.2	5.3	1.1	0.2
	low and middle	1.8	0.6	6.7	9.7	4.0	1.4	0.6
Western Pacific Region	all	3.7	0.3	3.8	24.7	16.5	5.9	1.5
	high	1.8	1.1	6.6	25.0	13.3	5.4	0.8
	low and middle	4.0	0.3	3.7	24.7	16.7	5.9	1.7

TABLE A.3

Estimated mortality caused by homicide,[a] by sex, age group, WHO region and income level, 2000

Absolute numbers (in thousands)[b]

WHO region	Income level	Total[c]	Males						
			All ages	0–4 years	5–14 years	15–29 years	30–44 years	45–59 years	⩾60 years
All	all	520	401	18	13	155	120	60	35
	high	26	19	1	<1	8	6	3	1
	low and middle	494	382	18	13	147	114	57	34
African Region[d]	low and middle	116	82	10	4	30	19	10	9
Region of the Americas	all	159	142	1	2	72	44	17	7
	high	19	15	<1	<1	7	4	2	1
	low and middle	140	128	1	2	65	39	15	6
South-East Asia Region[d]	low and middle	78	54	3	4	13	14	11	9
European Region	all	78	58	<1	1	15	23	13	6
	high	4	3	<1	<1	1	1	1	<1
	low and middle	74	56	<1	<1	14	22	13	6
Eastern Mediterranean Region	all	31	20	2	1	8	5	2	2
	high	<1	<1	<1	<1	<1	<1	<1	<1
	low and middle	30	19	2	1	8	5	2	2
Western Pacific Region	all	59	45	1	2	17	15	6	3
	high	2	1	<1	<1	<1	<1	<1	<1
	low and middle	57	44	1	2	17	15	6	3

Rate per 100 000 population

WHO region	Income level	Total[c, e]	Males						
			All ages[e]	0–4 years	5–14 years	15–29 years	30–44 years	45–59 years	⩾60 years
All	all	8.8	13.6	5.8	2.1	19.4	18.7	14.8	13.0
	high	2.9	4.3	2.2	0.7	8.4	5.5	3.3	1.9
	low and middle	10.1	15.6	6.1	2.3	20.9	21.3	17.9	17.3
African Region[d]	low and middle	22.2	33.4	17.9	4.0	34.1	39.6	39.6	63.3
Region of the Americas	all	19.3	34.7	3.5	2.4	68.6	49.1	28.9	16.4
	high	6.5	9.9	4.0	1.2	21.4	11.6	6.7	3.7
	low and middle	27.5	51.0	3.3	2.9	89.7	76.4	50.4	31.9
South-East Asia Region[d]	low and middle	5.8	8.1	3.9	2.2	6.0	8.8	11.6	16.9
European Region	all	8.4	13.0	1.7	0.8	15.1	23.5	18.1	9.3
	high	1.0	1.4	0.9	0.3	1.7	2.1	1.6	1.1
	low and middle	14.8	23.2	2.2	1.2	23.9	42.6	34.8	19.7
Eastern Mediterranean Region	all	7.1	9.4	5.0	2.0	11.3	11.1	9.8	13.6
	high	4.2	6.0	1.4	0.6	10.1	9.1	4.1	5.7
	low and middle	7.2	9.4	5.1	2.0	11.3	11.1	10.0	13.7
Western Pacific Region	all	3.4	5.1	1.9	1.5	7.9	7.4	4.9	3.4
	high	1.1	1.3	1.1	0.5	1.5	2.0	1.6	1.1
	low and middle	3.8	5.6	2.0	1.5	8.6	8.0	5.5	3.9

Proportion of all deaths due to injury (%)

WHO region	Income level	Total[c]	Males						
			All ages	0–4 years	5–14 years	15–29 years	30–44 years	45–59 years	⩾60 years
All	all	10.3	11.7	6.7	4.8	17.6	14.5	10.1	6.2
	high	5.5	6.0	12.7	6.9	12.2	8.0	4.4	1.4
	low and middle	10.8	12.3	6.6	4.8	18.0	15.1	10.8	7.2
African Region[d]	low and middle	15.4	16.0	13.6	4.6	23.7	17.9	14.5	14.9
Region of the Americas	all	28.4	32.6	8.0	12.5	47.5	36.7	24.7	9.9
	high	11.4	12.6	19.6	9.9	23.7	13.7	8.7	2.8
	low and middle	35.8	39.9	6.2	13.1	53.2	45.1	32.5	15.4
South-East Asia Region[d]	low and middle	5.7	6.1	5.1	4.6	5.3	6.8	7.3	6.6
European Region	all	9.5	9.6	4.2	3.1	11.7	12.8	9.1	4.8
	high	2.2	2.3	8.1	3.9	3.0	3.8	2.6	0.9
	low and middle	11.7	11.4	3.7	3.0	13.6	14.3	10.3	7.1

Absolute numbers (in thousands)[b]

WHO region	Income level	Females						
		All ages	0–4 years	5–14 years	15–29 years	30–44 years	45–59 years	⩾60 years
All	all	119	14	12	33	27	18	15
	high	7	<1	<1	2	2	1	1
	low and middle	112	14	11	32	25	17	14
African Region[d]	low and middle	34	7	2	12	7	4	2
Region of the Americas	all	17	1	1	7	5	2	1
	high	5	<1	<1	1	2	1	<1
	low and middle	12	1	1	5	4	1	1
South-East Asia Region[d]	low and middle	24	3	4	3	4	5	4
European Region	all	20	<1	<1	4	6	4	5
	high	1	<1	<1	<1	<1	<1	<1
	low and middle	18	<1	<1	4	5	4	5
Eastern Mediterranean Region	all	11	2	2	4	2	1	1
	high	<1	<1	<1	<1	<1	<1	<1
	low and middle	11	2	2	3	2	1	1
Western Pacific Region	all	14	1	1	4	4	2	2
	high	1	<1	<1	<1	<1	<1	<1
	low and middle	13	1	1	4	4	2	1

Rate per 100 000 population

WHO region	Income level	Females						
		All ages[e]	0–4 years	5–14 years	15–29 years	30–44 years	45–59 years	⩾60 years
All	all	4.0	4.8	2.0	4.4	4.3	4.5	4.5
	high	1.5	1.8	0.5	2.0	2.1	1.2	1.0
	low and middle	4.6	5.1	2.1	4.7	4.7	5.4	6.1
African Region[d]	low and middle	11.8	12.7	2.9	14.1	13.8	14.6	11.8
Region of the Americas	all	4.0	2.6	1.2	6.4	5.7	3.3	2.6
	high	3.0	3.2	1.0	4.4	4.2	2.2	1.7
	low and middle	4.8	2.3	1.3	7.3	6.6	4.3	3.8
South-East Asia Region[d]	low and middle	3.5	3.5	2.6	1.6	2.5	5.7	7.3
European Region	all	3.9	1.2	0.7	4.0	5.7	5.6	5.3
	high	0.6	0.7	0.2	0.7	0.8	0.7	0.7
	low and middle	6.8	1.6	1.0	6.1	9.9	10.1	10.3
Eastern Mediterranean Region	all	4.8	5.5	3.6	5.4	4.3	3.8	5.9
	high	1.2	0.4	0.0	1.5	1.3	1.4	2.6
	low and middle	4.8	5.5	3.6	5.4	4.4	3.8	5.9
Western Pacific Region	all	1.7	2.2	1.0	1.9	2.0	1.4	1.6
	high	0.8	1.3	0.4	0.8	1.1	0.8	0.8
	low and middle	1.8	2.3	1.0	2.0	2.1	1.6	1.9

Proportion of all deaths due to injury (%)

WHO region	Income level	Females						
		All ages	0–4 years	5–14 years	15–29 years	30–44 years	45–59 years	⩾60 years
All	all	7.2	6.4	5.6	9.4	9.5	8.8	4.1
	high	4.4	14.7	10.2	10.4	10.4	5.2	1.1
	low and middle	7.5	6.3	5.5	9.3	9.5	9.2	5.0
African Region[d]	low and middle	14.3	11.0	5.4	23.7	19.4	16.7	8.9
Region of the Americas	all	13.7	8.7	11.8	25.6	23.0	12.7	3.3
	high	8.8	22.4	13.5	17.2	15.3	8.3	2.1
	low and middle	17.4	6.5	11.4	29.3	29.6	17.0	5.0
South-East Asia Region[d]	low and middle	4.9	6.4	4.6	2.6	4.3	9.5	5.4
European Region	all	9.3	4.4	6.2	13.8	15.9	11.6	5.3
	high	2.0	8.9	6.0	4.6	5.7	3.5	0.7
	low and middle	12.8	3.8	6.2	16.0	18.2	13.7	9.7

TABLE A.3 *(continued)*

Proportion of all deaths due to injury (%) *(continued)*

WHO region	Income level	Total[c]	Males						
			All ages	0–4 years	5–14 years	15–29 years	30–44 years	45–59 years	⩾60 years
Eastern Mediterranean Region	all	9.0	9.2	5.2	4.9	12.9	11.8	8.4	7.0
	high	8.3	8.7	5.6	3.0	11.4	11.8	5.0	4.7
	low and middle	9.1	9.2	5.2	4.9	12.9	11.8	8.5	7.0
Western Pacific Region	all	4.8	5.9	1.9	3.9	10.1	8.7	4.9	1.8
	high	2.0	1.8	5.0	4.5	2.5	2.9	1.7	0.7
	low and middle	5.1	6.4	1.8	3.9	10.8	9.3	5.5	2.1

Proportion of all deaths (%)

WHO region	Income level	Total[c]	Males						
			All ages	0–4 years	5–14 years	15–29 years	30–44 years	45–59 years	⩾60 years
All	all	0.9	1.4	0.3	1.8	8.2	4.0	1.4	0.3
	high	0.3	0.5	1.4	3.4	8.7	2.9	0.6	0.0
	low and middle	1.0	1.5	0.3	1.8	8.2	4.0	1.5	0.3
African Region[d]	low and middle	1.1	1.5	0.4	1.6	5.8	2.2	1.7	0.9
Region of the Americas	all	2.7	4.5	0.5	5.3	33.2	14.8	3.6	0.4
	high	0.7	1.1	2.2	5.5	18.1	5.3	1.0	0.1
	low and middle	4.4	7.0	0.4	5.2	36.4	18.5	5.3	0.7
South-East Asia Region[d]	low and middle	0.5	0.7	0.2	1.4	2.4	1.8	0.9	0.3
European Region	all	0.8	1.2	0.3	1.7	8.3	5.8	1.6	0.2
	high	0.1	0.1	0.7	1.6	2.0	1.2	0.3	0.0
	low and middle	1.3	1.8	0.3	1.7	9.8	6.9	2.1	0.3
Eastern Mediterranean Region	all	0.8	0.9	0.2	1.6	5.9	2.9	0.9	0.2
	high	1.0	1.4	0.5	1.7	8.6	5.0	0.7	0.2
	low and middle	0.8	0.9	0.2	1.6	5.9	2.9	0.9	0.2
Western Pacific Region	all	0.5	0.7	0.2	1.9	6.0	3.1	0.7	0.1
	high	0.2	0.2	0.8	2.2	1.8	1.2	0.3	0.0
	low and middle	0.6	0.8	0.2	1.9	6.3	3.3	0.7	0.1

Source: WHO Global Burden of Disease project for 2000, Version 1.

[a] Homicide = ICD-10 X85–Y09 (ICD-9 E960–E969).

[b] Absolute numbers are rounded to the nearest 1000. Any apparent discrepancies in total sums are a result of rounding.

[c] Combined total for males and females.

[d] No high-income countries in the region.

[e] Age-standardized.

Proportion of all deaths due to injury (%) *(continued)*

WHO region	Income level	Females						
		All ages	**0–4 years**	**5–14 years**	**15–29 years**	**30–44 years**	**45–59 years**	**⩾60 years**
Eastern Mediterranean Region	all	8.8	5.1	10.5	12.6	11.6	9.0	5.4
	high	5.9	2.9	0.2	9.3	5.5	6.3	6.0
	low and middle	8.8	5.1	10.5	12.6	11.7	9.0	5.4
Western Pacific Region	all	3.0	2.3	4.1	4.0	4.4	2.7	1.3
	high	2.4	7.4	7.6	4.6	5.6	3.0	0.8
	low and middle	3.0	2.2	4.0	4.0	4.4	2.7	1.4

Proportion of all deaths (%)

WHO region	Income level	Females						
		All ages	**0–4 years**	**5–14 years**	**15–29 years**	**30–44 years**	**45–59 years**	**⩾60 years**
All	all	0.5	0.3	1.6	1.9	1.3	0.7	0.1
	high	0.2	1.4	4.0	5.4	2.3	0.4	0.0
	low and middle	0.5	0.3	1.6	1.8	1.3	0.7	0.1
African Region[d]	low and middle	0.7	0.3	1.1	1.6	0.8	0.9	0.2
Region of the Americas	all	0.6	0.5	3.3	8.3	3.5	0.7	0.1
	high	0.3	2.2	6.3	9.5	3.7	0.6	0.0
	low and middle	0.9	0.3	2.9	8.0	3.5	0.8	0.1
South-East Asia Region[d]	low and middle	0.4	0.2	1.5	0.7	0.7	0.6	0.2
European Region	all	0.4	0.3	2.3	6.1	3.9	1.2	0.1
	high	0.1	0.6	1.9	2.1	1.1	0.2	0.0
	low and middle	0.7	0.2	2.4	7.1	4.8	1.6	0.2
Eastern Mediterranean Region	all	0.6	0.2	2.8	2.7	1.3	0.5	0.1
	high	0.3	0.2	0.1	3.9	1.1	0.4	0.1
	low and middle	0.6	0.2	2.8	2.7	1.4	0.5	0.1
Western Pacific Region	all	0.3	0.3	1.5	1.9	1.3	0.3	0.0
	high	0.1	1.1	2.9	2.5	1.4	0.3	0.0
	low and middle	0.3	0.3	1.5	1.9	1.3	0.3	0.1

TABLE A.4

Estimated mortality caused by suicide,[a] by sex, age group, WHO region and income level, 2000

Absolute numbers (in thousands)[b]

WHO region	Income level	Total[c]	Males						
			All ages	0–4 years	5–14 years	15–29 years	30–44 years	45–59 years	≥60 years
All	all	815	509	0	10	124	138	115	122
	high	122	91	0	<1	16	25	24	25
	low and middle	692	418	0	10	108	113	91	96
African Region[d]	low and middle	27	21	0	1	6	5	5	4
Region of the Americas	all	65	52	0	1	14	15	11	10
	high	36	29	0	<1	6	9	7	6
	low and middle	29	22	0	<1	8	6	4	4
South-East Asia Region[d]	low and middle	168	107	0	5	37	30	21	14
European Region	all	186	149	0	1	30	46	39	33
	high	51	38	0	<1	6	10	9	12
	low and middle	135	111	0	1	24	35	29	21
Eastern Mediterranean Region	all	24	12	0	1	5	3	2	1
	high	<1	<1	0	<1	<1	<1	<1	<1
	low and middle	23	12	0	1	5	3	2	1
Western Pacific Region	all	344	169	0	2	32	39	38	59
	high	35	24	0	<1	4	6	8	7
	low and middle	309	144	0	2	28	33	30	52

Rate per 100 000 population

WHO region	Income level	Total[c, e]	Males						
			All ages[e]	0–4 years	5–14 years	15–29 years	30–44 years	45–59 years	≥60 years
All	all	14.5	18.9	0.0	1.7	15.6	21.5	28.4	44.9
	high	11.4	17.7	0.0	0.8	17.0	23.6	27.9	33.8
	low and middle	15.5	19.5	0.0	1.8	15.4	21.1	28.6	49.2
African Region[d]	low and middle	6.7	10.6	0.0	1.4	6.4	11.2	18.1	26.6
Region of the Americas	all	8.1	13.2	0.0	0.7	13.7	17.1	18.7	26.0
	high	10.6	17.4	0.0	1.2	19.9	24.1	23.8	29.9
	low and middle	6.3	10.2	0.0	0.5	11.0	12.1	13.9	21.2
South-East Asia Region[d]	low and middle	12.0	15.7	0.0	3.1	16.9	18.5	23.3	26.1
European Region	all	19.1	32.2	0.0	1.8	30.2	46.7	52.3	51.3
	high	10.5	16.4	0.0	0.4	14.8	22.6	25.1	33.2
	low and middle	26.6	46.8	0.0	2.6	40.3	68.2	79.9	74.1
Eastern Mediterranean Region	all	5.9	6.3	0.0	0.8	7.6	7.6	8.5	10.8
	high	3.4	4.1	0.0	0.4	5.2	5.6	4.1	7.3
	low and middle	5.9	6.4	0.0	0.8	7.6	7.7	8.6	10.8
Western Pacific Region	all	20.8	21.2	0.0	1.1	14.7	19.0	28.7	69.2
	high	14.3	20.9	0.0	0.7	17.1	25.8	39.7	40.7
	low and middle	22.3	21.8	0.0	1.2	14.4	18.2	26.7	76.2

Proportion of all deaths due to injury (%)

WHO region	Income level	Total[c]	Males						
			All ages	0–4 years	5–14 years	15–29 years	30–44 years	45–59 years	≥60 years
All	all	16.1	14.9	0.0	3.8	14.1	16.7	19.5	21.3
	high	25.9	28.8	0.0	7.7	24.7	34.4	37.2	24.7
	low and middle	15.1	13.5	0.0	3.7	13.2	15.0	17.3	20.5
African Region[d]	low and middle	3.6	4.0	0.0	1.6	4.5	5.1	6.6	6.3
Region of the Americas	all	11.7	11.8	0.0	3.5	9.5	12.8	16.1	15.7
	high	21.5	24.9	0.0	9.6	22.1	28.5	30.9	22.8
	low and middle	7.4	7.0	0.0	2.1	6.5	7.1	8.9	10.2
South-East Asia Region[d]	low and middle	12.3	12.1	0.0	6.6	15.0	14.3	14.6	10.2
European Region	all	22.8	24.5	0.0	6.6	23.5	25.4	26.2	26.5
	high	27.2	31.3	0.0	6.1	25.8	40.1	40.2	26.2
	low and middle	21.5	22.8	0.0	6.7	23.0	22.9	23.6	26.6

Absolute numbers (in thousands)[b]

WHO region	Income level	Females						
		All ages	0–4 years	5–14 years	15–29 years	30–44 years	45–59 years	⩾60 years
All	all	305	0	12	93	77	50	74
	high	31	0	<1	4	7	8	11
	low and middle	274	0	11	88	70	43	63
African Region[d]	low and middle	7	0	1	2	2	1	1
Region of the Americas	all	14	0	<1	4	4	3	2
	high	7	0	<1	1	3	2	1
	low and middle	7	0	<1	3	1	1	1
South-East Asia Region[d]	low and middle	61	0	8	30	15	5	4
European Region	all	37	0	<1	5	8	9	15
	high	13	0	<1	1	3	3	5
	low and middle	24	0	<1	4	5	5	10
Eastern Mediterranean Region	all	11	0	1	6	2	1	1
	high	<1	0	<1	<1	<1	<1	<1
	low and middle	11	0	1	6	2	1	1
Western Pacific Region	all	175	0	2	46	46	31	50
	high	10	0	<1	2	2	2	4
	low and middle	164	0	1	45	44	29	46

Rate per 100 000 population

WHO region	Income level	Females						
		All ages[e]	0–4 years	5–14 years	15–29 years	30–44 years	45–59 years	⩾60 years
All	all	10.6	0.0	2.0	12.2	12.4	12.6	22.1
	high	5.4	0.0	0.4	4.7	7.1	9.0	11.3
	low and middle	11.9	0.0	2.1	13.2	13.4	13.5	26.8
African Region[d]	low and middle	3.1	0.0	0.7	1.7	4.8	4.1	7.5
Region of the Americas	all	3.3	0.0	0.6	4.0	4.3	5.0	4.4
	high	4.1	0.0	0.4	3.9	6.6	7.1	4.9
	low and middle	2.7	0.0	0.6	4.1	2.8	3.1	3.9
South-East Asia Region[d]	low and middle	8.3	0.0	4.7	14.5	9.9	5.7	7.2
European Region	all	6.8	0.0	0.4	5.8	8.1	11.4	15.7
	high	5.0	0.0	0.2	3.8	6.6	9.0	11.0
	low and middle	8.4	0.0	0.5	7.0	9.4	13.6	20.6
Eastern Mediterranean Region	all	5.4	0.0	2.0	8.6	6.2	4.4	7.0
	high	2.1	0.0	0.1	3.2	3.5	1.7	2.0
	low and middle	5.4	0.0	2.0	8.6	6.2	4.4	7.0
Western Pacific Region	all	20.7	0.0	1.1	22.6	23.3	25.1	51.7
	high	8.0	0.0	0.5	7.6	8.9	12.0	20.2
	low and middle	23.2	0.0	1.1	24.3	25.0	27.7	60.9

Proportion of all deaths due to injury (%)

WHO region	Income level	Females						
		All ages	0–4 years	5–14 years	15–29 years	30–44 years	45–59 years	⩾60 years
All	all	18.5	0.0	5.6	26.0	27.4	24.6	19.7
	high	20.0	0.0	6.6	24.7	34.9	37.9	12.6
	low and middle	18.4	0.0	5.6	26.0	26.8	23.1	22.0
African Region[d]	low and middle	2.8	0.0	1.2	2.9	6.7	4.6	5.6
Region of the Americas	all	11.2	0.0	5.6	16.1	17.6	19.3	5.6
	high	13.8	0.0	5.9	15.3	23.8	26.7	6.0
	low and middle	9.3	0.0	5.5	16.5	12.4	12.2	5.0
South-East Asia Region[d]	low and middle	12.6	0.0	8.2	23.2	17.2	9.5	5.3
European Region	all	17.9	0.0	3.7	19.9	22.5	23.6	15.8
	high	19.7	0.0	6.2	26.4	45.0	44.4	11.8
	low and middle	17.1	0.0	3.4	18.4	17.2	18.3	19.4

TABLE A.4 *(continued)*

Proportion of all deaths due to injury (%) *(continued)*

WHO region	Income level	Total[c]	Males						
			All ages	0–4 years	5–14 years	15–29 years	30–44 years	45–59 years	≥60 years
Eastern Mediterranean Region	all	7.0	5.8	0.0	2.0	8.6	8.1	7.2	5.6
	high	6.5	5.8	0.0	2.3	5.9	7.3	5.0	6.0
	low and middle	7.0	5.8	0.0	2.0	8.6	8.1	7.3	5.5
Western Pacific Region	all	28.1	22.3	0.0	3.0	18.9	22.5	28.6	37.2
	high	31.0	31.6	0.0	6.0	29.7	38.3	42.0	24.4
	low and middle	27.8	21.2	0.0	2.9	18.1	21.0	26.3	40.0

Proportion of all deaths (%)

WHO region	Income level	Total[c]	Males						
			All ages	0–4 years	5–14 years	15–29 years	30–44 years	45–59 years	≥60 years
All	all	1.5	1.7	0.0	1.4	6.6	4.6	2.6	0.9
	high	1.5	2.2	0.0	3.8	17.5	12.7	4.6	0.8
	low and middle	1.5	1.6	0.0	1.4	6.0	4.0	2.4	0.9
African Region[d]	low and middle	0.3	0.4	0.0	0.6	1.1	0.6	0.8	0.4
Region of the Americas	all	1.1	1.6	0.0	1.5	6.6	5.2	2.3	0.6
	high	1.3	2.2	0.0	5.4	16.8	11.1	3.7	0.7
	low and middle	0.9	1.2	0.0	0.8	4.5	2.9	1.5	0.4
South-East Asia Region[d]	low and middle	1.2	1.4	0.0	2.1	6.8	3.7	1.7	0.4
European Region	all	1.9	3.0	0.0	3.6	16.6	11.6	4.7	1.0
	high	1.3	1.9	0.0	2.4	16.8	13.3	4.3	0.8
	low and middle	2.3	3.7	0.0	3.8	16.5	11.1	4.9	1.2
Eastern Mediterranean Region	all	0.6	0.6	0.0	0.7	4.0	2.0	0.8	0.2
	high	0.8	0.9	0.0	1.3	4.5	3.1	0.7	0.2
	low and middle	0.6	0.6	0.0	0.7	4.0	2.0	0.8	0.2
Western Pacific Region	all	3.0	2.7	0.0	1.5	11.1	8.1	3.9	1.5
	high	2.4	3.1	0.0	3.0	20.9	15.2	7.0	1.1
	low and middle	3.1	2.6	0.0	1.5	10.5	7.5	3.4	1.5

Source: WHO Global Burden of Disease project for 2000, Version 1.

[a] Suicide = ICD-10 X60–X84 (ICD-9 E950–E959).

[b] Absolute numbers are rounded to the nearest 1000. Any apparent discrepancies in total sums are a result of rounding.

[c] Combined total for males and females.

[d] No high-income countries in the region.

[e] Age-standardized.

Proportion of all deaths due to injury (%) *(continued)*

WHO region	Income level	Females						
		All ages	**0–4 years**	**5–14 years**	**15–29 years**	**30–44 years**	**45–59 years**	**≥60 years**
Eastern Mediterranean Region	all	9.0	0.0	5.8	20.0	16.5	10.4	6.3
	high	10.8	0.0	0.9	19.3	15.1	7.7	4.5
	low and middle	9.0	0.0	5.8	20.0	16.5	10.4	6.3
Western Pacific Region	all	37.7	0.0	4.6	48.3	51.7	47.7	41.7
	high	29.7	0.0	9.4	41.7	46.5	45.1	21.9
	low and middle	38.3	0.0	4.5	48.5	52.0	47.9	45.7

Proportion of all deaths (%)

WHO region	Income level	Females						
		All ages	**0–4 years**	**5–14 years**	**15–29 years**	**30–44 years**	**45–59 years**	**≥60 years**
All	all	1.2	0.0	1.6	5.3	3.7	1.9	0.5
	high	0.8	0.0	2.6	12.7	7.7	2.9	0.3
	low and middle	1.2	0.0	1.6	5.1	3.5	1.8	0.6
African Region[d]	low and middle	0.1	0.0	0.3	0.2	0.3	0.3	0.1
Region of the Americas	all	0.5	0.0	1.6	5.2	2.7	1.0	0.1
	high	0.5	0.0	2.8	8.4	5.7	1.9	0.1
	low and middle	0.5	0.0	1.4	4.5	1.5	0.5	0.1
South-East Asia Region[d]	low and middle	0.9	0.0	2.7	6.0	2.7	0.6	0.2
European Region	all	0.8	0.0	1.4	8.9	5.5	2.4	0.4
	high	0.7	0.0	2.0	12.1	8.3	3.1	0.3
	low and middle	0.9	0.0	1.3	8.1	4.6	2.2	0.4
Eastern Mediterranean Region	all	0.6	0.0	1.5	4.4	1.9	0.5	0.2
	high	0.5	0.0	0.3	8.0	3.1	0.5	0.0
	low and middle	0.6	0.0	1.6	4.3	1.9	0.5	0.2
Western Pacific Region	all	3.5	0.0	1.7	22.7	15.1	5.5	1.5
	high	1.6	0.0	3.7	22.5	11.9	5.0	0.8
	low and middle	3.7	0.0	1.7	22.8	15.3	5.6	1.6

TABLE A.5

Estimated mortality caused by war-related injuries,[a] by sex, age group, WHO region and income level, 2000

Absolute numbers (in thousands)[b]

WHO region	Income level	Total[c]	Males						
			All ages	0–4 years	5–14 years	15–29 years	30–44 years	45–59 years	⩾60 years
All	all	310	233	22	30	69	58	29	25
	high	<1	<1	<1	<1	<1	<1	<1	<1
	low and middle	310	233	22	30	69	58	29	25
African Region[d]	low and middle	167	122	7	18	36	33	16	13
Region of the Americas	all	2	2	<1	<1	<1	<1	<1	<1
	high	<1	<1	0	0	0	0	<1	<1
	low and middle	2	2	<1	<1	<1	<1	<1	<1
South-East Asia Region[d]	low and middle	63	49	2	6	18	13	5	5
European Region	all	37	30	1	3	8	9	5	4
	high	<1	<1	0	0	<1	<1	<1	<1
	low and middle	37	30	1	3	8	9	5	4
Eastern Mediterranean Region	all	39	29	12	3	7	3	2	2
	high	<1	<1	<1	<1	<1	<1	<1	<1
	low and middle	39	28	12	3	7	3	2	2
Western Pacific Region	all	2	1	0	<1	<1	<1	0	<1
	high	0	0	0	0	0	0	0	0
	low and middle	2	1	0	<1	<1	<1	0	<1

Rate per 100 000 population

WHO region	Income level	Total[c, e]	Males						
			All ages[e]	0–4 years	5–14 years	15–29 years	30–44 years	45–59 years	⩾60 years
All	all	5.2	7.8	7.1	4.9	8.6	9.1	7.1	9.2
	high	0.0	0.0	0.0	0.0	0.0	0.0	0.0	0.0
	low and middle	6.2	9.4	7.8	5.4	9.8	10.9	9.0	12.7
African Region[d]	low and middle	32.0	50.6	13.3	20.4	40.4	67.2	62.1	92.6
Region of the Americas	all	0.2	0.4	0.3	0.3	0.4	0.5	0.3	0.6
	high	0.0	0.0	0.0	0.0	0.0	0.0	0.0	0.1
	low and middle	0.4	0.7	0.4	0.4	0.6	0.9	0.5	1.3
South-East Asia Region[d]	low and middle	4.4	6.6	1.9	3.3	8.0	8.2	5.9	10.0
European Region	all	4.2	7.0	4.2	5.3	8.0	8.7	7.2	6.3
	high	0.0	0.0	0.0	0.0	0.0	0.0	0.0	0.0
	low and middle	7.6	13.0	7.1	8.5	13.3	16.5	14.5	14.3
Eastern Mediterranean Region	all	8.1	11.2	34.6	4.1	9.8	7.5	8.2	15.4
	high	2.7	3.7	2.5	2.3	3.6	2.9	4.1	7.2
	low and middle	8.2	11.3	34.8	4.2	9.9	7.6	8.3	15.6
Western Pacific Region	all	0.1	0.2	0.0	0.3	0.1	0.2	0.0	0.3
	high	0.0	0.0	0.0	0.0	0.0	0.0	0.0	0.0
	low and middle	0.1	0.2	0.0	0.3	0.1	0.2	0.0	0.4

Proportion of all deaths due to injury (%)

WHO region	Income level	Total[c]	Males						
			All ages	0–4 years	5–14 years	15–29 years	30–44 years	45–59 years	⩾60 years
All	all	6.1	6.8	8.2	11.0	7.8	7.1	4.9	4.3
	high	0.0	0.1	0.1	0.2	0.0	0.0	0.1	0.0
	low and middle	6.8	7.5	8.3	11.3	8.4	7.7	5.4	5.3
African Region[d]	low and middle	22.3	23.9	10.1	23.4	28.1	30.4	22.7	21.8
Region of the Americas	all	0.4	0.4	0.7	1.5	0.3	0.4	0.2	0.4
	high	0.0	0.0	0.0	0.0	0.0	0.0	0.0	0.0
	low and middle	0.5	0.5	0.8	1.8	0.4	0.5	0.3	0.6
South-East Asia Region[d]	low and middle	4.6	5.5	2.6	7.0	7.1	6.3	3.7	3.9
European Region	all	4.5	5.0	10.2	19.7	6.2	4.8	3.6	3.3
	high	0.0	0.0	0.0	0.0	0.0	0.0	0.0	0.0
	low and middle	5.8	6.2	11.5	21.8	7.6	5.5	4.3	5.1

Absolute numbers (in thousands)[b]

WHO region	Income level	Females						
		All ages	0–4 years	5–14 years	15–29 years	30–44 years	45–59 years	⩾60 years
All	all	77	8	14	26	14	8	8
	high	<1	<1	<1	<1	<1	<1	<1
	low and middle	77	8	14	26	14	8	8
African Region[d]	low and middle	45	5	10	18	6	4	3
Region of the Americas	all	<1	<1	<1	<1	<1	<1	<1
	high	0	0	0	0	0	0	0
	low and middle	<1	<1	<1	<1	<1	<1	<1
South-East Asia Region[d]	low and middle	14	<1	1	4	4	2	3
European Region	all	6	<1	1	1	3	1	<1
	high	<1	0	<1	0	<1	0	<1
	low and middle	6	<1	1	1	3	1	<1
Eastern Mediterranean Region	all	10	2	2	3	1	1	2
	high	<1	<1	<1	<1	<1	<1	<1
	low and middle	10	2	2	3	1	1	2
Western Pacific Region	all	1	0	<1	0	<1	0	0
	high	0	0	0	0	0	0	0
	low and middle	1	0	<1	0	<1	0	0

Rate per 100 000 population

WHO region	Income level	Females						
		All ages[e]	0–4 years	5–14 years	15–29 years	30–44 years	45–59 years	⩾60 years
All	all	2.6	2.6	2.3	3.4	2.2	1.9	2.4
	high	0.0	0.0	0.0	0.0	0.0	0.0	0.0
	low and middle	3.0	2.9	2.6	3.9	2.7	2.4	3.4
African Region[d]	low and middle	14.7	9.2	11.0	20.3	12.9	13.5	17.1
Region of the Americas	all	0.1	0.2	0.1	0.1	0.1	0.1	0.1
	high	0.0	0.0	0.0	0.0	0.0	0.0	0.0
	low and middle	0.1	0.2	0.1	0.1	0.1	0.1	0.2
South-East Asia Region[d]	low and middle	2.2	0.6	0.9	1.8	2.5	2.6	4.8
European Region	all	1.5	0.7	1.0	1.5	3.0	1.2	0.4
	high	0.0	0.0	0.0	0.0	0.0	0.0	0.0
	low and middle	2.6	1.3	1.5	2.4	5.6	2.4	0.8
Eastern Mediterranean Region	all	4.9	6.6	2.8	4.8	2.0	3.0	13.7
	high	1.0	1.6	0.6	0.9	1.3	0.9	1.5
	low and middle	4.9	6.7	2.8	4.8	2.1	3.0	13.8
Western Pacific Region	all	0.1	0.0	0.3	0.0	0.1	0.0	0.0
	high	0.0	0.0	0.0	0.0	0.0	0.0	0.0
	low and middle	0.1	0.0	0.4	0.0	0.1	0.0	0.0

Proportion of all deaths due to injury (%)

WHO region	Income level	Females						
		All ages	0–4 years	5–14 years	15–29 years	30–44 years	45–59 years	⩾60 years
All	all	4.7	3.5	6.6	7.3	5.0	3.7	2.1
	high	0.0	0.1	0.3	0.0	0.0	0.0	0.0
	low and middle	5.2	3.6	6.7	7.7	5.4	4.1	2.8
African Region[d]	low and middle	18.8	8.0	20.6	34.2	18.1	15.5	12.9
Region of the Americas	all	0.3	0.5	0.7	0.4	0.3	0.2	0.1
	high	0.0	0.0	0.0	0.0	0.0	0.0	0.0
	low and middle	0.5	0.6	0.9	0.5	0.6	0.5	0.3
South-East Asia Region[d]	low and middle	3.0	1.1	1.5	2.9	4.3	4.4	3.5
European Region	all	3.1	2.6	8.5	5.1	8.3	2.6	0.4
	high	0.0	0.0	0.6	0.0	0.0	0.0	0.0
	low and middle	4.5	2.9	9.5	6.4	10.2	3.2	0.8

TABLE A.5 *(continued)*

Proportion of all deaths due to injury (%) *(continued)*

WHO region	Income level	Total[c]	Males						
			All ages	0–4 years	5–14 years	15–29 years	30–44 years	45–59 years	⩾60 years
Eastern Mediterranean Region	all	11.5	13.4	35.6	10.1	11.2	8.0	7.0	7.9
	high	5.0	4.9	10.2	11.9	4.1	3.8	5.1	5.9
	low and middle	11.6	13.5	35.6	10.1	11.3	8.0	7.0	8.0
Western Pacific Region	all	0.2	0.2	0.0	0.7	0.2	0.2	0.0	0.2
	high	0.0	0.0	0.0	0.0	0.0	0.0	0.0	0.0
	low and middle	0.2	0.2	0.0	0.7	0.2	0.3	0.0	0.2

Proportion of all deaths (%)

WHO region	Income level	Total[c]	Males						
			All ages	0–4 years	5–14 years	15–29 years	30–44 years	45–59 years	⩾60 years
All	all	0.6	0.8	0.4	4.1	3.7	1.9	0.7	0.2
	high	0.0	0.0	0.0	0.1	0.0	0.0	0.0	0.0
	low and middle	0.7	0.9	0.4	4.2	3.8	2.1	0.7	0.2
African Region[d]	low and middle	1.6	2.3	0.3	8.3	6.9	3.7	2.6	1.4
Region of the Americas	all	0.0	0.1	0.0	0.6	0.2	0.2	0.0	0.0
	high	0.0	0.0	0.0	0.0	0.0	0.0	0.0	0.0
	low and middle	0.1	0.1	0.1	0.7	0.3	0.2	0.1	0.0
South-East Asia Region[d]	low and middle	0.4	0.6	0.1	2.2	3.2	1.6	0.4	0.2
European Region	all	0.4	0.6	0.8	10.8	4.4	2.2	0.6	0.1
	high	0.0	0.0	0.0	0.0	0.0	0.0	0.0	0.0
	low and middle	0.6	1.0	0.9	12.4	5.4	2.7	0.9	0.2
Eastern Mediterranean Region	all	1.0	1.3	1.5	3.4	5.2	1.9	0.8	0.3
	high	0.6	0.8	0.8	6.7	3.1	1.6	0.7	0.2
	low and middle	1.0	1.3	1.5	3.4	5.2	1.9	0.8	0.3
Western Pacific Region	all	0.0	0.0	0.0	0.3	0.1	0.1	0.0	0.0
	high	0.0	0.0	0.0	0.0	0.0	0.0	0.0	0.0
	low and middle	0.0	0.0	0.0	0.3	0.1	0.1	0.0	0.0

Source: WHO Global Burden of Disease project for 2000, Version 1.

[a] War-related injuries = ICD-10 Y36 (ICD-9 E990–E999).

[b] Absolute numbers are rounded to the nearest 1000. Any apparent discrepancies in total sums are a result of rounding.

[c] Combined total for males and females.

[d] No high-income countries in the region.

[e] Age-standardized.

Proportion of all deaths due to injury (%) *(continued)*

WHO region	Income level	Females						
		All ages	0–4 years	5–14 years	15–29 years	30–44 years	45–59 years	⩾60 years
Eastern Mediterranean Region	all	8.4	6.2	8.0	11.3	5.5	7.1	12.5
	high	5.6	10.6	8.2	5.6	5.4	4.0	3.4
	low and middle	8.4	6.2	8.0	11.3	5.5	7.1	12.5
Western Pacific Region	all	0.1	0.0	1.4	0.0	0.1	0.0	0.0
	high	0.0	0.0	0.0	0.0	0.0	0.0	0.0
	low and middle	0.1	0.0	1.4	0.0	0.2	0.0	0.0

Proportion of all deaths (%)

WHO region	Income level	Females						
		All ages	0–4 years	5–14 years	15–29 years	30–44 years	45–59 years	⩾60 years
All	all	0.3	0.1	1.9	1.5	0.7	0.3	0.1
	high	0.0	0.0	0.1	0.0	0.0	0.0	0.0
	low and middle	0.4	0.2	1.9	1.5	0.7	0.3	0.1
African Region[d]	low and middle	0.9	0.2	4.3	2.3	0.8	0.9	0.3
Region of the Americas	all	0.0	0.0	0.2	0.1	0.1	0.0	0.0
	high	0.0	0.0	0.0	0.0	0.0	0.0	0.0
	low and middle	0.0	0.0	0.2	0.1	0.1	0.0	0.0
South East Asia Region[d]	low and middle	0.2	0.0	0.5	0.7	0.7	0.3	0.1
European Region	all	0.1	0.2	3.1	2.3	2.0	0.3	0.0
	high	0.0	0.0	0.2	0.0	0.0	0.0	0.0
	low and middle	0.2	0.2	3.6	2.8	2.7	0.4	0.0
Eastern Mediterranean Region	all	0.5	0.3	2.1	2.4	0.6	0.4	0.3
	high	0.3	0.6	2.5	2.3	1.1	0.2	0.0
	low and middle	0.5	0.3	2.1	2.4	0.6	0.4	0.3
Western Pacific Region	all	0.0	0.0	0.5	0.0	0.0	0.0	0.0
	high	0.0	0.0	0.0	0.0	0.0	0.0	0.0
	low and middle	0.0	0.0	0.5	0.0	0.0	0.0	0.0

TABLE A.6

The ten leading causes of death and DALYs, and rankings for violence-related deaths and DALYs, by WHO region, 2000

ALL MEMBER STATES

Total

Rank	Cause	Proportion of total (%)
Deaths		
1	Ischaemic heart disease	12.4
2	Cerebrovascular disease	9.2
3	Lower respiratory infections	6.9
4	HIV/AIDS	5.3
5	Chronic obstructive pulmonary disease	4.5
6	Perinatal conditions	4.4
7	Diarrhoeal diseases	3.8
8	Tuberculosis	3.0
9	Road traffic injuries	2.3
10	Trachea, bronchus, lung cancers	2.2
13	Suicide	1.5
22	Homicide	0.9
30	War	0.6

Rank	Cause	Proportion of total (%)
DALYs		
1	Lower respiratory infections	6.4
2	Perinatal conditions	6.2
3	HIV/AIDS	6.1
4	Unipolar depressive disorders	4.4
5	Diarrhoeal diseases	4.2
6	Ischaemic heart disease	3.8
7	Cerebrovascular disease	3.1
8	Road traffic injuries	2.8
9	Malaria	2.7
10	Tuberculosis	2.4
17	Self-inflicted injuries	1.3
21	Interpersonal violence	1.1
32	War	0.7

Males

Rank	Cause	Proportion of total (%)
Deaths		
1	Ischaemic heart disease	12.2
2	Cerebrovascular disease	8.1
3	Lower respiratory infections	7.0
4	HIV/AIDS	5.0
5	Chronic obstructive pulmonary disease	4.6
6	Perinatal conditions	4.4
7	Diarrhoeal diseases	4.0
8	Tuberculosis	3.5
9	Road traffic injuries	3.1
10	Trachea, bronchus, lung cancers	3.0
13	Suicide	1.7
17	Homicide	1.4
27	War	0.8

Rank	Cause	Proportion of total (%)
DALYs		
1	Perinatal conditions	6.4
2	Lower respiratory infections	6.4
3	HIV/AIDS	5.8
4	Diarrhoeal diseases	4.2
5	Ischaemic heart disease	4.2
6	Road traffic injuries	4.0
7	Unipolar depressive disorders	3.4
8	Cerebrovascular disease	3.0
9	Tuberculosis	2.9
10	Malaria	2.5
16	Interpersonal violence	1.6
19	Self-inflicted injuries	1.5
26	War	1.0

Females

Rank	Cause	Proportion of total (%)
Deaths		
1	Ischaemic heart disease	12.6
2	Cerebrovascular disease	10.4
3	Lower respiratory infections	6.9
4	HIV/AIDS	5.6
5	Chronic obstructive pulmonary disease	4.4
6	Perinatal conditions	4.4
7	Diarrhoeal diseases	3.6
8	Tuberculosis	2.4
9	Malaria	2.1
10	Hypertensive heart disease	1.9
17	Suicide	1.2
37	Homicide	0.5
46	War	0.3

Rank	Cause	Proportion of total (%)
DALYs		
1	HIV/AIDS	6.5
2	Lower respiratory infections	6.4
3	Perinatal conditions	6.0
4	Unipolar depressive disorders	5.5
5	Diarrhoeal diseases	4.2
6	Ischaemic heart disease	3.4
7	Cerebrovascular disease	3.2
8	Malaria	3.0
9	Congenital anomalies	2.2
10	Chronic obstructive pulmonary disease	2.1
18	Self-inflicted injuries	1.1
43	Interpersonal violence	0.5
49	War	0.4

TABLE A.6 *(continued)*

ALL MEMBER STATES *(continued)*

High-income countries

Rank	Cause	Proportion of total (%)
Deaths		
1	Ischaemic heart disease	17.9
2	Cerebrovascular disease	10.7
3	Trachea, bronchus, lung cancers	5.6
4	Lower respiratory infections	4.7
5	Chronic obstructive pulmonary disease	3.5
6	Colon and rectum cancers	3.2
7	Diabetes mellitus	2.3
8	Stomach cancer	2.0
9	Breast cancer	2.0
10	Alzheimer and other dementias	1.8
13	Suicide	1.5
35	Homicide	0.3
61	War	0.0

Rank	Cause	Proportion of total (%)
DALYs		
1	Unipolar depressive disorders	8.8
2	Ischaemic heart disease	6.7
3	Alcohol use disorders	5.4
4	Cerebrovascular disease	4.9
5	Alzheimer and other dementias	4.3
6	Road traffic injuries	3.1
7	Trachea, bronchus, lung cancers	3.0
8	Osteoarthritis	2.7
9	Chronic obstructive pulmonary disease	2.5
10	Hearing loss, adult onset	2.5
12	Self-inflicted injuries	2.0
31	Interpersonal violence	0.7
88	War	0.0

Low-income and middle-income countries

Rank	Cause	Proportion of total (%)
Deaths		
1	Ischaemic heart disease	11.5
2	Cerebrovascular disease	8.9
3	Lower respiratory infections	7.3
4	HIV/AIDS	6.1
5	Perinatal conditions	5.1
6	Chronic obstructive pulmonary disease	4.7
7	Diarrhoeal diseases	4.4
8	Tuberculosis	3.4
9	Road traffic injuries	2.4
10	Malaria	2.3
14	Suicide	1.5
21	Homicide	1.0
27	War	0.7

Rank	Cause	Proportion of total (%)
DALYs		
1	Lower respiratory infections	6.8
2	Perinatal conditions	6.7
3	HIV/AIDS	6.6
4	Meningitis	4.6
5	Diarrhoeal diseases	4.6
6	Unipolar depressive disorders	4.0
7	Ischaemic heart disease	3.5
8	Malaria	3.0
9	Cerebrovascular disease	2.9
10	Road traffic injuries	2.8
19	Self-inflicted injuries	1.2
21	Interpersonal violence	1.1
31	War	0.8

Source: WHO Global Burden of Disease project for 2000, Version 1.

TABLE A.6 *(continued)*

AFRICAN REGION

Total

Rank	Cause	Proportion of total (%)
Deaths		
1	HIV/AIDS	22.6
2	Lower respiratory infections	10.1
3	Malaria	9.1
4	Diarrhoeal diseases	6.7
5	Perinatal conditions	5.5
6	Measles	4.3
7	Tuberculosis	3.6
8	Ischaemic heart disease	3.1
9	Cerebrovascular disease	2.9
10	Road traffic injuries	1.6
11	War	1.6
14	Homicide	1.1
42	Suicide	0.3

Rank	Cause	Proportion of total (%)
DALYs		
1	HIV/AIDS	20.6
2	Malaria	10.1
3	Lower respiratory infections	8.6
4	Perinatal conditions	6.3
5	Diarrhoeal diseases	6.1
6	Measles	4.5
7	Tuberculosis	2.8
8	Whooping cough	1.8
9	Road traffic injuries	1.6
10	Protein–energy malnutrition	1.6
11	War	1.6
15	Interpersonal violence	1.0
58	Self-inflicted injuries	0.2

Males

Rank	Cause	Proportion of total (%)
Deaths		
1	HIV/AIDS	20.9
2	Lower respiratory infections	11.2
3	Malaria	8.4
4	Diarrhoeal diseases	7.2
5	Perinatal conditions	6.1
6	Tuberculosis	4.8
7	Measles	4.2
8	Ischaemic heart disease	2.9
9	War	2.3
10	Cerebrovascular disease	2.1
13	Homicide	1.5
28	Suicide	0.4

Rank	Cause	Proportion of total (%)
DALYs		
1	HIV/AIDS	18.7
2	Lower respiratory infections	9.6
3	Malaria	9.5
4	Perinatal conditions	7.2
5	Diarrhoeal diseases	6.7
6	Measles	4.5
7	Tuberculosis	3.6
8	Road traffic injuries	2.1
9	War	2.1
10	Whooping cough	1.8
12	Interpersonal violence	1.4
44	Self-inflicted injuries	0.3

Females

Rank	Cause	Proportion of total (%)
Deaths		
1	HIV/AIDS	24.4
2	Malaria	9.9
3	Lower respiratory infections	8.9
4	Diarrhoeal diseases	6.1
5	Perinatal conditions	4.8
6	Measles	4.4
7	Cerebrovascular disease	3.7
8	Ischaemic heart disease	3.3
9	Tuberculosis	2.4
10	Whooping cough	1.6
17	War	0.9
22	Homicide	0.7
53	Suicide	0.1

Rank	Cause	Proportion of total (%)
DALYs		
1	HIV/AIDS	22.4
2	Malaria	10.7
3	Lower respiratory infections	7.6
4	Diarrhoeal diseases	5.5
5	Perinatal conditions	5.4
6	Measles	4.5
7	Tuberculosis	1.9
8	Whooping cough	1.9
9	Protein–energy malnutrition	1.5
10	Unipolar depressive disorders	1.4
18	War	1.0
25	Interpersonal violence	0.7
69	Self-inflicted injuries	0.1

TABLE A.6 *(continued)*

AFRICAN REGION[a] *(continued)*
Low-income and middle-income countries

Rank	Cause	Proportion of total (%)	Rank	Cause	Proportion of total (%)
Deaths			DALYs		
1	HIV/AIDS	22.6	1	HIV/AIDS	20.6
2	Lower respiratory infections	10.1	2	Malaria	10.1
3	Malaria	9.1	3	Lower respiratory infections	8.6
4	Diarrhoeal diseases	6.7	4	Perinatal conditions	6.3
5	Perinatal conditions	5.5	5	Diarrhoeal diseases	6.1
6	Measles	4.3	6	Measles	4.5
7	Tuberculosis	3.6	7	Tuberculosis	2.8
8	Ischaemic heart disease	3.1	8	Whooping cough	1.8
9	Cerebrovascular disease	2.9	9	Road traffic injuries	1.6
10	Road traffic injuries	1.6	10	Protein–energy malnutrition	1.6
11	War	1.6	11	War	1.6
14	Homicide	1.1	15	Interpersonal violence	1.0
42	Suicide	0.3	58	Self-inflicted injuries	0.2

Source: WHO Global Burden of Disease project for 2000, Version 1.

[a] No high-income countries in the region.

TABLE A.6 *(continued)*

REGION OF THE AMERICAS
Total

Rank	Cause	Proportion of total (%)	Rank	Cause	Proportion of total (%)
Deaths			**DALYs**		
1	Ischaemic heart disease	15.6	1	Unipolar depressive disorders	8.1
2	Cerebrovascular disease	7.7	2	Alcohol use disorders	4.4
3	Lower respiratory infections	4.4	3	Ischaemic heart disease	4.4
4	Trachea, bronchus and lung cancers	3.9	4	Perinatal conditions	3.9
5	Diabetes mellitus	3.7	5	Interpersonal violence	3.8
6	Chronic obstructive pulmonary disease	3.5	6	Cerebrovascular disease	3.3
7	Homicide	2.7	7	Road traffic injuries	3.2
8	Perinatal conditions	2.6	8	Lower respiratory infections	2.7
9	Road traffic injuries	2.4	9	Congenital anomalies	2.6
10	Hypertensive heart disease	2.3	10	Hearing loss, adult onset	2.6
21	Suicide	1.1	26	Self-inflicted injuries	1.1
62	War	0.0	86	War	0.0

Males

Rank	Cause	Proportion of total (%)	Rank	Cause	Proportion of total (%)
Deaths			**DALYs**		
1	Ischaemic heart disease	15.5	1	Alcohol use disorders	6.6
2	Cerebrovascular disease	6.5	2	Interpersonal violence	6.2
3	Trachea, bronchus and lung cancers	4.6	3	Unipolar depressive disorders	5.5
4	Homicide	4.5	4	Ischaemic heart disease	4.9
5	Lower respiratory infections	4.1	5	Road traffic injuries	4.5
6	Chronic obstructive pulmonary disease	3.6	6	Perinatal conditions	4.1
7	Road traffic injuries	3.3	7	Cerebrovascular disease	2.8
8	Diabetes mellitus	3.1	8	Lower respiratory infections	2.7
9	Perinatal conditions	2.8	9	Hearing loss, adult onset	2.6
10	Cirrhosis of the liver	2.4	10	Congenital anomalies	2.5
15	Suicide	1.6	19	Self-inflicted injuries	1.5
51	War	0.1	73	War	0.1

Females

Rank	Cause	Proportion of total (%)	Rank	Cause	Proportion of total (%)
Deaths			**DALYs**		
1	Ischaemic heart disease	15.7	1	Unipolar depressive disorders	11.2
2	Cerebrovascular disease	9.1	2	Ischaemic heart disease	3.8
3	Lower respiratory infections	4.7	3	Cerebrovascular disease	3.8
4	Diabetes mellitus	4.5	4	Perinatal conditions	3.7
5	Chronic obstructive pulmonary disease	3.4	5	Diabetes mellitus	2.8
6	Trachea, bronchus and lung cancers	3.2	6	Congenital anomalies	2.8
7	Breast cancer	3.2	7	Lower respiratory infections	2.7
8	Hypertensive heart disease	2.7	8	Hearing loss, adult onset	2.6
9	Perinatal conditions	2.3	9	Diarrhoeal diseases	2.0
10	Colon and rectum cancers	2.0	10	Anaemia	2.0
30	Homicide	0.6	27	Interpersonal violence	0.9
32	Suicide	0.5	42	Self-inflicted injuries	0.6
66	War	0.3	87	War	0.0

TABLE A.6 *(continued)*

REGION OF THE AMERICAS *(continued)*

High-income countries

Rank	Cause	Proportion of total (%)
Deaths		
1	Ischaemic heart disease	20.8
2	Cerebrovascular disease	7.0
3	Trachea, bronchus and lung cancers	6.6
4	Chronic obstructive pulmonary disease	4.5
5	Lower respiratory infections	4.0
6	Colon and rectum cancers	2.8
7	Diabetes mellitus	2.8
8	Alzheimer and other dementias	2.2
9	Breast cancer	2.0
10	Hypertensive heart disease	1.8
14	Suicide	1.3
22	Homicide	0.7
66	War	0.0

Rank	Cause	Proportion of total (%)
DALYs		
1	Unipolar depressive disorders	11.0
2	Ischaemic heart disease	7.1
3	Alcohol use disorders	6.7
4	Cerebrovascular disease	3.4
5	Road traffic injuries	3.3
6	Trachea, bronchus and lung cancers	3.2
7	Alzheimer and other dementias	3.1
8	Diabetes mellitus	2.8
9	Chronic obstructive pulmonary disease	2.8
10	Hearing loss, adult onset	2.6
12	Self-inflicted injuries	1.7
18	Interpersonal violence	1.4
87	War	0.0

Low-income and middle-income countries

Rank	Cause	Proportion of total (%)
Deaths		
1	Ischaemic heart disease	11.2
2	Cerebrovascular disease	8.2
3	Lower respiratory infections	4.7
4	Diabetes mellitus	4.5
5	Homicide	4.4
6	Perinatal conditions	4.2
7	Road traffic injuries	2.9
8	Chronic obstructive pulmonary disease	2.7
9	Hypertensive heart disease	2.6
10	Diarrhoeal diseases	2.4
24	Suicide	0.9
60	War	0.1

Rank	Cause	Proportion of total (%)
DALYs		
1	Unipolar depressive disorders	6.7
2	Perinatal conditions	5.1
3	Interpersonal violence	4.8
4	Alcohol use disorders	3.4
5	Lower respiratory infections	3.4
6	Road traffic injuries	3.2
7	Cerebrovascular disease	3.2
8	Congenital anomalies	3.1
9	Ischaemic heart disease	3.1
10	Diarrhoeal diseases	2.8
30	Self-inflicted injuries	0.8
82	War	0.1

Source: WHO Global Burden of Disease project for 2000, Version 1.

TABLE A.6 *(continued)*

SOUTH-EAST ASIA REGION

Total

Rank	Cause	Proportion of total (%)	Rank	Cause	Proportion of total (%)
Deaths			DALYs		
1	Ischaemic heart disease	13.7	1	Perinatal conditions	8.9
2	Lower respiratory infections	9.5	2	Lower respiratory infections	7.4
3	Perinatal conditions	7.1	3	Diarrhoeal diseases	5.5
4	Diarrhoeal diseases	6.7	4	Unipolar depressive disorders	4.7
5	Cerebrovascular disease	5.7	5	Ischaemic heart disease	4.4
6	Tuberculosis	4.8	6	Tuberculosis	3.5
7	Road traffic injuries	3.1	7	Road traffic injuries	3.3
8	HIV/AIDS	2.6	8	Congenital anomalies	3.0
9	Chronic obstructive pulmonary disease	2.2	9	HIV/AIDS	2.7
10	Congenital anomalies	1.9	10	Anaemia	2.3
16	Suicide	1.2	19	Self-inflicted injuries	1.2
28	Homicide	0.5	38	Interpersonal violence	0.5
34	War	0.4	41	War	0.5

Males

Rank	Cause	Proportion of total (%)	Rank	Cause	Proportion of total (%)
Deaths			DALYs		
1	Ischaemic heart disease	13.6	1	Perinatal conditions	9.0
2	Lower respiratory infections	9.8	2	Lower respiratory infections	7.2
3	Diarrhoeal diseases	7.1	3	Diarrhoeal diseases	5.4
4	Perinatal conditions	6.8	4	Road traffic injuries	5.0
5	Cerebrovascular disease	5.3	5	Ischaemic heart disease	4.8
6	Tuberculosis	5.1	6	Tuberculosis	4.0
7	Road traffic injuries	4.3	7	Unipolar depressive disorders	3.7
8	HIV/AIDS	3.1	8	HIV/AIDS	3.3
9	Chronic obstructive pulmonary disease	2.1	9	Congenital anomalies	3.1
10	Cirrhosis of the liver	1.9	10	Hearing loss, adult onset	2.1
14	Suicide	1.4	17	Self-inflicted injuries	1.3
22	Homicide	0.7	27	War	0.8
25	War	0.6	32	Interpersonal violence	0.7

Females

Rank	Cause	Proportion of total (%)	Rank	Cause	Proportion of total (%)
Deaths			DALYs		
1	Ischaemic heart disease	13.9	1	Perinatal conditions	8.7
2	Lower respiratory infections	9.0	2	Lower respiratory infections	7.6
3	Perinatal conditions	7.5	3	Unipolar depressive disorders	5.7
4	Diarrhoeal diseases	6.3	4	Diarrhoeal diseases	5.6
5	Cerebrovascular disease	6.2	5	Ischaemic heart disease	4.1
6	Tuberculosis	4.3	6	Tuberculosis	3.1
7	Chronic obstructive pulmonary disease	2.3	7	Congenital anomalies	2.9
8	Congenital anomalies	2.0	8	Anaemia	2.7
9	HIV/AIDS	2.0	9	Cerebrovascular disease	2.1
10	Cervix uteri cancer	1.8	10	HIV/AIDS	2.1
20	Suicide	0.9	25	Self-inflicted injuries	1.0
37	Homicide	0.4	51	Interpersonal violence	0.3
48	War	0.2	63	War	0.2

TABLE A.6 *(continued)*

SOUTH-EAST ASIA REGION[a] *(continued)*
Low-income and middle-income countries

Rank	Cause	Proportion of total (%)	Rank	Cause	Proportion of total (%)
Deaths			DALYs		
1	Ischaemic heart disease	13.7	1	Perinatal conditions	8.9
2	Lower respiratory infections	9.5	2	Lower respiratory infections	7.4
3	Perinatal conditions	7.1	3	Diarrhoeal diseases	5.5
4	Diarrhoeal diseases	6.7	4	Unipolar depressive disorders	4.7
5	Cerebrovascular disease	5.7	5	Ischaemic heart disease	4.4
6	Tuberculosis	4.8	6	Tuberculosis	3.5
7	Road traffic injuries	3.1	7	Road traffic injuries	3.3
8	HIV/AIDS	2.6	8	Congenital anomalies	3.0
9	Chronic obstructive pulmonary disease	2.2	9	HIV/AIDS	2.7
10	Congenital anomalies	1.9	10	Anaemia	2.3
16	Suicide	1.2	19	Self-inflicted injuries	1.2
28	Homicide	0.5	38	Interpersonal violence	0.5
34	War	0.4	41	War	0.5

Source: WHO Global Burden of Disease project for 2000, Version 1.

[a] No high-income countries in the region.

TABLE A.6 *(continued)*

EUROPEAN REGION

Total

Rank	Cause	Proportion of total (%)
Deaths		
1	Ischaemic heart disease	24.3
2	Cerebrovascular disease	15.4
3	Trachea, bronchus and lung cancers	3.9
4	Lower respiratory infections	3.0
5	Chronic obstructive pulmonary disease	2.8
6	Colon and rectum cancers	2.5
7	Suicide	1.9
8	Stomach cancer	1.9
9	Cirrhosis of the liver	1.8
10	Hypertensive heart disease	1.6
18	Homicide	0.8
34	War	0.4

Rank	Cause	Proportion of total (%)
DALYs		
1	Ischaemic heart disease	10.1
2	Cerebrovascular disease	6.8
3	Unipolar depressive disorders	6.0
4	Alcohol use disorders	3.4
5	Alzheimer and other dementias	3.0
6	Self-inflicted injuries	2.6
7	Road traffic injuries	2.5
8	Lower respiratory infections	2.4
9	Hearing loss, adult onset	2.3
10	Trachea, bronchus and lung cancers	2.2
18	Interpersonal violence	1.4
33	War	0.7

Males

Rank	Cause	Proportion of total (%)
Deaths		
1	Ischaemic heart disease	23.4
2	Cerebrovascular disease	11.6
3	Trachea, bronchus and lung cancers	6.0
4	Chronic obstructive pulmonary disease	3.6
5	Suicide	3.0
6	Lower respiratory infections	3.0
7	Colon and rectum cancers	2.4
8	Stomach cancer	2.2
9	Cirrhosis of the liver	2.2
10	Prostate cancer	1.9
14	Homicide	1.2
29	War	0.6

Rank	Cause	Proportion of total (%)
DALYs		
1	Ischaemic heart disease	11.0
2	Cerebrovascular disease	5.6
3	Alcohol use disorders	5.1
4	Unipolar depressive disorders	4.0
5	Self-inflicted injuries	3.7
6	Road traffic injuries	3.4
7	Trachea, bronchus and lung cancers	3.2
8	Chronic obstructive pulmonary disease	2.6
9	Lower respiratory infections	2.5
10	Poisonings	2.1
15	Interpersonal violence	1.9
26	War	1.0

Females

Rank	Cause	Proportion of total (%)
Deaths		
1	Ischaemic heart disease	25.2
2	Cerebrovascular disease	19.3
3	Breast cancer	3.3
4	Lower respiratory infections	3.1
5	Colon and rectum cancers	2.5
6	Chronic obstructive pulmonary disease	2.0
7	Hypertensive heart disease	2.0
8	Diabetes mellitus	1.8
9	Stomach cancer	1.6
10	Trachea, bronchus and lung cancers	1.6
16	Suicide	0.8
28	Homicide	0.4
44	War	0.1

Rank	Cause	Proportion of total (%)
DALYs		
1	Ischaemic heart disease	9.0
2	Unipolar depressive disorders	8.6
3	Cerebrovascular disease	8.3
4	Alzheimer and other dementias	4.2
5	Osteoarthritis	2.9
6	Breast cancer	2.8
7	Hearing loss, adult onset	2.5
8	Lower respiratory infections	2.3
9	Diabetes mellitus	2.0
10	Perinatal conditions	1.8
21	Self-inflicted injuries	1.1
34	Interpersonal violence	0.7
58	War	0.3

TABLE A.6 *(continued)*

EUROPEAN REGION *(continued)*

High-income countries

Rank	Cause	Proportion of total (%)
Deaths		
1	Ischaemic heart disease	18.4
2	Cerebrovascular disease	11.3
3	Trachea, bronchus and lung cancers	5.1
4	Lower respiratory infections	4.1
5	Colon and rectum cancers	3.4
6	Chronic obstructive pulmonary disease	3.4
7	Breast cancer	2.3
8	Diabetes mellitus	2.1
9	Alzheimer and other dementias	1.9
10	Prostate cancer	1.8
15	Suicide	1.3
44	Homicide	0.1
68	War	0.0

Rank	Cause	Proportion of total (%)
DALYs		
1	Unipolar depressive disorders	7.9
2	Ischaemic heart disease	7.5
3	Alzheimer and other dementias	6.1
4	Alcohol use disorders	5.3
5	Cerebrovascular disease	5.1
6	Trachea, bronchus and lung cancers	3.1
7	Osteoarthritis	2.9
8	Road traffic injuries	2.7
9	Hearing loss, adult onset	2.5
10	Chronic obstructive pulmonary disease	2.4
14	Self-inflicted injuries	1.9
53	Interpersonal violence	0.2
86	War	0.0

Low-income and middle-income countries

Rank	Cause	Proportion of total (%)
Deaths		
1	Ischaemic heart disease	28.3
2	Cerebrovascular disease	18.1
3	Trachea, bronchus and lung cancers	3.1
4	Chronic obstructive pulmonary disease	2.4
5	Suicide	2.3
6	Lower respiratory infections	2.3
7	Stomach cancer	2.1
8	Cirrhosis of the liver	1.8
9	Poisonings	1.8
10	Colon and rectum cancers	1.8
13	Homicide	1.3
21	War	0.6

Rank	Cause	Proportion of total (%)
DALYs		
1	Ischaemic heart disease	11.4
2	Cerebrovascular disease	7.7
3	Unipolar depressive disorders	5.1
4	Lower respiratory infections	3.0
5	Self-inflicted injuries	2.9
6	Alcohol use disorders	2.5
7	Perinatal conditions	2.4
8	Road traffic injuries	2.3
9	Hearing loss, adult onset	2.2
10	Poisonings	2.1
12	Interpersonal violence	1.9
24	War	1.0

Source: WHO Global Burden of Disease project for 2000, Version 1.

TABLE A.6 *(continued)*

EASTERN MEDITERRANEAN REGION

Total

Rank	Cause	Proportion of total (%)	Rank	Cause	Proportion of total (%)
Deaths			DALYs		
1	Ischaemic heart disease	10.5	1	Perinatal conditions	8.4
2	Lower respiratory infections	9.1	2	Lower respiratory infections	8.4
3	Perinatal conditions	7.5	3	Diarrhoeal diseases	6.9
4	Diarrhoeal diseases	7.1	4	Unipolar depressive disorders	3.5
5	Cerebrovascular disease	5.3	5	Congenital anomalies	3.3
6	Tuberculosis	3.4	6	Ischaemic heart disease	3.1
7	Road traffic injuries	2.3	7	Road traffic injuries	2.5
8	Congenital anomalies	2.2	8	Tuberculosis	2.2
9	Measles	2.0	9	Measles	2.2
10	Hypertensive heart disease	1.8	10	Cerebrovascular disease	2.0
18	War	1.0	20	War	1.0
21	Homicide	0.8	29	Interpersonal violence	0.7
25	Suicide	0.6	34	Self-inflicted injuries	0.5

Males

Rank	Cause	Proportion of total (%)	Rank	Cause	Proportion of total (%)
Deaths			DALYs		
1	Ischaemic heart disease	11.7	1	Perinatal conditions	8.9
2	Lower respiratory infections	8.6	2	Lower respiratory infections	8.3
3	Perinatal conditions	7.6	3	Diarrhoeal diseases	6.7
4	Diarrhoeal diseases	6.7	4	Road traffic injuries	3.7
5	Cerebrovascular disease	5.0	5	Ischaemic heart disease	3.6
6	Tuberculosis	4.3	6	Congenital anomalies	3.3
7	Road traffic injuries	3.2	7	Tuberculosis	2.8
8	Congenital anomalies	2.1	8	Unipolar depressive disorders	2.8
9	Measles	1.9	9	Measles	2.1
10	Nephritis and nephrosis	1.8	10	Cerebrovascular disease	2.0
15	War	1.3	15	War	1.5
21	Homicide	0.9	25	Interpersonal violence	0.9
26	Suicide	0.6	37	Self-inflicted injuries	0.5

Females

Rank	Cause	Proportion of total (%)	Rank	Cause	Proportion of total (%)
Deaths			DALYs		
1	Lower respiratory infections	9.6	1	Lower respiratory infections	8.4
2	Ischaemic heart disease	9.2	2	Perinatal conditions	7.9
3	Diarrhoeal diseases	7.5	3	Diarrhoeal diseases	7.1
4	Perinatal conditions	7.4	4	Unipolar depressive disorders	4.2
5	Cerebrovascular disease	5.7	5	Congenital anomalies	3.2
6	Tuberculosis	2.3	6	Ischaemic heart disease	2.6
7	Congenital anomalies	2.2	7	Anaemia	2.3
8	Measles	2.1	8	Measles	2.2
9	Hypertensive heart disease	2.0	9	Cerebrovascular disease	2.0
10	Diabetes mellitus	1.7	10	Whooping cough	1.7
26	Suicide	0.6	36	Self-inflicted injuries	0.6
27	Homicide	0.6	39	War	0.6
29	War	0.5	40	Interpersonal violence	0.5

TABLE A.6 *(continued)*

EASTERN MEDITERRANEAN REGION *(continued)*

High-income countries

Rank	Cause	Proportion of total (%)
Deaths		
1	Ischaemic heart disease	20.7
2	Cerebrovascular disease	11.3
3	Road traffic injuries	6.3
4	Hypertensive heart disease	4.2
5	Trachea, bronchus and lung cancers	3.1
6	Nephritis and nephrosis	2.3
7	Diabetes mellitus	2.3
8	Lower respiratory infections	2.2
9	Congenital anomalies	1.8
10	Chronic obstructive pulmonary disease	1.6
16	Homicide	1.0
22	Suicide	0.8
27	War	0.6

Rank	Cause	Proportion of total (%)
DALYs		
1	Ischaemic heart disease	7.5
2	Road traffic injuries	7.2
3	Unipolar depressive disorders	6.9
4	Hearing loss, adult onset	5.5
5	Cerebrovascular disease	3.4
6	Congenital anomalies	3.1
7	Anaemia	2.7
8	Diabetes mellitus	2.5
9	Drug use disorders	2.3
10	Falls	2.3
22	Interpersonal violence	1.0
31	Self-inflicted injuries	0.7
35	War	0.6

Low-income and middle-income countries

Rank	Cause	Proportion of total (%)
Deaths		
1	Ischaemic heart disease	10.4
2	Lower respiratory infections	9.1
3	Perinatal conditions	7.6
4	Diarrhoeal diseases	7.1
5	Cerebrovascular disease	5.3
6	Tuberculosis	3.4
7	Road traffic injuries	2.2
8	Congenital anomalies	2.2
9	Measles	2.0
10	Hypertensive heart disease	1.8
18	War	1.0
20	Homicide	0.8
26	Suicide	0.6

Rank	Cause	Proportion of total (%)
DALYs		
1	Perinatal conditions	8.5
2	Lower respiratory infections	8.4
3	Diarrhoeal diseases	6.9
4	Unipolar depressive disorders	3.5
5	Congenital anomalies	3.3
6	Ischaemic heart disease	3.1
7	Road traffic injuries	2.5
8	Tuberculosis	2.2
9	Measles	2.2
10	Cerebrovascular disease	2.0
20	War	1.0
29	Interpersonal violence	0.7
34	Self-inflicted injuries	0.5

Source: WHO Global Burden of Disease project for 2000, Version 1.

TABLE A.6 *(continued)*

WESTERN PACIFIC REGION
Total

Rank	Cause	Proportion of total (%)
Deaths		
1	Cerebrovascular disease	16.2
2	Chronic obstructive pulmonary disease	13.8
3	Ischaemic heart disease	8.2
4	Lower respiratory infections	4.7
5	Trachea, bronchus and lung cancers	3.5
6	Liver cancer	3.5
7	Stomach cancer	3.2
8	Suicide	3.0
9	Tuberculosis	3.0
10	Perinatal conditions	2.8
27	Homicide	0.5
66	War	0.0

Rank	Cause	Proportion of total (%)
DALYs		
1	Chronic obstructive pulmonary disease	7.3
2	Cerebrovascular disease	5.8
3	Unipolar depressive disorders	5.8
4	Lower respiratory infections	5.2
5	Perinatal conditions	4.6
6	Road traffic injuries	3.7
7	Anaemia	3.2
8	Ischaemic heart disease	3.0
9	Self-inflicted injuries	2.8
10	Falls	2.6
33	Interpersonal violence	0.7
85	War	0.1

Males

Rank	Cause	Proportion of total (%)
Deaths		
1	Cerebrovascular disease	15.8
2	Chronic obstructive pulmonary disease	13.1
3	Ischaemic heart disease	8.3
4	Liver cancer	4.5
5	Trachea, bronchus and lung cancers	4.5
6	Lower respiratory infections	4.0
7	Stomach cancer	3.8
8	Road traffic injuries	3.4
9	Tuberculosis	3.3
10	Suicide	2.7
23	Homicide	0.7
56	War	0.0

Rank	Cause	Proportion of total (%)
DALYs		
1	Chronic obstructive pulmonary disease	7.3
2	Cerebrovascular disease	6.1
3	Road traffic injuries	4.9
4	Unipolar depressive disorders	4.8
5	Lower respiratory infections	4.6
6	Perinatal conditions	4.3
7	Ischaemic heart disease	3.2
8	Anaemia	3.1
9	Falls	2.8
10	Liver cancer	2.7
13	Self-inflicted injuries	2.3
27	Interpersonal violence	0.9
75	War	0.1

Females

Rank	Cause	Proportion of total (%)
Deaths		
1	Cerebrovascular disease	16.6
2	Chronic obstructive pulmonary disease	14.6
3	Ischaemic heart disease	8.1
4	Lower respiratory infections	5.6
5	Suicide	3.5
6	Perinatal conditions	3.2
7	Hypertensive heart disease	2.8
8	Tuberculosis	2.7
9	Stomach cancer	2.5
10	Trachea, bronchus and lung cancers	2.3
39	Homicide	0.3
67	War	0.0

Rank	Cause	Proportion of total (%)
DALYs		
1	Chronic obstructive pulmonary disease	7.2
2	Unipolar depressive disorders	7.1
3	Lower respiratory infections	5.9
4	Cerebrovascular disease	5.5
5	Perinatal conditions	4.9
6	Self-inflicted injuries	3.5
7	Anaemia	3.3
8	Ischaemic heart disease	2.6
9	Osteoarthritis	2.5
10	Congenital anomalies	2.4
51	Interpersonal violence	0.4
86	War	0.0

TABLE A.6 *(continued)*

WESTERN PACIFIC REGION *(continued)*

High-income countries

Rank	Cause	Proportion of total (%)
Deaths		
1	Cerebrovascular disease	15.7
2	Ischaemic heart disease	10.8
3	Lower respiratory infections	7.4
4	Trachea, bronchus and lung cancers	5.3
5	Stomach cancer	5.1
6	Colon and rectum cancers	3.4
7	Liver cancer	3.3
8	Suicide	2.4
9	Road traffic injuries	2.2
10	Diabetes mellitus	2.1
43	Homicide	0.2
—[a]	War	—[a]

Rank	Cause	Proportion of total (%)
DALYs		
1	Cerebrovascular disease	7.6
2	Unipolar depressive disorders	6.4
3	Ischaemic heart disease	4.2
4	Osteoarthritis	3.4
5	Road traffic injuries	3.4
6	Alcohol use disorders	3.1
7	Self-inflicted injuries	2.9
8	Stomach cancer	2.7
9	Diabetes mellitus	2.7
10	Trachea, bronchus, lung cancers	2.6
52	Interpersonal violence	0.3
—[a]	War	—[a]

Low-income and middle-income countries

Rank	Cause	Proportion of total (%)
Deaths		
1	Cerebrovascular disease	16.2
2	Chronic obstructive pulmonary disease	15.5
3	Ischaemic heart disease	7.8
4	Lower respiratory infections	4.4
5	Liver cancer	3.5
6	Tuberculosis	3.3
7	Trachea, bronchus and lung cancers	3.3
8	Perinatal conditions	3.2
9	Suicide	3.1
10	Stomach cancer	3.0
26	Homicide	6.0
64	War	0.0

Rank	Cause	Proportion of total (%)
DALYs		
1	Chronic obstructive pulmonary disease	7.7
2	Unipolar depressive disorders	5.8
3	Cerebrovascular disease	5.7
4	Lower respiratory infections	5.5
5	Perinatal conditions	5.0
6	Road traffic injuries	3.7
7	Anaemia	3.3
8	Ischaemic heart disease	2.8
9	Self-inflicted injuries	2.8
10	Falls	2.6
32	Interpersonal violence	0.7
83	War	0.1

Source: WHO Global Burden of Disease project for 2000, Version 1.

[a] No war-related deaths or injuries reported.

TABLE A.7

Mortality caused by intentional injury,[a] by sex, age group and country, most recent year available between 1990 and 2000[b]

Country or area	Year	Measure[c]	Total[d, e]	Males						
				All ages[d]	0–4 years	5–14 years	15–29 years	30–44 years	45–59 years	⩾60 years
Albania	1998	No.	846	689	4	16	333	193	103	39
		Rate	26.7	46.4	—	—	93.1	53.2	45.9	27.8
Argentina	1996	No.	3 980	3 145	37	85	936	720	689	678
		Rate	11.4	19.0	2.1	1.7	21.0	21.9	28.5	34.1
Armenia	1999	No.	167	128	2	3	29	45	27	22
		Rate	4.3	6.9	—	—	5.9	10.4	12.0	10.3
Australia	1998	No.	2 954	2 325	9	23	727	803	435	328
		Rate	14.9	23.6	—	1.1	34.6	37.4	25.7	24.0
Austria	1999	No.	1 629	1 161	3	7	174	304	279	394
		Rate	16.3	25.0	—	—	22.1	29.6	36.7	60.4
Azerbaijan	1999	No.	430	367	0	10	185	107	41	24
		Rate	5.8	10.0	—	—	17.5	12.6	10.9	8.3
Bahamas	1995–1997	No.	47	40	1	2	21	11	3	2
		Rate	16.0	28.4	—	—	50.4	—	—	—
Barbados	1993–1995	No.	36	28	0	0	11	9	4	3
		Rate	14.0	22.1	—	—	—	—	—	—
Belarus	1999	No.	4 537	3 664	3	27	755	1 226	968	685
		Rate	41.4	72.5	—	2.7	67.6	105.9	125.6	101.5
Belgium	1995	No.	2 330	1 653	3	14	276	505	395	460
		Rate	19.5	28.9	—	—	26.6	42.7	44.4	50.4
Brazil	1995	No.	43 866	39 046	99	573	20 183	12 011	4 344	1 835
		Rate	27.7	50.2	1.2	2.2	89.1	71.9	49.5	35.8
Bulgaria	1999	No.	1 550	1 143	4	12	156	227	293	451
		Rate	14.9	23.5	—	—	17.0	27.2	37.0	57.9
Canada	1997	No.	4 145	3 222	14	65	784	1 091	758	510
		Rate	12.8	20.1	—	2.1	24.8	28.4	28.7	23.8
Chile	1994	No.	1 226	1 070	10	16	365	329	191	159
		Rate	9.0	16.5	—	—	19.7	21.5	22.2	28.1
China (Hong Kong SAR)	1996	No.	863	548	5	14	105	181	103	141
		Rate	12.3	15.9	—	—	15.0	19.8	20.0	33.6
Selected urban and rural areas	1999	No.	19 276	9 719	16	143	1 766	2 702	1 944	3 148
		Rate	15.5	15.9	—	1.1	10.1	17.2	20.7	47.7
Colombia	1995	No.	24 728	22 685	56	310	12 169	7 272	2 141	737
		Rate	65.1	122.4	2.3	4.6	220.5	191.3	116.5	65.1
Costa Rica	1995	No.	394	330	3	9	124	124	50	21
		Rate	12.0	20.1	—	—	24.9	32.9	27.0	18.3
Croatia	1999	No.	1 134	825	1	8	131	207	197	281
		Rate	21.4	34.8	—	—	27.1	39.6	49.8	86.2
Cuba	1997	No.	2 819	2 024	7	17	511	581	375	533
		Rate	23.5	33.9	—	—	35.7	44.4	42.7	78.0
Czech Republic	1999	No.	1 769	1 386	3	7	245	335	426	370
		Rate	14.4	24.1	—	—	19.9	31.8	39.6	49.1
Denmark	1996	No.	955	670	2	4	92	178	184	210
		Rate	14.8	21.6	—	—	16.7	29.9	34.6	47.1
Ecuador	1996	No.	2 242	1 905	5	34	872	643	234	117
		Rate	20.8	36.0	—	1.6	50.7	58.5	41.5	32.6
El Salvador	1991	No.	2 776	2 491	2	31	1 464	552	250	192
		Rate	61.9	119.2	—	2.9	204.9	143.2	106.3	125.2
Estonia	1999	No.	701	546	2	4	102	156	167	115
		Rate	42.9	74.0	—	—	63.6	101.8	138.7	112.8
Finland	1998	No.	1 355	1 053	1	5	188	334	312	213
		Rate	23.3	37.3	—	—	38.1	57.3	57.2	52.8

Country or area	Year	Measure[c]	Females						
			All ages[d]	0–4 years	5–14 years	15–29 years	30–44 years	45–59 years	≥60 years
Albania	1998	No.	156	5	10	76	39	16	11
		Rate	9.1	—	—	17.4	10.8	—	—
Argentina	1996	No.	835	35	60	214	176	160	190
		Rate	4.4	2.1	1.2	4.9	5.2	6.2	7.1
Armenia	1999	No.	39	0	2	3	10	8	16
		Rate	1.9	—	—	—	—	—	—
Australia	1998	No.	629	10	13	161	209	118	117
		Rate	6.2	—	—	7.9	9.7	7.2	7.1
Austria	1999	No.	468	3	4	50	101	109	201
		Rate	8.4	—	—	6.5	10.3	14.3	20.6
Azerbaijan	1999	No.	63	1	3	14	22	12	11
		Rate	1.8	—	—	—	2.4	—	—
Bahamas	1995–1997	No.	7	0	1	2	3	1	0
		Rate	—	—	—	—	—	—	—
Barbados	1993–1995	No.	9	0	0	3	2	2	1
		Rate	—	—	—	—	—	—	—
Belarus	1999	No.	873	3	13	143	215	219	279
		Rate	14.2	—	—	13.2	18.1	24.9	22.8
Belgium	1995	No.	677	3	9	73	195	156	241
		Rate	10.7	—	—	—	17.0	17.5	19.2
Brazil	1995	No.	4820	84	302	1977	1518	569	370
		Rate	6.0	1.0	1.2	8.7	8.8	6.0	6.0
Bulgaria	1999	No.	407	1	5	44	64	86	207
		Rate	7.1	—	—	5.0	7.7	10.1	20.7
Canada	1997	No.	923	10	32	189	303	233	156
		Rate	5.6	—	1.1	6.2	8.0	8.7	5.7
Chile	1994	No.	156	5	12	50	42	25	22
		Rate	2.2	—	—	2.7	2.7	2.7	2.9
China									
Hong Kong SAR	1996	No.	315	4	13	65	83	39	110
		Rate	8.6	—	—	9.0	8.8	8.9	23.4
Selected urban and rural areas	1999	No.	9557	19	120	2117	2587	1757	2957
		Rate	15.2	—	1.0	13.1	17.5	19.6	40.5
Colombia	1995	No.	2043	34	151	982	575	218	83
		Rate	10.4	1.5	2.3	17.8	14.2	10.9	6.0
Costa Rica	1995	No.	64	1	4	31	20	7	1
		Rate	3.7	—	—	6.5	5.3	—	—
Croatia	1999	No.	309	1	3	21	50	74	160
		Rate	9.9	—	—	4.5	9.9	17.1	31.1
Cuba	1997	No.	795	4	14	208	212	164	193
		Rate	13.4	—	—	15.1	16.1	18.1	26.3
Czech Republic	1999	No.	383	4	6	54	64	99	156
		Rate	5.7	—	—	4.6	6.3	8.9	14.0
Denmark	1996	No.	285	1	1	21	73	90	99
		Rate	8.3	—	—	4.0	12.8	17.2	16.8
Ecuador	1996	No.	337	6	28	185	70	24	24
		Rate	5.8	—	1.4	11.0	6.4	4.2	5.9
El Salvador	1991	No.	285	1	23	164	50	29	18
		Rate	11.5	—	2.2	21.6	11.6	11.4	—
Estonia	1999	No.	155	3	4	14	35	43	56
		Rate	16.3	—	—	9.2	22.7	29.7	29.7
Finland	1998	No.	302	1	3	43	77	99	79
		Rate	9.9	—	—	9.1	13.7	18.4	13.2

TABLE A.7 *(continued)*

Country or area	Year	Measure[c]	Total[d, e]	Males						
				All ages[d]	0–4 years	5–14 years	15–29 years	30–44 years	45–59 years	⩾60 years
France	1998	No.	10 997	8 058	14	36	1 092	2 358	1 938	2 620
		Rate	15.6	24.1	—	0.6	17.8	36.6	36.7	51.7
Georgia	1992	No.	214	160	0	0	38	42	30	50
		Rate	4.1	6.8	—	—	7.0	8.4	8.6	16.9
Germany	1999	No.	11 928	8 532	27	65	1 185	2 348	2 133	2 774
		Rate	11.5	17.7	1.3	1.0	15.9	22.6	26.9	36.4
Greece	1998	No.	548	425	1	1	82	107	100	134
		Rate	4.3	6.9	—	—	6.9	9.5	10.6	12.4
Guyana	1994–1996	No.	126	99	0	0	43	32	16	8
		Rate	19.1	32.3	—	—	37.1	47.8	—	—
Hungary	1999	No.	3 628	2 724	4	19	302	747	873	780
		Rate	29.5	49.0	—	—	25.9	72.8	90.5	102.3
Iceland	1994–1996	No.	29	24	0	0	8	6	5	4
		Rate	10.6	17.8	—	—	—	—	—	—
Ireland	1997	No.	498	398	1	5	156	118	76	42
		Rate	13.4	21.6	—	—	33.8	31.2	25.8	16.9
Israel	1997	No.	430	335	0	2	108	82	48	95
		Rate	7.3	12.1	—	—	14.6	15.1	12.4	28.4
Italy	1997	No.	5 416	4 108	0	11	748	933	873	1 543
		Rate	7.3	11.8	—	—	12.1	14.6	16.2	27.4
Japan	1997	No.	24 300	16 376	32	86	2 036	3 145	5 963	5 114
		Rate	15.1	21.4	1.1	0.9	14.9	26.1	43.2	43.1
Kazakhstan	1992	No.	5 844	4 569	14	99	1 470	1 706	845	434
		Rate	36.7	60.3	—	3.7	68.8	91.6	86.3	74.3
Kuwait	1999	No.	97	71	1	3	24	38	3	2
		Rate	4.2	5.1	—	—	7.5	7.9	—	—
Kyrgyzstan	1999	No.	906	727	1	16	201	272	153	84
		Rate	22.6	38.1	—	—	30.1	56.2	74.3	52.7
Latvia	1999	No.	1 075	806	0	1	132	256	246	171
		Rate	38.6	64.4	—	—	50.5	96.4	122.4	99.1
Lithuania	1999	No.	1 856	1 498	2	13	282	482	468	251
		Rate	45.8	80.5	—	—	68.7	115.1	163.3	100.9
Luxembourg	1995–1997	No.	75	55	0	0	8	17	14	16
		Rate	15.4	23.4	—	—	—	—	—	—
Malta	1997–1999	No.	25	19	0	0	4	8	2	4
		Rate	6.1	—	—	—	—	—	—	—
Mauritius	1999	No.	214	144	2	3	40	66	22	11
		Rate	17.5	23.6	—	—	26.2	45.6	27.5	—
Mexico	1997	No.	17 153	15 131	129	434	6 636	4 540	2 116	1 276
		Rate	19.8	36.5	2.2	2.6	46.6	53.5	46.3	45.0
Netherlands	1999	No.	1 729	1 166	4	15	202	380	308	257
		Rate	9.5	13.1	—	—	12.9	19.5	19.5	20.9
New Zealand	1998	No.	638	479	5	16	180	132	77	69
		Rate	16.6	25.3	—	—	44.0	30.8	24.0	26.5
Nicaragua	1996	No.	522	398	2	13	193	108	51	30
		Rate	14.4	23.8	—	—	30.1	31.7	32.2	32.9
Norway	1997	No.	575	416	1	6	94	114	91	110
		Rate	11.8	17.4	—	—	20.4	23.0	22.6	29.6
Panama (excluding Canal Zone)	1997	No.	453	401	5	8	186	125	44	32
		Rate	17.0	30.1	—	—	48.5	45.3	28.0	31.1
Paraguay	1994	No.	577	508	3	11	203	162	76	53
		Rate	15.9	28.6	—	—	31.8	37.2	39.8	50.4

Country or area	Year	Measure[c]	Females						
			All ages[d]	0–4 years	5–14 years	15–29 years	30–44 years	45–59 years	≥60 years
France	1998	No.	2 939	8	23	308	721	781	1 098
		Rate	7.9	—	0.4	5.1	11.1	14.7	15.8
Georgia	1992	No.	54	0	0	12	13	9	20
		Rate	1.9	—	—	—	—	—	4.4
Germany	1999	No.	3 396	16	42	303	685	783	1 567
		Rate	5.9	—	0.7	4.3	7.0	10.0	14.3
Greece	1998	No.	123	0	1	15	26	37	44
		Rate	1.9	—	—	—	2.3	3.8	3.4
Guyana	1994–1996	No.	27	0	1	13	8	4	2
		Rate	7.5	—	—	—	—	—	—
Hungary	1999	No.	904	5	9	73	173	222	422
		Rate	12.7	—	—	6.6	16.9	20.8	34.8
Iceland	1994–1996	No.	5	0	0	1	0	1	2
		Rate	—	—	—	—	—	—	—
Ireland	1997	No.	100	1	1	26	24	24	24
		Rate	5.1	—	—	5.8	6.2	8.3	7.8
Israel	1997	No.	95	0	3	14	25	8	45
		Rate	3.0	—	—	—	4.4	—	10.4
Italy	1997	No.	1 308	2	14	173	252	279	588
		Rate	3.3	—	—	2.9	4.0	5.0	7.8
Japan	1997	No.	7 923	42	82	903	1 139	2 078	3 679
		Rate	9.0	1.5	0.9	6.9	9.6	14.9	23.7
Kazakhstan	1992	No.	1 275	18	40	299	354	239	325
		Rate	15.1	—	1.5	14.6	18.6	21.8	30.1
Kuwait	1999	No.	26	0	0	6	18	1	1
		Rate	3.2	—	—	—	—	—	—
Kyrgyzstan	1999	No.	179	5	10	56	39	21	48
		Rate	8.2	—	—	8.5	7.9	9.4	20.9
Latvia	1999	No.	269	3	6	27	63	66	103
		Rate	16.7	—	—	10.7	23.5	27.3	31.8
Lithuania	1999	No.	358	5	9	44	78	87	135
		Rate	15.1	—	—	11.0	18.4	25.6	31.4
Luxembourg	1995–1997	No.	20	0	0	3	7	5	5
		Rate	8.3	—	—	—	—	—	—
Malta	1997–1999	No.	6	0	0	2	1	1	2
		Rate	—	—	—	—	—	—	—
Mauritius	1999	No.	70	2	3	29	26	7	3
		Rate	11.4	—	—	19.7	18.8	—	—
Mexico	1997	No.	2 022	109	236	825	467	195	190
		Rate	4.2	2.0	1.5	5.7	5.2	4.0	5.7
Netherlands	1999	No.	563	1	10	96	156	147	153
		Rate	6.1	—	—	6.3	8.3	9.6	9.4
New Zealand	1998	No.	159	2	7	58	51	22	19
		Rate	8.1	—	—	14.2	11.3	6.8	—
Nicaragua	1996	No.	124	2	18	71	17	10	6
		Rate	5.7	—	—	10.9	—	—	—
Norway	1997	No.	159	0	1	28	46	47	37
		Rate	6.4	—	—	6.3	9.7	12.1	7.5
Panama (excluding Canal Zone)	1997	No.	52	3	6	22	10	5	6
		Rate	3.7	—	—	5.9	—	—	—
Paraguay	1994	No.	69	2	4	25	19	9	10
		Rate	3.7	—	—	4.0	—	—	—

TABLE A.7 *(continued)*

Country or area	Year	Measure[c]	Total[d, e]	Males						
				All ages[d]	0–4 years	5–14 years	15–29 years	30–44 years	45–59 years	≥60 years
Philippines	1993	No.	8 677	7 770	20	80	3 296	3 039	1 041	294
		Rate	15.9	28.5	0.4	0.6	34.9	53.4	35.4	20.0
Poland	1995	No.	6 619	5 364	12	82	944	1 919	1 485	922
		Rate	16.0	27.3	—	1.8	21.8	42.1	50.2	37.9
Portugal	1999	No.	671	494	3	4	70	98	85	234
		Rate	5.2	8.3	—	—	6.0	9.3	10.0	27.0
Puerto Rico	1998	No.	1 129	1 022	1	11	557	238	125	89
		Rate	28.6	53.7	—	—	112.6	65.2	45.1	38.1
Republic of Korea	1997	No.	7 061	4 794	17	71	1 141	1 646	1 125	794
		Rate	14.9	21.3	—	1.3	17.2	26.3	33.9	45.3
Republic of Moldova	1999	No.	999	794	4	15	150	255	221	149
		Rate	26.7	46.2	—	—	33.6	66.0	82.9	76.3
Romania	1999	No.	3 560	2 817	10	57	479	763	843	665
		Rate	14.1	23.3	—	2.6	17.2	32.3	44.5	37.2
Russian Federation	1998	No.	85 511	68 013	98	581	15 476	25 190	16 695	9 973
		Rate	53.7	91.9	2.9	4.0	95.7	146.3	143.5	111.7
Singapore	1998	No.	446	280	0	3	67	97	57	56
		Rate	13.9	17.4	—	—	19.3	21.4	21.3	37.2
Slovakia	1999	No.	825	680	0	5	111	208	215	141
		Rate	13.8	24.1	—	—	16.3	34.9	46.4	42.9
Slovenia	1999	No.	623	476	1	5	65	125	135	145
		Rate	26.0	42.4	—	—	29.5	55.0	68.8	97.7
Spain	1998	No.	3 620	2 757	2	9	561	636	489	1 060
		Rate	7.3	11.7	—	—	11.8	14.3	14.9	29.2
Saint Lucia	1993–1995	No.	21	17	0	0	9	5	2	1
		Rate	16.0	—	—	—	—	—	—	—
Sweden	1996	No.	1 367	947	0	1	147	239	274	286
		Rate	13.0	18.4	—	—	17.0	25.8	31.3	33.7
Switzerland	1996	No.	1 513	1 060	2	10	197	265	262	324
		Rate	17.8	26.5	—	—	28.5	30.8	38.6	55.7
Tajikistan	1995	No.	557	451	4	6	149	175	74	43
		Rate	13.7	22.4	—	—	19.6	37.2	36.3	28.7
Thailand	1994	No.	6 530	5 133	21	106	1 881	1 866	885	375
		Rate	11.6	18.5	0.8	1.3	20.6	29.9	27.7	19.5
The former Yugoslav Republic of Macedonia	1997	No.	202	153	0	1	18	53	31	50
		Rate	9.7	15.0	—	—	—	23.5	19.7	39.1
Trinidad and Tobago	1994	No.	313	243	0	4	82	78	52	27
		Rate	26.1	39.0	—	—	45.3	53.1	64.5	48.1
Turkmenistan	1998	No.	742	603	2	19	249	215	94	23
		Rate	18.9	31.4	—	—	38.1	47.9	53.0	20.1
Ukraine	1999	No.	20 762	16 255	28	148	2 862	5 133	4 710	3 373
		Rate	36.9	63.8	2.5	3.2	51.8	96.7	117.4	93.5
United Kingdom	1999	No.	4 920	3 803	20	34	886	1 329	868	666
		Rate	7.6	12.0	1.1	0.6	15.1	19.3	15.9	12.7
England and Wales	1999	No.	4 015	3 077	19	29	667	1 050	736	576
		Rate	6.9	10.8	—	0.6	12.9	17.2	15.2	12.3
Northern Ireland	1999	No.	145	123	0	1	49	50	15	8
		Rate	8.8	14.9	—	—	25.9	27.6	—	—

Country or area	Year	Measure[c]	Females						
			All ages[d]	0–4 years	5–14 years	15–29 years	30–44 years	45–59 years	⩾60 years
Philippines	1993	No.	907	11	46	403	226	136	86
		Rate	3.3	—	0.4	4.4	4.0	4.6	4.7
Poland	1995	No.	1 255	14	25	168	379	301	368
		Rate	5.6	—	0.6	4.0	8.4	9.4	10.1
Portugal	1999	No.	177	3	8	18	33	25	90
		Rate	2.5	—	—	—	3.0	2.7	7.6
Puerto Rico	1998	No.	107	3	4	43	30	13	14
		Rate	5.1	—	—	8.9	7.2	—	—
Republic of Korea	1997	No.	2 267	19	72	663	690	363	460
		Rate	9.2	—	1.5	10.5	11.6	10.8	17.2
Republic of Moldova	1999	No.	205	5	11	28	49	48	64
		Rate	9.9	—	—	6.3	11.8	15.4	21.3
Romania	1999	No.	743	11	20	114	157	177	264
		Rate	5.5	—	1.0	4.2	6.7	8.8	11.1
Russian Federation	1998	No.	17 498	90	303	3 000	4 342	3 862	5 902
		Rate	19.2	2.8	2.2	19.3	24.8	28.6	34.5
Singapore	1998	No.	166	0	0	50	30	29	56
		Rate	10.4	—	—	14.5	6.7	11.1	32.4
Slovakia	1999	No.	145	0	1	18	42	40	44
		Rate	4.5	—	—	—	7.2	8.0	8.8
Slovenia	1999	No.	147	0	0	15	28	48	56
		Rate	11.4	—	—	—	12.3	24.6	24.6
Spain	1998	No.	863	1	5	122	174	162	399
		Rate	3.2	—	—	2.7	4.0	4.8	8.3
Saint Lucia	1993–1995	No.	3	0	0	2	0	0	0
		Rate	—	—	—	—	—	—	—
Sweden	1996	No.	420	3	8	48	90	132	139
		Rate	7.7			5.8	10.2	15.5	12.7
Switzerland	1996	No.	453	3	5	53	102	114	176
		Rate	9.9	—	—	7.7	12.2	16.9	21.8
Tajikistan	1995	No.	106	0	0	38	31	15	21
		Rate	5.3	—	—	5.0	6.4	—	11.0
Thailand	1994	No.	1 397	15	78	550	418	210	126
		Rate	4.9	—	1.0	6.2	6.7	6.3	5.3
The former Yugoslav Republic of Macedonia	1997	No.	49	0	1	6	18	5	19
		Rate	4.7	—	—	—	—	—	—
Trinidad and Tobago	1994	No.	70	2	2	33	19	6	8
		Rate	11.6	—	—	21.2	—	—	—
Turkmenistan	1998	No.	139	1	4	59	35	18	21
		Rate	7.1	—	—	9.1	7.6	—	13.5
Ukraine	1999	No.	4 507	22	72	559	983	1 100	1 771
		Rate	13.6	2.0	1.6	10.5	17.7	22.9	27.4
United Kingdom	1999	No.	1 117	7	14	195	330	261	310
		Rate	3.2	—	—	3.5	4.9	4.7	4.5
England and Wales	1999	No.	938	7	13	152	272	219	275
		Rate	3.0	—	—	3.1	4.6	4.5	4.5
Northern Ireland	1999	No.	22	0	0	11	8	1	2
		Rate	2.7	—	—	—	—	—	—

TABLE A.7 *(continued)*

Country or area	Year	Measure[c]	Total[d, e]	Males						
				All ages[d]	0–4 years	5–14 years	15–29 years	30–44 years	45–59 years	≥60 years
Scotland	1999	No.	760	603	1	4	170	229	117	82
		Rate	14.1	22.9	—	—	33.4	38.7	25.3	18.7
United States of America	1998	No.	49 586	38 974	396	894	12 511	11 688	6 885	6 600
		Rate	17.4	28.3	4.1	3.0	44.2	36.4	30.1	34.6
Uruguay	1990	No.	457	357	1	5	64	90	86	111
		Rate	14.0	23.5	—	—	17.8	31.5	36.7	50.3
Uzbekistan	1998	No.	2 414	1 821	2	73	585	690	315	156
		Rate	12.1	19.0	—	1.6	17.6	29.7	33.0	22.2
Venezuela	1994	No.	4 704	4 254	16	104	2 435	1 109	357	232
		Rate	23.2	42.0	—	2.6	80.8	53.1	33.4	38.6

Source: WHO mortality database as of September 2001.

[a] Intentional injury = ICD-10 X60–Y09, Y35, Y36 (ICD-9 E950–E978, E990–E999).

[b] Or average of the three most recent years available between 1990 and 2000 for countries with populations under 1 million.

[c] No. = number of deaths; rate = number of deaths per 100 000 population. Deaths where the age of the deceased person was not known were proportionally distributed across age groups based on the distribution of intentional injury deaths in the population. The numbers of deaths have therefore been rounded to the nearest whole number. Any apparent discrepancy in the total sums is due to rounding. The rate was not calculated if fewer than 20 deaths were reported. The population counts on which the rates are based are available from the World Health Organization at http://www3.who.int/whosis/whsa/ftp/download.htm.

[d] Age-standardized.

[e] Combined total for males and females.

Country or area	Year	Measure[c]	Females						
			All ages[d]	0–4 years	5–14 years	15–29 years	30–44 years	45–59 years	⩾60 years
Scotland	1999	No.	157	0	1	32	50	41	33
		Rate	5.4	—	—	6.5	8.4	8.5	5.4
United States of America	1998	No.	10 612	326	613	2 297	3 524	2 170	1 682
		Rate	7.1	3.5	2.2	8.3	10.8	9.0	6.6
Uruguay	1990	No.	100	2	6	25	14	13	39
		Rate	5.6	—	—	7.1	—	—	13.6
Uzbekistan	1998	No.	593	2	17	266	147	77	84
		Rate	5.7	—	—	8.1	6.2	7.8	8.7
Venezuela	1994	No.	450	16	43	202	116	38	35
		Rate	4.4	—	1.1	6.9	5.6	3.5	5.1

TABLE A.8

Mortality caused by homicide,[a] by sex, age group and country, most recent year available between 1990 and 2000[b]

Country or area	Year	Measure[c]	Total[d, e]	Males						
				All ages[d]	0–4 years	5–14 years	15–29 years	30–44 years	45–59 years	≥60 years
Albania	1998	No.	660	573	2	9	286	165	84	27
		Rate	21.0	38.7	—	—	79.9	45.5	37.2	19.4
Argentina	1996	No.	1 611	1 347	37	35	514	371	239	152
		Rate	4.7	8.1	2.1	1.0	11.5	11.3	9.9	7.6
Armenia	1999	No.	98	77	2	1	20	29	16	9
		Rate	2.6	4.2	—	—	4.1	6.7	—	—
Australia	1998	No.	295	201	9	8	59	66	42	17
		Rate	1.6	2.1	—	—	2.8	3.1	2.5	—
Austria	1999	No.	68	32	3	2	3	15	4	5
		Rate	0.8	0.8	—	—	—	—	—	—
Azerbaijan	1999	No.	375	323	0	10	176	86	32	19
		Rate	5.0	8.7	—	—	16.6	10.1	8.5	—
Bahamas	1995–1997	No.	43	37	1	1	20	10	3	2
		Rate	14.9	26.1	—	—	48.4	—	—	—
Belarus	1999	No.	1 123	784	3	2	203	303	171	102
		Rate	10.5	15.6	—	—	18.2	26.2	22.1	15.1
Belgium	1995	No.	169	100	3	1	24	34	22	16
		Rate	1.6	1.9	—	—	2.3	2.9	2.5	—
Brazil	1995	No.	37 076	33 751	99	436	18 400	10 352	3 393	1 071
		Rate	23.0	42.5	1.2	2.5	81.2	61.9	38.7	20.9
Bulgaria	1999	No.	238	174	4	1	38	47	48	36
		Rate	2.6	4.0	—	—	4.1	5.6	6.1	4.6
Canada	1997	No.	431	285	14	12	100	76	48	35
		Rate	1.4	1.9	—	—	3.2	2.0	1.8	1.6
Chile	1994	No.	410	356	10	4	125	118	58	41
		Rate	3.0	5.4	—	—	6.7	7.7	6.7	7.2
China										
Hong Kong SAR	1996	No.	63	39	5	3	8	10	3	9
		Rate	1.0	1.3	—	—	—	—	—	—
Selected urban and rural areas	1999	No.	2 405	1 655	16	44	514	684	264	133
		Rate	1.8	2.5	—	0.5	3.0	4.4	2.8	2.0
Colombia	1995	No.	23 443	21 705	56	239	11 730	7 039	2 016	625
		Rate	61.6	116.8	2.3	5.5	212.5	185.1	109.7	55.2
Costa Rica	1995	No.	179	153	3	1	57	62	22	7
		Rate	5.4	9.3	—	—	11.5	16.6	12.2	—
Croatia	1999	No.	128	95	1	1	17	33	22	21
		Rate	2.6	4.0	—	—	—	6.3	5.6	6.4
Cuba	1997	No.	747	584	7	5	263	210	63	36
		Rate	6.2	9.6	—	—	18.4	16.0	7.2	5.3
Czech Republic	1999	No.	151	97	3	1	22	36	27	8
		Rate	1.4	1.8	—	—	1.8	3.4	2.5	—
Denmark	1996	No.	59	36	2	1	12	14	4	3
		Rate	1.1	1.4	—	—	—	—	—	—
Ecuador	1996	No.	1 632	1 501	5	21	684	535	178	78
		Rate	15.3	28.2	—	1.5	39.8	48.7	31.5	21.8
El Salvador	1993	No.	2 480	2 290	8	35	1 043	659	344	201
		Rate	55.6	108.4	—	5.1	133.1	165.4	139.5	122.7
Estonia	1999	No.	227	168	2	0	29	59	56	23
		Rate	14.8	23.1	—	—	18.0	38.4	46.3	22.2
Finland	1998	No.	125	90	1	1	15	38	22	13
		Rate	2.2	3.3	—	—	—	6.5	4.0	—
France	1998	No.	436	269	14	12	56	80	75	32
		Rate	0.7	0.9	—	—	0.9	1.2	1.4	0.6

Country or area	Year	Measure[c]	Females						
			All ages[d]	0–4 years	5–14 years	15–29 years	30–44 years	45–59 years	≥60 years
Albania	1998	No.	87	4	3	31	30	12	6
		Rate	5.3	—	—	7.2	8.3	—	—
Argentina	1996	No.	264	36	15	86	63	30	35
		Rate	1.5	2.1	—	2.0	1.9	1.2	1.3
Armenia	1999	No.	21	0	2	3	6	5	5
		Rate	1.0	—	—	—	—	—	—
Australia	1998	No.	94	10	1	26	26	15	16
		Rate	1.0	—	—	1.3	1.2	—	—
Austria	1999	No.	36	3	0	4	16	8	5
		Rate	0.8	—	—	—	—	—	—
Azerbaijan	1999	No.	52	1	2	12	19	9	9
		Rate	1.4	—	—	—	—	—	—
Bahamas	1995–1997	No.	7	0	1	2	3	1	0
		Rate	—	—	—	—	—	—	—
Belarus	1999	No.	339	3	6	60	102	78	90
		Rate	5.8	—	—	5.5	8.6	8.8	7.3
Belgium	1995	No.	69	3	3	12	24	9	18
		Rate	1.2	—	—	—	2.1	—	—
Brazil	1995	No.	3 325	85	183	1 484	1 089	308	177
		Rate	4.1	1.1	1.1	6.5	6.3	3.3	2.8
Bulgaria	1999	No.	64	1	1	12	13	15	22
		Rate	1.3	—	—	—	—	—	2.2
Canada	1997	No.	146	10	10	33	48	25	20
		Rate	1.0	—	—	1.1	1.3	0.9	0.7
Chile	1994	No.	54	5	3	17	17	5	7
		Rate	0.8						
China									
Hong Kong SAR	1996	No.	24	4	4	4	9	3	0
		Rate	0.8	—	—	—	—	—	—
Selected urban and rural areas	1999	No.	750	19	37	218	283	117	76
		Rate	1.2	—	0.4	1.4	1.9	1.3	1.0
Colombia	1995	No.	1 738	33	106	827	511	189	72
		Rate	9.0	1.4	2.5	15.0	12.6	9.4	5.2
Costa Rica	1995	No.	26	1	2	15	7	1	0
		Rate	1.4	—	—	—	—	—	—
Croatia	1999	No.	33	1	1	3	7	9	12
		Rate	1.2	—	—	—	—	—	—
Cuba	1997	No.	163	4	4	78	55	13	9
		Rate	2.7	—	—	5.7	4.2	—	—
Czech Republic	1999	No.	54	4	2	14	9	13	12
		Rate	1.0	—	—	—	—	—	—
Denmark	1996	No.	23	1	0	7	7	5	3
		Rate	0.8	—	—	—	—	—	—
Ecuador	1996	No.	131	5	5	54	40	9	18
		Rate	2.5	—	—	3.2	3.7	—	—
El Salvador	1993	No.	190	3	4	72	56	34	20
		Rate	8.4	—	—	8.8	12.4	12.9	9.8
Estonia	1999	No.	59	3	1	4	19	21	11
		Rate	7.4	—	—	—	—	14.4	—
Finland	1998	No.	35	1	0	3	12	14	5
		Rate	1.2	—	—	—	—	—	—
France	1998	No.	167	8	6	31	42	41	39
		Rate	0.5	—	—	0.5	0.6	0.8	0.6

TABLE A.8 *(continued)*

Country or area	Year	Measure[c]	Total[d, e]	Males						
				All ages[d]	0–4 years	5–14 years	15–29 years	30–44 years	45–59 years	⩾60 years
Germany	1999	No.	720	418	27	12	95	127	101	56
		Rate	0.9	1.0	1.3	—	1.3	1.2	1.3	0.7
Greece	1998	No.	144	109	1	0	21	38	31	18
		Rate	1.2	1.9	—	—	1.8	3.4	3.3	—
Guyana	1994–1996	No.	42	35	0	0	14	12	6	3
		Rate	6.6	11.8	—	—	—	—	—	—
Hungary	1999	No.	291	170	4	4	19	54	58	31
		Rate	2.6	3.2	—	—	—	5.3	6.0	4.1
Ireland	1997	No.	30	21	1	0	8	6	5	1
		Rate	0.8	1.2	—	—	—	—	—	—
Israel	1997	No.	30	24	0	0	11	8	3	2
		Rate	0.5	0.9	—	—	—	—	—	—
Italy	1997	No.	720	561	0	6	170	207	101	77
		Rate	1.1	1.8	—	—	2.7	3.2	1.9	1.4
Japan	1997	No.	719	435	32	19	72	80	132	99
		Rate	0.6	0.7	1.1	—	0.5	0.7	1.0	0.8
Kazakhstan	1999	No.	2 448	1 841	14	17	483	738	380	209
		Rate	17.1	27.4	—	—	24.8	45.5	42.4	36.1
Kuwait	1999	No.	39	26	1	1	9	12	2	1
		Rate	2.2	2.4	—	—	—	—	—	—
Kyrgyzstan	1999	No.	341	266	1	3	63	110	59	30
		Rate	8.6	14.2	—	—	9.4	22.7	28.7	18.8
Latvia	1999	No.	308	213	0	0	47	69	61	36
		Rate	11.6	17.3	—	—	18.0	26.0	30.4	20.9
Lithuania	1999	No.	297	209	2	3	45	72	55	32
		Rate	7.5	11.3	—	—	11.0	17.2	19.2	12.9
Mauritius	1999	No.	33	19	2	0	3	9	2	3
		Rate	2.9	—	—	—	—	—	—	—
Mexico	1997	No.	13 542	12 170	129	224	5 281	3 810	1 751	975
		Rate	15.9	29.6	2.3	2.1	37.1	44.9	38.3	34.4
Netherlands	1999	No.	203	144	4	4	36	58	31	11
		Rate	1.3	1.7	—	—	2.3	3.0	2.0	—
New Zealand	1998	No.	57	32	5	2	10	6	6	3
		Rate	1.5	1.7	—	—	—	—	—	—
Nicaragua	1996	No.	285	246	2	5	117	66	37	19
		Rate	8.4	15.1	—	—	18.2	19.3	23.3	—
Norway	1997	No.	41	28	1	2	7	11	6	1
		Rate	0.9	1.3	—	—	—	—	—	—
Panama (excluding Canal Zone)	1997	No.	293	265	5	2	136	75	29	18
		Rate	10.9	19.8	—	—	35.3	27.1	18.5	—
Paraguay	1994	No.	459	420	3	4	171	144	61	37
		Rate	12.6	23.4	—	—	26.8	33.0	31.9	35.9
Philippines	1993	No.	7 726	7 181	20	59	3 020	2 845	977	260
		Rate	14.2	26.4	0.4	0.7	31.9	49.9	33.2	17.7
Poland	1995	No.	1 088	785	12	10	132	292	211	128
		Rate	2.7	4.0	—	—	3.0	6.4	7.1	5.3
Portugal	1999	No.	118	82	3	0	30	19	14	16
		Rate	1.1	1.6	—	—	2.6	—	—	—
Puerto Rico	1998	No.	804	731	1	7	500	149	59	15
		Rate	20.6	38.1	—	—	101.0	40.8	21.3	—
Republic of Korea	1997	No.	987	602	17	23	168	243	112	39
		Rate	2.0	2.4	—	0.7	2.5	3.9	3.4	2.2
Republic of Moldova	1999	No.	410	307	4	5	78	106	65	49
		Rate	11.2	18.0	—	—	17.5	27.4	24.4	25.1

Country or area	Year	Measure[c]	Females						
			All ages[d]	0–4 years	5–14 years	15–29 years	30–44 years	45–59 years	≥60 years
Germany	1999	No.	302	16	17	53	98	58	60
		Rate	0.7	—	—	0.7	1.0	0.7	0.5
Greece	1998	No.	35	0	0	4	6	9	16
		Rate	0.5	—	—	—	—	—	—
Guyana	1994–1996	No.	7	0	0	3	3	1	0
		Rate	—	—	—	—	—	—	—
Hungary	1999	No.	121	5	3	19	35	23	36
		Rate	2.0	—	—	—	3.4	2.2	3.0
Ireland	1997	No.	9	1	0	2	1	3	2
		Rate	—	—	—	—	—	—	—
Israel	1997	No.	6	0	0	2	3	0	1
		Rate	—	—	—	—	—	—	—
Italy	1997	No.	159	2	6	36	28	27	60
		Rate	0.5	—	—	0.6	0.4	0.5	0.8
Japan	1997	No.	284	42	21	37	29	64	91
		Rate	0.4	1.5	0.3	0.3	0.2	0.5	0.6
Kazakhstan	1999	No.	607	2	19	130	184	117	156
		Rate	7.9	—	—	6.8	11.0	11.2	15.4
Kuwait	1999	No.	13	0	0	4	7	1	1
		Rate	—	—	—	—	—	—	—
Kyrgyzstan	1999	No.	75	5	3	22	17	12	16
		Rate	3.5	—	—	3.4	—	—	—
Latvia	1999	No.	95	3	3	8	31	23	27
		Rate	6.6	—	—	—	11.5	9.5	8.3
Lithuania	1999	No.	88	5	3	10	21	16	33
		Rate	4.0	—	—	—	5.0	—	7.7
Mauritius	1999	No.	14	2	1	1	6	2	2
		Rate	—	—	—	—	—	—	—
Mexico	1997	No.	1 372	110	97	496	360	148	161
		Rate	3.1	2.0	0.9	3.4	4.0	3.0	4.8
Netherlands	1999	No.	59	1	4	21	16	7	10
		Rate	0.8	—	—	1.4	—	—	—
New Zealand	1998	No.	25	2	1	9	11	2	0
		Rate	1.3	—	—	—	—	—	—
Nicaragua	1996	No.	39	2	4	16	7	6	4
		Rate	2.2	—	—	—	—	—	—
Norway	1997	No.	13	0	1	3	3	4	2
		Rate	—	—	—	—	—	—	—
Panama (excluding Canal Zone)	1997	No.	28	3	3	13	5	1	3
		Rate	2.0	—	—	—	—	—	—
Paraguay	1994	No.	39	2	0	16	10	6	5
		Rate	2.2	—	—	—	—	—	—
Philippines	1993	No.	545	11	33	173	160	108	59
		Rate	2.1	—	0.4	1.9	2.8	3.6	3.3
Poland	1995	No.	303	14	5	46	93	56	89
		Rate	1.4	—	—	1.1	2.1	1.8	2.4
Portugal	1999	No.	36	3	2	6	10	9	6
		Rate	0.7	—	—	—	—	—	—
Puerto Rico	1998	No.	73	3	1	33	23	7	6
		Rate	3.7	—	—	6.8	5.6	—	—
Republic of Korea	1997	No.	385	19	19	100	141	59	47
		Rate	1.6	—	—	1.6	2.4	1.8	1.8
Republic of Moldova	1999	No.	103	4	6	13	31	19	30
		Rate	5.2	—	—	—	7.5	—	10.0

TABLE A.8 *(continued)*

Country or area	Year	Measure[c]	Total[d, e]	Males						
				All ages[d]	0–4 years	5–14 years	15–29 years	30–44 years	45–59 years	≥60 years
Romania	1999	No.	803	572	10	12	122	164	140	124
		Rate	3.3	4.8	—	—	4.4	6.9	7.4	6.9
Russian Federation	1998	No.	33 553	25 130	99	147	6 067	10 595	5 792	2 429
		Rate	21.6	34.0	2.9	1.3	37.5	61.5	49.8	27.2
Singapore	1998	No.	45	29	0	0	9	13	5	2
		Rate	1.3	1.7	—	—	—	—	—	—
Slovakia	1999	No.	132	89	0	0	21	38	18	12
		Rate	2.3	3.2	—	—	3.1	6.4	—	—
Slovenia	1999	No.	30	20	1	0	3	6	7	3
		Rate	1.3	1.8	—	—	—	—	—	—
Spain	1998	No.	355	255	2	3	70	91	50	39
		Rate	0.8	1.2	—	—	1.5	2.1	1.5	1.1
Sweden	1996	No.	110	74	0	0	11	28	21	14
		Rate	1.2	1.5	—	—	—	3.0	2.4	—
Switzerland	1996	No.	77	48	2	4	10	17	11	4
		Rate	1.1	1.4	—	—	—	—	—	—
Tajikistan	1995	No.	354	301	4	2	107	129	38	21
		Rate	8.5	14.3	—	—	14.0	27.4	18.6	14.0
Thailand	1994	No.	4 161	3 481	21	83	1 138	1 394	628	217
		Rate	7.5	12.6	0.8	1.4	12.5	22.3	19.7	11.3
The former Yugoslav Republic of Macedonia	1997	No.	47	38	0	0	5	19	7	7
		Rate	2.2	3.7	—	—	—	—	—	—
Trinidad and Tobago	1994	No.	146	108	0	2	39	35	23	9
		Rate	12.1	17.1	—	—	21.6	23.8	28.5	—
Turkmenistan	1998	No.	333	279	2	2	116	114	32	12
		Rate	8.6	14.6	—	—	17.8	25.5	18.2	—
Ukraine	1999	No.	6 260	4 421	28	41	941	1 674	1 196	541
		Rate	11.7	17.8	2.5	1.2	17.0	31.6	29.8	15.0
United Kingdom	1999	No.	440	335	20	10	108	109	60	28
		Rate	0.8	1.2	1.1	—	1.8	1.6	1.1	0.5
England and Wales	1999	No.	295	214	19	8	68	61	34	24
		Rate	0.6	0.9	—	—	1.3	1.0	0.7	0.5
Northern Ireland	1999	No.	24	20	0	1	4	11	3	1
		Rate	1.4	2.4	—	—	—	—	—	—
Scotland	1999	No.	121	101	1	1	36	37	23	3
		Rate	2.4	4.1	—	—	7.1	6.3	5.0	—
United States of America	1998	No.	17 893	13 652	396	257	6 670	3 984	1 609	736
		Rate	6.9	10.7	4.1	1.3	23.6	12.4	7.0	3.9
Uruguay	1990	No.	136	105	1	1	22	36	22	24
		Rate	4.4	7.1	—	—	6.0	12.6	9.2	10.8
Uzbekistan	1998	No.	790	567	2	18	178	222	100	47
		Rate	4.1	6.0	—	—	5.3	9.6	10.5	6.7
Venezuela	1994	No.	3 353	3 120	15	60	1 926	787	232	100
		Rate	16.0	29.7	—	2.3	63.9	37.7	21.7	16.7

Source: WHO mortality database as of September 2001.

[a] Homicide = ICD-10 X85–Y09 (ICD-9 E960–E969).

[b] Or average of the three most recent years available between 1990 and 2000 for countries with populations under 1 million.

[c] No. = number of deaths; rate = number of deaths per 100 000 population. Deaths where the age of the deceased person was not known were proportionally distributed across age groups based on the distribution of homicides in the population. The numbers of deaths have therefore been rounded to the nearest whole number. Any apparent discrepancy in the total sums is due to rounding. The rate was not calculated if fewer than 20 deaths were reported. The population counts on which the rates are based are available from the World Health Organization at http://www3.who.int/whosis/whsa/ftp/download.htm.

[d] Age-standardized.

[e] Combined total for males and females.

Country or area	Year	Measure[c]	Females						
			All ages[d]	0–4 years	5–14 years	15–29 years	30–44 years	45–59 years	≥60 years
Romania	1999	No.	231	11	5	37	56	48	74
		Rate	1.8	—	—	1.4	2.4	2.4	3.1
Russian Federation	1998	No.	8 423	90	135	1 632	2 452	1 907	2 207
		Rate	9.8	2.8	1.3	10.5	14.0	14.1	12.9
Singapore	1998	No.	16	0	0	5	4	3	3
		Rate	—	—	—	—	—	—	—
Slovakia	1999	No.	43	0	1	4	14	11	13
		Rate	1.4	—	—	—	—	—	—
Slovenia	1999	No.	10	0	0	1	4	0	5
		Rate	—	—	—	—	—	—	—
Spain	1998	No.	100	1	0	24	22	15	38
		Rate	0.4	—	—	0.5	0.5	—	0.8
Sweden	1996	No.	36	3	3	5	14	6	5
		Rate	0.8	—	—	—	—	—	—
Switzerland	1996	No.	29	3	2	6	5	4	9
		Rate	0.8	—	—	—	—	—	—
Tajikistan	1995	No.	53	0	0	16	18	7	11
		Rate	2.8	—	—	—	—	—	—
Thailand	1994	No.	680	15	62	208	216	109	71
		Rate	2.5	—	1.1	2.4	3.4	3.3	3.0
The former Yugoslav Republic of Macedonia	1997	No.	9	0	1	0	5	1	2
		Rate	—	—	—	—	—	—	—
Trinidad and Tobago	1994	No.	38	2	0	15	11	5	5
		Rate	6.6	—	—	—	—	—	—
Turkmenistan	1998	No.	54	1	0	13	21	8	11
		Rate	3.0	—	—	—	4.5	—	—
Ukraine	1999	No.	1 839	22	36	285	500	454	541
		Rate	6.1	2.0	1.1	5.3	9.0	9.5	8.4
United Kingdom	1999	No.	105	7	6	26	38	15	13
		Rate	0.4	—	—	0.5	0.6	—	—
England and Wales	1999	No.	81	7	6	19	28	11	10
		Rate	0.3	—	—	—	0.5	—	—
Northern Ireland	1999	No.	4	0	0	2	2	0	0
		Rate	—	—	—	—	—	—	—
Scotland	1999	No.	20	0	0	5	8	4	3
		Rate	0.7	—	—	—	—	—	—
United States of America	1998	No.	4 241	327	202	1 268	1 446	542	457
		Rate	3.1	3.5	1.1	4.6	4.4	2.2	1.8
Uruguay	1990	No.	31	2	1	12	5	2	9
		Rate	1.9	—	—	—	—	—	—
Uzbekistan	1998	No.	223	2	8	58	67	49	39
		Rate	2.4	—	—	1.8	2.8	4.9	4.0
Venezuela	1994	No.	233	16	18	103	67	14	15
		Rate	2.3	—	—	3.5	3.2	—	—

TABLE A.9

Mortality caused by suicide,[a] by sex, age group and country, most recent year available between 1990 and 2000[b]

Country or area	Year	Measure[c]	Total[d, e]	Males						
				All ages[d]	0–4 years	5–14 years	15–29 years	30–44 years	45–59 years	⩾60 years
Albania	1998	No.	165	104	0	2	46	28	18	10
		Rate	5.3	7.1	—	—	12.7	7.8	—	—
Argentina	1996	No.	2 245	1 709	0	14	402	328	442	523
		Rate	6.5	10.6	—	—	9.0	10.0	18.3	26.3
Armenia	1999	No.	67	49	0	0	9	16	11	13
		Rate	1.7	2.6	—	—	—	—	—	—
Australia	1998	No.	2 633	2 108	0	6	666	732	393	311
		Rate	13.3	21.4	—	—	31.7	34.1	23.2	22.7
Austria	1999	No.	1 555	1 126	0	2	171	289	275	389
		Rate	15.5	24.2	—	—	21.7	28.2	36.1	59.7
Azerbaijan	1999	No.	54	44	0	0	9	21	9	5
		Rate	0.8	1.3	—	—	—	2.5	—	—
Belarus	1999	No.	3 408	2 877	0	22	552	923	797	583
		Rate	30.9	56.9	—	2.9	49.4	79.7	103.4	86.3
Belgium	1995	No.	2 155	1 550	0	10	252	471	373	444
		Rate	17.9	27.1	—	—	24.3	39.9	41.9	48.7
Bosnia and Herzegovina	1991	No.	531	457	0	15	167	151	83	41
		Rate	11.3	19.4	—	—	27.0	29.4	22.9	20.4
Brazil	1995	No.	6 584	5 174	0	38	1 812	1 649	935	740
		Rate	4.7	7.6	—	0.2	8.0	9.9	10.7	14.4
Bulgaria	1999	No.	1 307	965	0	7	118	180	245	415
		Rate	12.3	19.6	—	—	12.8	21.5	30.9	53.3
Canada	1997	No.	3 681	2 914	0	39	682	1 010	708	475
		Rate	11.3	18.1	—	1.9	21.6	26.3	26.8	22.1
Chile	1994	No.	801	704	0	2	240	211	133	118
		Rate	6.1	11.1	—	—	12.9	13.8	15.5	20.9
China										
Hong Kong SAR	1996	No.	788	501	0	6	96	168	99	131
		Rate	11.2	14.6	—	—	13.8	18.5	19.4	31.2
Selected urban and rural areas	1999	No.	16 836	8 048	0	83	1 252	2 018	1 680	3 015
		Rate	13.7	13.5	—	0.9	7.2	12.9	17.9	45.7
Colombia	1995	No.	1 172	905	0	15	427	230	123	110
		Rate	3.4	5.5	—	—	7.7	6.1	6.7	9.7
Costa Rica	1995	No.	211	174	0	5	66	61	27	14
		Rate	6.6	10.9	—	—	13.4	16.4	14.8	—
Croatia	1999	No.	989	716	0	5	112	170	171	258
		Rate	18.5	30.2	—	—	23.2	32.5	43.2	79.1
Cuba	1997	No.	2 029	1 401	0	5	235	355	310	496
		Rate	17.1	23.8	—	—	16.4	27.1	35.3	72.6
Czech Republic	1999	No.	1 610	1 285	0	3	223	298	399	362
		Rate	13.0	22.3	—	—	18.1	28.2	37.1	48.1
Denmark	1996	No.	892	631	0	1	80	163	180	207
		Rate	13.6	20.2	—	—	14.5	27.4	33.8	46.5
Ecuador	1996	No.	593	396	0	7	188	107	56	38
		Rate	5.5	7.8	—	—	10.9	9.7	9.9	10.5
El Salvador	1993	No.	429	276	0	4	168	56	26	21
		Rate	8.5	12.1	—	—	21.5	14.0	10.7	13.0
Estonia	1999	No.	469	376	0	2	73	97	111	92
		Rate	28.1	50.9	—	—	45.5	63.6	92.5	90.3
Finland	1998	No.	1 228	962	0	3	173	296	290	200
		Rate	21.1	34.0	—	—	35.1	50.8	53.2	49.6

Country or area	Year	Measure[c]	Females						
			All ages[d]	0–4 years	5–14 years	15–29 years	30–44 years	45–59 years	≥60 years
Albania	1998	No.	61	0	1	42	9	4	4
		Rate	3.6	—	—	9.7	—	—	—
Argentina	1996	No.	536	0	9	129	113	130	155
		Rate	3.0	—	—	2.9	3.3	5.1	5.8
Armenia	1999	No.	18	0	0	0	4	3	11
		Rate	—	—	—	—	—	—	—
Australia	1998	No.	525	0	2	135	183	103	101
		Rate	5.2	—	—	6.6	8.5	6.3	6.1
Austria	1999	No.	429	0	1	46	85	101	196
		Rate	7.6	—	—	6.0	8.6	13.2	20.1
Azerbaijan	1999	No.	10	0	0	2	3	3	2
		Rate	—	—	—	—	—	—	—
Belarus	1999	No.	531	0	4	83	113	142	189
		Rate	8.5	—	—	7.7	9.5	16.1	15.4
Belgium	1995	No.	605	0	3	61	171	147	223
		Rate	9.4	—	—	6.1	14.9	16.5	17.8
Bosnia and Herzegovina	1991	No.	74	0	4	19	17	16	18
		Rate	3.3	—	—	—	—	—	—
Brazil	1995	No.	1 410	0	36	496	430	258	190
		Rate	1.9	—	0.2	2.2	2.5	2.7	3.1
Bulgaria	1999	No.	342	0	3	32	51	71	185
		Rate	5.8	—	—	3.6	6.1	8.4	18.5
Canada	1997	No.	767	0	12	156	255	208	136
		Rate	4.6	—	—	5.1	6.7	7.8	5.0
Chile	1994	No.	97	0	4	33	25	20	15
		Rate	1.4	—	—	1.8	1.6	2.2	—
China									
Hong Kong SAR	1996	No.	287	0	5	61	74	36	110
		Rate	7.9	—	—	8.5	7.9	8.2	23.4
Selected urban and rural areas	1999	No.	8 788	0	64	1 899	2 304	1 640	2 881
		Rate	14.0	—	0.8	11.8	15.6	18.3	39.5
Colombia	1995	No.	267	0	10	153	63	29	11
		Rate	1.4	—	—	2.8	1.6	1.4	—
Costa Rica	1995	No.	37	0	1	16	12	6	1
		Rate	2.3	—	—	—	—	—	—
Croatia	1999	No.	273	0	1	18	41	65	148
		Rate	8.6	—	—	—	8.1	15.0	28.8
Cuba	1997	No.	628	0	6	130	157	151	184
		Rate	10.6	—	—	9.5	11.9	16.6	25.1
Czech Republic	1999	No.	325	0	0	40	55	86	144
		Rate	4.7	—	—	3.4	5.4	7.7	12.9
Denmark	1996	No.	261	0	0	14	66	85	96
		Rate	7.5	—	—	—	11.6	16.2	16.3
Ecuador	1996	No.	197	0	17	130	30	14	6
		Rate	3.2	—	—	7.7	2.7	—	—
El Salvador	1993	No.	153	0	13	103	18	11	8
		Rate	5.3	—	—	12.5	—	—	—
Estonia	1999	No.	93	0	0	10	17	22	44
		Rate	8.9	—	—	—	—	15.3	23.4
Finland	1998	No.	266	0	2	40	65	85	74
		Rate	8.8	—	—	8.5	11.6	15.8	12.3

TABLE A.9 *(continued)*

Country or area	Year	Measure[c]	Total[d, e]	Males						
				All ages[d]	0–4 years	5–14 years	15–29 years	30–44 years	45–59 years	⩾60 years
France	1998	No.	10 534	7 771	0	10	1 036	2 278	1 863	2 584
		Rate	14.8	23.2	—	—	16.9	35.3	35.3	51.0
Georgia	1992	No.	204	151	0	0	35	37	29	50
		Rate	3.9	6.4	—	—	6.4	7.4	8.3	16.9
Germany	1999	No.	11 160	8 082	0	26	1 087	2 221	2 032	2 716
		Rate	10.6	16.7	—	0.6	14.6	21.3	25.6	35.6
Greece	1998	No.	403	315	0	0	61	69	69	116
		Rate	3.1	4.9	—	—	5.2	6.1	7.3	10.7
Guyana	1994–1996	No.	84	64	0	0	28	20	10	5
		Rate	12.5	20.5	—	—	24.6	30.2	—	—
Hungary	1999	No.	3 328	2 550	0	11	283	693	815	749
		Rate	26.9	45.7	—	—	24.3	67.5	84.5	98.2
Iceland	1994–1996	No.	28	24	0	0	8	6	5	4
		Rate	10.4	17.5	—	—	—	—	—	—
Ireland	1997	No.	466	376	0	4	148	112	71	41
		Rate	12.5	20.4	—	—	32.0	29.6	24.1	16.5
Israel	1997	No.	379	301	0	2	95	70	44	90
		Rate	6.5	10.8	—	—	12.8	12.9	11.4	26.9
Italy	1997	No.	4 694	3 547	0	5	578	726	772	1 466
		Rate	6.2	9.9	—	—	9.3	11.4	14.3	26.0
Japan	1997	No.	23 502	15 906	0	34	1 964	3 064	5 829	5 015
		Rate	14.5	20.7	—	0.5	14.4	25.4	42.2	42.3
Kazakhstan	1999	No.	4 004	3 340	0	49	963	1 172	711	445
		Rate	27.9	50.3	—	3.2	49.4	72.2	79.3	76.9
Kuwait	1999	No.	47	34	0	1	11	21	1	0
		Rate	1.5	1.8	—	—	—	4.3	—	—
Kyrgyzstan	1999	No.	559	460	0	12	138	162	94	54
		Rate	14.0	23.9	—	—	20.6	33.5	45.6	34.0
Latvia	1999	No.	764	593	0	1	85	187	185	135
		Rate	27.0	47.1	—	—	32.5	70.4	92.1	78.3
Lithuania	1999	No.	1 552	1 287	0	8	237	410	413	219
		Rate	38.4	69.2	—	—	57.8	97.9	144.1	88.1
Luxembourg	1995–1997	No.	72	53	0	0	8	16	14	15
		Rate	14.7	22.5	—	—	—	—	—	—
Mauritius	1999	No.	174	120	0	1	35	56	20	8
		Rate	14.3	19.7	—	—	23.0	38.7	25.0	—
Mexico	1997	No.	3 369	2 828	0	81	1 350	731	365	300
		Rate	3.9	6.9	—	0.8	9.5	8.6	8.0	10.6
Netherlands	1999	No.	1 517	1 015	0	7	165	321	276	246
		Rate	8.3	11.3	—	—	10.5	16.5	17.5	20.0
New Zealand	1998	No.	574	442	0	9	170	126	71	66
		Rate	15.0	23.6	—	—	41.5	29.4	22.1	25.3
Nicaragua	1996	No.	230	147	0	6	76	41	13	11
		Rate	5.9	8.4	—	—	11.8	12.0	—	—
Norway	1997	No.	533	387	0	3	87	103	85	109
		Rate	10.9	16.1	—	—	18.8	20.8	21.1	29.3
Panama (excluding Canal Zone)	1997	No.	145	124	0	1	48	46	15	14
		Rate	5.8	9.8	—	—	12.5	16.7	—	—
Paraguay	1994	No.	109	82	0	4	30	18	14	15
		Rate	3.2	5.1	—	—	4.8	—	—	—
Philippines	1993	No.	851	509	0	0	256	163	59	31
		Rate	1.5	1.9	—	—	2.7	2.9	2.0	2.1

Country or area	Year	Measure[c]	Females						
			All ages[d]	0–4 years	5–14 years	15–29 years	30–44 years	45–59 years	≥60 years
France	1998	No.	2 763	0	9	277	679	740	1 058
		Rate	7.4	—	—	4.6	10.4	14.0	15.3
Georgia	1992	No.	53	0	0	11	13	9	20
		Rate	1.9	—	—	—	—	—	4.4
Germany	1999	No.	3 078	0	9	250	587	725	1 507
		Rate	5.1	—	—	3.5	6.0	9.2	13.7
Greece	1998	No.	88	0	1	11	20	28	28
		Rate	1.4	—	—	—	1.8	2.9	2.1
Guyana	1994–1996	No.	20	0	1	10	5	3	1
		Rate	5.6	—	—	—	—	—	—
Hungary	1999	No.	778	0	1	54	138	199	386
		Rate	10.7	—	—	4.8	13.5	18.6	31.8
Iceland	1994–1996	No.	5	0	0	1	0	1	2
		Rate	—	—	—	—	—	—	—
Ireland	1997	No.	90	0	0	24	23	21	22
		Rate	4.7	—	—	5.4	5.9	7.3	7.1
Israel	1997	No.	78	0	0	12	20	7	39
		Rate	2.4	—	—	—	3.5	—	9.0
Italy	1997	No.	1 147	0	6	137	224	252	528
		Rate	2.9	—	—	2.3	3.5	4.5	7.0
Japan	1997	No.	7 596	0	19	866	1 110	2 013	3 588
		Rate	8.5	—	—	6.6	9.4	14.4	23.2
Kazakhstan	1999	No.	664	0	10	187	163	136	167
		Rate	8.7	—	—	9.8	9.7	13.1	16.6
Kuwait	1999	No.	13	0	0	2	11	0	0
		Rate	—	—	—	—	—	—	—
Kyrgyzstan	1999	No.	99	0	2	34	22	9	32
		Rate	4.7	—	—	5.2	4.5	—	13.9
Latvia	1999	No.	171	0	0	19	32	43	76
		Rate	10.0	—	—	—	11.9	17.9	23.5
Lithuania	1999	No.	265	0	1	34	57	71	102
		Rate	11.2	—	—	8.5	13.4	20.9	23.7
Luxembourg	1995–1997	No.	19	0	0	3	7	5	5
		Rate	—	—	—	—	—	—	—
Mauritius	1999	No.	54	0	0	28	20	5	1
		Rate	8.9	—	—	19.0	14.5	—	—
Mexico	1997	No.	541	0	30	327	107	47	29
		Rate	1.1	—	0.3	2.3	1.2	1.0	0.9
Netherlands	1999	No.	502	0	5	75	140	139	143
		Rate	5.4	—	—	4.9	7.5	9.1	8.8
New Zealand	1998	No.	132	0	4	49	40	20	19
		Rate	6.8	—	—	12.0	8.9	6.2	—
Nicaragua	1996	No.	83	0	12	55	10	4	2
		Rate	3.5	—	—	8.5	—	—	—
Norway	1997	No.	146	0	0	25	43	43	35
		Rate	5.9	—	—	5.6	9.1	11.0	7.1
Panama (excluding Canal Zone)	1997	No.	21	0	0	9	5	4	3
		Rate	1.7	—	—	—	—	—	—
Paraguay	1994	No.	27	0	2	9	8	3	5
		Rate	1.5	—	—	—	—	—	—
Philippines	1993	No.	342	0	0	226	64	27	24
		Rate	1.2	—	—	2.5	1.1	0.9	1.3

TABLE A.9 *(continued)*

Country or area	Year	Measure[c]	Total[d, e]	Males						
				All ages[d]	0–4 years	5–14 years	15–29 years	30–44 years	45–59 years	⩾60 years
Poland	1995	No.	5 499	4 562	0	60	809	1 625	1 274	794
		Rate	13.4	23.2	—	1.9	18.7	35.7	43.0	32.7
Portugal	1999	No.	545	407	0	1	39	78	71	218
		Rate	4.0	6.7	—	—	3.3	7.4	8.3	25.1
Puerto Rico	1998	No.	321	290	0	3	58	89	66	74
		Rate	8.1	15.6	—	—	11.7	24.4	23.7	31.6
Republic of Korea	1997	No.	6 024	4 162	0	31	966	1 398	1 012	755
		Rate	12.8	18.8	—	0.9	14.6	22.3	30.5	43.1
Republic of Moldova	1999	No.	579	482	0	6	72	149	155	100
		Rate	15.5	28.1	—	—	16.1	38.6	58.2	51.2
Romania	1999	No.	2 736	2 235	0	35	357	599	703	541
		Rate	10.8	18.5	—	2.2	12.8	25.4	37.1	30.3
Russian Federation	1998	No.	51 770	42 785	0	335	9 414	14 614	10 898	7 524
		Rate	32.1	57.9	—	3.0	58.2	84.9	93.7	84.3
Singapore	1998	No.	371	221	0	3	50	66	50	52
		Rate	11.7	14.1	—	—	14.4	14.5	18.8	34.7
Slovakia	1999	No.	692	590	0	5	90	170	197	128
		Rate	11.5	20.8	—	—	13.2	28.5	42.5	38.9
Slovenia	1999	No.	590	453	0	4	61	119	128	141
		Rate	24.6	40.3	—	—	27.7	52.3	65.3	95.0
Spain	1998	No.	3 261	2 499	0	4	490	545	439	1 021
		Rate	6.5	10.5	—	—	10.3	12.3	13.3	28.1
Sweden	1996	No.	1 253	872	0	1	135	211	253	272
		Rate	11.8	16.9	—	—	15.6	22.8	28.9	32.0
Switzerland	1996	No.	1 431	1 010	0	4	187	248	251	320
		Rate	16.7	25.1	—	—	27.0	28.9	37.0	55.0
Tajikistan	1995	No.	199	146	0	0	42	46	36	22
		Rate	5.2	8.1	—	—	5.5	9.8	17.7	14.7
Thailand	1994	No.	2 333	1 631	0	1	743	473	257	158
		Rate	4.1	5.9	—	—	8.1	7.6	8.1	8.2
The former Yugoslav Republic of Macedonia	1997	No.	155	115	0	1	13	34	24	43
		Rate	7.4	11.3	—	—	—	15.1	15.3	33.6
Trinidad and Tobago	1994	No.	148	118	0	2	35	35	28	18
		Rate	12.6	19.5	—	—	19.3	23.8	34.7	—
Turkmenistan	1998	No.	406	322	0	15	133	101	62	11
		Rate	10.4	16.9	—	—	20.3	22.5	34.8	—
Ukraine	1999	No.	14 452	11 806	0	80	1 922	3 460	3 514	2 830
		Rate	25.2	46.0	—	2.3	34.8	65.2	87.6	78.4
United Kingdom	1999	No.	4 448	3 443	0	4	777	1 220	806	636
		Rate	6.8	10.8	—	—	13.2	17.7	14.8	12.1
England and Wales	1999	No.	3 690	2 840	0	2	598	989	700	551
		Rate	6.3	9.9	—	—	11.5	16.2	14.4	11.8
Northern Ireland	1999	No.	121	103	0	0	45	39	12	7
		Rate	7.3	12.5	—	—	23.8	21.5	—	—
Scotland	1999	No.	637	500	0	2	134	192	94	78
		Rate	11.7	18.8	—	—	26.3	32.5	20.3	17.8
United States of America	1998	No.	30 575	24 538	0	241	5 718	7 523	5 218	5 838
		Rate	10.4	17.3	—	1.2	20.2	23.4	22.8	30.6

Country or area	Year	Measure[c]	Females						
			All ages[d]	0–4 years	5–14 years	15–29 years	30–44 years	45–59 years	≥60 years
Poland	1995	No.	937	0	6	121	286	245	279
		Rate	4.2	—	—	2.9	6.3	7.7	7.6
Portugal	1999	No.	138	0	3	12	23	16	84
		Rate	1.9	—	—	—	2.1	—	7.1
Puerto Rico	1998	No.	31	0	0	10	7	6	8
		Rate	1.5	—	—	—	—	—	—
Republic of Korea	1997	No.	1 862	0	34	563	549	303	413
		Rate	7.6	—	1.1	8.9	9.3	9.0	15.5
Republic of Moldova	1999	No.	97	1	0	15	18	29	34
		Rate	4.7	—	—	—	—	9.3	11.3
Romania	1999	No.	501	0	4	77	101	129	190
		Rate	3.6	—	—	2.9	4.3	6.4	8.0
Russian Federation	1998	No.	8 985	0	79	1 369	1 893	1 955	3 689
		Rate	9.4	—	0.8	8.8	10.8	14.5	21.6
Singapore	1998	No.	150	0	0	45	26	26	53
		Rate	9.4	—	—	12.9	5.8	9.9	30.5
Slovakia	1999	No.	102	0	0	14	28	29	31
		Rate	3.2	—	—	—	4.8	5.8	6.2
Slovenia	1999	No.	137	0	0	14	24	48	51
		Rate	10.6	—	—	—	10.5	24.6	22.4
Spain	1998	No.	762	0	4	98	152	147	361
		Rate	2.8	—	—	2.1	3.5	4.3	7.5
Sweden	1996	No.	381	0	2	43	76	126	134
		Rate	6.9	—	—	5.2	8.6	14.8	12.2
Switzerland	1996	No.	421	0	0	47	97	110	167
		Rate	9.1	—	—	6.8	11.6	16.3	20.7
Tajikistan	1995	No.	53	0	0	22	13	8	10
		Rate	2.5	—	—	2.8	—	—	—
Thailand	1994	No.	702	0	1	342	202	101	56
		Rate	2.4	—	—	3.9	3.2	3.0	2.4
The former Yugoslav Republic of Macedonia	1997	No.	40	0	0	6	13	4	17
		Rate	3.8	—	—	—	—	—	—
Trinidad and Tobago	1994	No.	30	0	0	18	8	1	3
		Rate	5.0	—	—	—	—	—	—
Turkmenistan	1998	No.	84	0	3	47	14	10	10
		Rate	4.1	—	—	7.1	—	—	—
Ukraine	1999	No.	2 646	0	14	275	484	645	1 228
		Rate	7.6	—	—	5.1	8.7	13.4	19.0
United Kingdom	1999	No.	1 005	0	1	169	292	246	297
		Rate	2.9	—	—	3.0	4.4	4.5	4.3
England and Wales	1999	No.	850	0	0	133	244	208	265
		Rate	2.7	—	—	2.7	4.1	4.3	4.3
Northern Ireland	1999	No.	18	0	0	9	6	1	2
		Rate	—	—	—	—	—	—	—
Scotland	1999	No.	137	0	1	27	42	37	30
		Rate	4.7	—	—	5.5	7.1	7.7	5.0
United States of America	1998	No.	6 037	0	83	1 029	2 076	1 624	1 225
		Rate	4.0	—	0.4	3.7	6.4	6.7	4.8

TABLE A.9 *(continued)*

Country or area	Year	Measure[c]	Total[d, e]	Males						
				All ages[d]	0–4 years	5–14 years	15–29 years	30–44 years	45–59 years	≥60 years
Uruguay	1990	No.	318	251	0	3	42	54	65	87
		Rate	9.6	16.4	—	—	11.8	19.0	27.5	39.4
Uzbekistan	1998	No.	1 620	1 252	0	53	407	468	215	109
		Rate	8.0	13.0	—	1.7	12.2	20.1	22.5	15.5
Venezuela	1994	No.	1 089	890	0	26	349	262	121	131
		Rate	6.1	10.3	—	1.0	11.6	12.6	11.3	21.8

Source: WHO mortality database as of September 2001.

[a] Suicide = ICD-10 X60–X84 (ICD-9 E950–E959).

[b] Or average of the three most recent years available between 1990 and 2000 for countries with populations under 1 million.

[c] No. = number of deaths; rate = number of deaths per 100 000 population. Deaths where the age of the deceased person was not known were proportionally distributed across age groups based on the distribution of suicides in the population. The numbers of deaths have therefore been rounded to the nearest whole number. Any apparent discrepancy in the total sums is due to rounding. The rate was not calculated if fewer than 20 deaths were reported. The population counts on which the rates are based are available from the World Health Organization at http://www3.who.int/whosis/whsa/ftp/download.htm.

[d] Age-standardized.

[e] Combined total for males and females.

Country or area	Year	Measure[c]	Females						
			All ages[d]	0–4 years	5–14 years	15–29 years	30–44 years	45–59 years	⩾60 years
Uruguay	1990	No.	67	0	3	13	9	11	30
		Rate	3.7	—	—	—	—	—	10.5
Uzbekistan	1998	No.	368	0	7	208	80	28	45
		Rate	3.3	—	—	6.3	3.3	2.8	4.7
Venezuela	1994	No.	199	0	9	98	49	23	20
		Rate	2.1	—	—	3.3	2.4	2.1	2.9

TABLE A.10

Firearm-related mortality, by manner of death[a] and country, most recent year available between 1990 and 2000[b]

Country or area	Year	Measure[c]	Total	Firearm-related deaths			
				Homicide	Suicide	Unintentional	Undetermined
Albania	1998	No.	741	591	98	50	2
		Rate	22.1	17.6	2.9	1.5	—
Australia	1998	No.	334	56	248	23	7
		Rate	1.8	0.3	1.3	0.1	—
Austria	1999	No.	293	17	272	3	1
		Rate	3.6	—	3.4	—	—
Belgium	1995	No.	379	59	289	2	29
		Rate	3.7	0.6	2.9	—	0.3
Bulgaria	1999	No.	133	51	55	20	7
		Rate	1.6	0.6	0.7	0.2	—
Canada	1997	No.	1 034	159	818	45	12
		Rate	3.4	0.5	2.7	0.1	—
China (Hong Kong SAR)	1996	No.	6	3	3	0	0
		Rate	—	—	—	—	—
Croatia	1999	No.	226	69	145	11	1
		Rate	5.0	1.5	3.2	—	—
Czech Republic	1999	No.	259	46	185	17	11
		Rate	2.5	0.4	1.8	—	—
Denmark	1996	No.	101	15	80	4	2
		Rate	1.9	—	1.5	—	—
Estonia	1999	No.	71	31	32	1	7
		Rate	4.9	2.1	2.2	—	—
Finland	1998	No.	295	22	267	3	3
		Rate	5.7	0.4	5.2	—	—
France	1998	No.	2 964	170	2 386	68	340
		Rate	5.0	0.3	4.1	0.1	0.6
Germany	1999	No.	1 201	155	906	16	124
		Rate	1.5	0.2	1.1	—	0.2
Greece	1998	No.	194	74	86	34	0
		Rate	1.8	0.7	0.8	0.3	—
Hungary	1999	No.	129	31	96	1	1
		Rate	1.3	0.3	1.0	—	—
Iceland	1994–1996	No.	7	1	5	0	1
		Rate	—	—	—	—	—
Ireland	1997	No.	54	7	44	3	0
		Rate	1.5	—	1.2	—	—
Israel	1997	No.	161	15	73	0	73
		Rate	2.8	—	1.3	—	1.3
Italy	1997	No.	1 171	463	626	38	44
		Rate	2.0	0.8	1.1	0.1	0.1
Japan	1997	No.	83	22	45	10	6
		Rate	0.1	0.0	0.0	—	—
Kuwait	1999	No.	16	16	0	0	0
		Rate	—	—	—	—	—
Latvia	1999	No.	92	34	47	5	6
		Rate	3.8	1.4	1.9	—	—
Lithuania	1999	No.	67	18	35	4	10
		Rate	1.8	—	0.9	—	—
Luxembourg	1995–1997	No.	12	1	9	0	2
		Rate	—	—	—	—	—
Malta	1997–1999	No.	7	4	2	1	0
		Rate	—	—	—	—	—
Netherlands	1999	No.	131	75	51	5	0
		Rate	0.8	0.5	0.3	—	—

TABLE A.10 *(continued)*

Country or area	Year	Measure[c]	Total	Firearm-related deaths			
				Homicide	Suicide	Unintentional[a]	Undetermined
New Zealand	1998	No.	84	4	72	6	2
		Rate	2.2	—	1.9	—	—
Norway	1997	No.	139	10	127	2	0
		Rate	3.2	—	2.9	—	—
Portugal	1999	No.	202	61	62	2	77
		Rate	2.0	0.6	0.6	—	0.8
Republic of Korea	1997	No.	59	19	22	9	9
		Rate	0.1	—	0.0	—	—
Republic of Moldova	1999	No.	68	45	7	9	7
		Rate	1.9	1.2	—	—	—
Romania	1999	No.	73	19	24	26	4
		Rate	0.3	—	0.1	0.1	—
Singapore	1998	No.	6	0	5	1	0
		Rate	—	—	—	—	—
Slovakia	1999	No.	171	43	88	20	20
		Rate	3.2	0.8	1.6	0.4	0.4
Slovenia	1999	No.	61	9	49	2	1
		Rate	3.1	—	2.5	—	—
Spain	1998	No.	352	85	224	43	0
		Rate	0.9	0.2	0.6	0.1	—
Sweden	1996	No.	183	11	163	3	6
		Rate	2.1	—	1.8	—	—
Thailand	1994	No.	2 434	2 184	158	84	8
		Rate	4.2	3.8	0.3	0.1	—
The former Yugoslav Republic of Macedonia	1997	No.	41	20	16	5	0
		Rate	2.1	1.0	—	—	—
United Kingdom	1999	No.	197	45	140	6	6
		Rate	0.3	0.1	0.2	—	—
England and Wales	1999	No.	159	23	115	6	15
		Rate	0.3	0.0	0.2	—	—
Northern Ireland	1999	No.	28	15	11	0	2
		Rate	1.7	—	—	—	—
Scotland	1999	No.	25	7	14	0	4
		Rate	0.5	—	—	—	—
United States of America	1998	No.	30 419	11 802	17 432	866	319
		Rate	11.3	4.4	6.4	0.3	0.1

Source: WHO mortality database as of September 2001.

[a] Homicide by firearm discharge = ICD-10 X93–X95 (ICD-9 E965); suicide by firearm discharge = ICD-10 X72–X74 (ICD-9 E955); firearm discharge, unintentional = ICD-10 W32–W34 (ICD-9 E922); firearm discharge, intent undetermined = ICD-10 Y22–Y24 (ICD-9 E985).

[b] Or average of the three most recent years available between 1990 and 2000 for countries with populations under 1 million.

[c] No. = number of deaths; rate = number of deaths per 100 000 population. The rate was not calculated if fewer than 20 deaths were reported. The population counts on which the rates are based are available from the World Health Organization at http://www3.who.int/whosis/whsa/ftp/download.htm.

Resources

The following is a listing of resources on violence-related topics, primarily Internet addresses of organizations involved in violence research, prevention and advocacy. In preparing this listing, the intention was to offer an illustrative sampling rather than a comprehensive listing of resources. Every effort was made to ensure that the web sites listed are reliable, current and content-rich. Section I contains a list of metasites, section II a list of web sites categorized according to type of violence, and section III a list of general web sites which may be of interest to those involved in violence research, prevention and advocacy.

Section I. Violence-related metasites

Included below are five metasites. Collectively, they offer access to hundreds of web sites of violence-related organizations from all over the world. A brief description is provided of each.

WHO Department of Injuries and Violence Prevention: external links

http://www.who.int/violence_injury_prevention/externalinks.htm

The WHO Department of Injuries and Violence Prevention offers an extensive listing of external links to organizations around the world involved in violence research, prevention and advocacy. The web sites of these agencies are listed by geographical region and country and by type of violence and other topics.

Economics of Civil Wars, Crime and Violence: related links

http://www.worldbank.org/research/conflict

Hosted on the web site of the World Bank, this link provides access to web sites dedicated to the study of conflict. The list includes data on political and economic variables for countries that have experienced internal violent conflicts; information on organizations and institutes that are working in the area of conflict resolution; and sites that provide historical background and analyses of specific cases of internal conflict.

Injury Control Resource Information Network

http://www.injurycontrol.com/icrin

The Injury Control Resource Information Network offers a dynamic list of key resources related to the field of injury and violence research and control that are accessible via the Internet. The sites are listed by categories, including data and statistics, recent research, and education and training. While the majority of sites are those of federal and state agencies in the United States, there are a handful of sites from other countries.

Injury Prevention Web

http://www.injuryprevention.org

The Injury Prevention Web contains more than 1400 links to injury and violence prevention web sites worldwide. The sites are listed alphabetically and by categories such as violence prevention, suicide prevention, and war and conflict. The site also offers a weekly literature update of recent journal articles and agency reports, book reviews, and listings of employment opportunities in the injury and violence research and prevention field.

Minnesota Center Against Violence and Abuse: electronic clearing house

http://www.mincava.umn.edu

The electronic clearing house of the Minnesota Center Against Violence and Abuse provides articles, fact sheets and other information resources, as well as links to web sites on a wide variety of violence-related topics, including child abuse, gang violence and abuse of the elderly. The site also provides searchable databases with over 700 training manuals, videos and other educational resources.

Section II. Violence-related web sites

Table 1 includes a list of web sites, primarily the home pages of organizations concerned with violence, categorized according to the type of violence. The web sites listed provide information not only about the organizations themselves, but also about violence-related topics in general.

TABLE 1

Violence-related web sites

Type of violence	Web site
Child abuse and neglect	
Casa Alianza: Covenant House Latin America	http://www.casa-alianza.org/EN/index-en.shtml
Child Abuse Prevention Network	http://child-abuse.com
Great Lakes Area Regional Resource Center: Early Prevention of Violence Database	http://www.glarrc.org/Resources/EPVD.cfm
International Society for Prevention of Child Abuse and Neglect	http://www.ispcan.org
Minnesota Center Against Violence and Abuse	http://www.mincava.umn.edu
Office of the United Nations High Commissioner for Human Rights: Convention on the Rights of the Child	http://www.unhchr.ch/html/menu2/6/crc.htm
United Nations Children's Fund Innocenti Research Centre	http://www.unicef.org http://www.unicef-icdc.org
Collective violence	
Centre for the Study of Violence and Reconciliation	http://www.wits.ac.za/csvr
Correlates of War Project	http://www.umich.edu/~cowproj
Global Internally Displaced Persons Project	http://www.idpproject.org
International Relations and Security Network: Security Watch	http://www.isn.ethz.ch/infoservice
Office for the Coordination of Humanitarian Affairs	http://www.reliefweb.int/ocha_ol
Office of the United Nations High Commissioner for Refugees	http://www.unhcr.ch
Stockholm International Peace Research Institute	http://www.sipri.se
Elder abuse	
Action on Elder Abuse	http://www.elderabuse.org.uk
Canadian Network for the Prevention of Elder Abuse	http://www.mun.ca/elderabuse
HelpAge International	http://www.helpage.org
International Network for the Prevention of Elder Abuse	http://www.inpea.net
National Center on Elder Abuse	http://www.elderabusecenter.org
National Committee for the Prevention of Elder Abuse	http://www.preventelderabuse.org/index.html

TABLE 1 *(continued)*

Type of violence	Web site
Suicide	
American Association of Suicidology	http://www.suicidology.org
Australian Institute for Suicide Research and Prevention	http://www.gu.edu.au/school/psy/aisrap
National Strategy for Suicide Prevention	http://www.mentalhealth.org/suicideprevention
Suicide Information and Education Centre/Suicide Prevention Training Programmes	http://www.suicideinfo.ca
The Suicidology Web: Suicide and Parasuicide	http://www.suicide-parasuicide.rumos.com
Violence against women	
Global Alliance Against Traffic in Women	http://www.inet.co.en/org/gaatw
International Center for Research on Women	http://www.icrw.org
Latin American and Caribbean Women's Health Network	http://www.reddesalud.web.cl
National Sexual Violence Resource Center	http://www.nsvrc.org
Network of East-West Women	http://www.neww.org/index.htm
Office of the United Nations High Commissioner for Human Rights: Women's Rights are Human Rights	http://www.unhchr.ch/women/index.html
Research, Action and Information Network for the Bodily Integrity of Women	http://www.rainbo.org
United Nations Development Fund for Women	http://www.undp.org/unifem
United Nations Development Programme: Gender in Development	http://www.undp.org/gender
Women Against Violence Europe	http://www.wave-network.org
Youth violence	
Center for the Prevention of School Violence	http://www.ncsu.edu/cpsv
Center for the Study and Prevention of Violence	http://www.colorado.edu/cspv
Inter-American Development Bank: Violence Prevention	http://www.iadb.org/sds/SOC/site_471_e.htm
National Center for Injury Prevention and Control	http://www.cdc.gov/ncipc
National Criminal Justice Reference Service	http://www.ncjrs.org/intlwww.html
Partnerships Against Violence Network	http://pavnet.org
TMR Network Project: Nature and Prevention of Bullying	http://www.goldsmiths.ac.uk/tmr
United Nations Crime and Justice Information Network	http://www.uncjin.org/Statistics/statistics.html

Section III. Other web sites

Table 2 lists other web sites that may be of interest to those involved in violence research, prevention and advocacy. They relate primarily to broad contextual issues such as economic and social development, human rights and crime, but also include some relevant tools for improving the understanding of violence-related injuries.

TABLE 2

Other web sites

Organization	Web site
Amnesty International	http://www.amnesty.org/
Campbell Collaboration's Crime and Justice Coordinating Group	http://www.aic.gov.au/campbellcj/
Centers for Disease Control and Prevention: National Center for Injury Prevention and Control	http://www.cdc.gov/ncipc http://www.cdc.gov/ncipc/pub_res/intimate.htm (*Intimate partner surveillance: uniform elements and recommended data elements*)
Centro Latino-Americano de Estudos sobre Violência e Saúde	http://www.ensp.fiocruz.br/claves.html
Economic and Social Research Council: Violence Research Programme	http://www1.rhbnc.ac.uk/sociopolitical-science/vrp/realhome.htm
Human Rights Watch	http://www.hrw.org/
Institute for Security Studies	http://www.iss.co.za
Inter-American Coalition for the Prevention of Violence	http://www.iacpv.org
International Action Network on Small Arms	http://www.iansa.org
International Campaign to Ban Landmines	http://www.icbl.org/
International Center for the Prevention of Crime	http://www.crime-prevention-intl.org
International Labour Organization	http://www.ilo.org
Medical Research Council of South Africa: Crime, Violence and Injury Lead Programme	http://www.mrc.ac.za/crime/crime.htm
National Library of Medicine: Entrez PubMed	http://www.ncbi.nlm.nih.gov/entrez/query.fcgi
Pan American Health Organization: Prevention of Violence and Injuries	http://www.paho.org/English/hcp/hcn/violence-unit-page.htm http://www.paho.org/English/HCP/HCN/guidelines-eng.htm (*Guidelines for the epidemiological surveillance of violence and injuries in the Americas*)
Red Andina de Prevención de Violencia	http://www.redandina.org
Trauma.org	http://www.trauma.org/trauma.html
United Nations Educational, Scientific and Cultural Organization	http://www.unesco.org
United Nations Human Settlements Programme	http://www.unhabitat.org/default.asp
United Nations Institute for Disarmament Research	http://www.unog.ch/unidir
United Nations Interregional Crime and Justice Research Institute	http://www.unicri.it
United Nations Office of Drug Control and Crime Prevention	http://www.odccp.org/crime_prevention.html
United Nations Population Fund	http://www.unfpa.org
United Nations Research Institute for Social Development	http://www.unrisd.org
University for Peace	http://www.upeace.org
World Health Organization	http://www.who.int/ http://www.who.int/violence_injury_prevention/pdf/injuryguidelines.pdf (*Injury surveillance guidelines*)

For readers without access to the Internet, the WHO Department of Injuries and Violence Prevention would be pleased to provide the full mailing address of the organizations listed. Kindly contact the Department at the following address:

Department of Injuries and Violence Prevention

World Health Organization

20 Avenue Appia

1211 Geneva 27

Switzerland

Tel.: +41 22 791 3480

Fax: +41 22 791 4332

Email: vip@who.int

Index

Note: Page numbers in bold type refer to main entries and definitions.